Manual of Infection Prevention and Control

THIRD EDITION

WITHDRAWN

Nizam Damani

MBBS, MSc (Lond.), FRCPath. (UK), FRCPI (Ireland),
CIC (USA), DipHIC (Lond.)

Clinical Director, Infection Prevention & Control
Craigavon Area Hospital
Portadown, UK

Honorary Lecturer, Department of Medical Microbiology
Queens University, Belfast, UK

Foreword by

Professor Didier Pittet

MD, MS

Director, Infection Control Programme
WHO Collaborating Centre on Patient Safety
University of Geneva Hospitals and Faculty of Medicine
Geneva, Switzerland

Lead: WHO First Global Patient Safety Challenge
Geneva, Switzerland

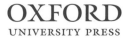

OXFORD
UNIVERSITY PRESS

OXFORD

UNIVERSITY PRESS

Great Clarendon Street, Oxford OX2 6DP

Oxford University Press is a department of the University of Oxford.
It furthers the University's objective of excellence in research, scholarship,
and education by publishing worldwide in

Oxford New York

Auckland Cape Town Dar es Salaam Hong Kong Karachi
Kuala Lumpur Madrid Melbourne Mexico City Nairobi
New Delhi Shanghai Taipei Toronto

With offices in

Argentina Austria Brazil Chile Czech Republic France Greece
Guatemala Hungary Italy Japan Poland Portugal Singapore
South Korea Switzerland Thailand Turkey Ukraine Vietnam

Oxford is a registered trade mark of Oxford University Press
in the UK and in certain other countries

Published in the United States
by Oxford University Press Inc., New York

© Oxford University Press, 2012

The moral rights of the author have been asserted
Database right Oxford University Press (maker)

First published 1997
Second edition published 2003

British Library Cataloguing in Publication Data
Data available

Library of Congress Cataloging in Publication Data
Data available

Typeset in Minion by Cenveo, Bangalore, India
Printed and bound by
CPI Group (UK) Ltd, Croyden, CR0 4YY

ISBN 978–0–19–969835–6

10 9 8 7 6 5 4 3 2 1

While the advice and information in this book is believed to be true and accurate, neither the authors
nor the publisher can accept any legal responsibility or liability for any loss or damage arising from
actions or decisions based in this book. The ultimate responsibility for the treatment of patients and
the interpretation lies with the medical practitioner. The opinions expressed are those of the authors
and the inclusion in this book of information relating to a particular product, method or technique
does not amount to an endorsement of its value or quality, or of the claims made by its manufacturer.
Every effort has been made to check drug dosages; however, it is still possible that errors have
occurred. Furthermore, dosage schedules are constantly being revised and new side-effects
recognised. For these reasons, the medical practitioner is strongly urged to consult the drug
companies' printed instructions before administering any of the drugs mentioned in this book.

To my parents, Gulbano and Noordin.

To my wife, Laila, and children Numair and Namiz
for their abiding love, understanding, and encouragement.

Foreword

It is an honour and a privilege to contribute the foreword to the third edition of this manual. When Professor G Ayliffe wrote the foreword of the first edition in 1997, he insisted on the high quality and practicality of the material presented: '. . . a number of useful tables, diagrams, definitions, and essential references'. He insisted also on the fact that the manual would 'allow health care workers to carry out individual procedures'. When Professor AM Emmerson wrote the foreword of the second edition in 2002, he emphasized that the material had been considerably revised, updated, extended, and even improved with the inclusion of several new chapters and additions. Strategic points were highlighted in the text and at the end of each section.

And the third edition? Not only has it built upon the strength and power of the first two editions, but again the content has been extensively revised, updated, and enriched with new material. This new edition is quite different from previous ones and most chapters have been completely rewritten. The title of the manual has changed to *Manual of Infection Prevention and Control* to reflect the shift in focus from mainly a procedure-oriented publication to one that really covers the entire field of infection prevention and control. In its new form, it now provides a very comprehensive overview, together with highly practical and easy-to-apply strategic advice and Nizam Damani should be warmly congratulated for such an achievement.

The manual addresses global issues and concerns in infection prevention and control and offers some fine-tuned practicalities for the reader. These include an extended glossary of infection control terms, multiple tables, and very well reproduced and highly educative schemas and figures to illustrate the main topics under discussion. Even the appendices are useful and pertinent for the daily routine of infection control practitioners, and include a very complete information resource and a table listing the incubation period of infectious diseases. Such information would be very helpful to organize the handling and control of the dreaded 'Friday afternoon outbreak of the hospital epidemiologist'.

Figures illustrating 'How to wear and remove a plastic apron', 'How to wear and remove a face mask properly', 'How to wear a respirator', or even 'How' and 'When' to cleanse hands during patient care, and 'Part of the hands most frequently missed during hand cleansing' are particularly useful for daily teaching in infection control. These should be used and reused worldwide to improve and facilitate our daily mission—to educate health care workers and support appropriate practices for basic infection control.

A large part of this manual is dedicated to the control of multi-resistant organisms, including antimicrobial stewardship, and a large variety of special pathogens and their management by the use of specific care bundles, infection control strategies, and barrier precautions. Major health care associated infections are discussed appropriately in terms of surveillance and control, as well as staff health and support services. Infection control in primary care is also addressed.

Last, but not least, each chapter is introduced by a very carefully selected citation ranging from '*The dream of a bacterium is to become two bacteria*' (F Jacob), '*What, will these hands ne'er be clean?*' (W Shakespeare) to '*If you think you're too small to make a difference, try sleeping in a closed room with a mosquito*' (Anonymous). In my opinion, the last citation is critical. It should be known by every single individual health care worker and repeated again and again by infection control practitioners and hospital epidemiologists worldwide. Infection control is everyone's priority during patient care and any improvement counts: the resulting impact can be minor or major . . . but we are all concerned.

Infection prevention and control is global and universal. It is our daily business and our daily mission. Each health care worker, from Kigali to Boston, Hong Kong to Stockholm, Sydney to Buenos Aires, and from Riyadh to Moscow, should embark on a revolution to make infection prevention a top priority of daily patient care and to improve universal access and safety of care. Infection control practices are at the heart of such improvement all around the globe. Politicians and stakeholders must adhere to a universal vision to improve patient safety and allocate sufficient support and resources to ensure that it becomes an everyday reality. The World Health Organization has designated the prevention of health care-associated infection as the first priority in patient safety by dedicating its First Global Patient Safety Challenge "Clean Care is Safer Care" to this cause. The *Manual of Infection Prevention and Control* is one of the great tools available to achieve our common mission: make health care safer together.

Professer Didier Pittet

Preface

In the nineteenth century, men lost their fear of God and acquired a fear of microbes.

Anonymous

Microbes are the simplest form of life, and having evolved over three billion years ago are arguably the most adaptable organisms, inhabiting nearly every corner of the globe and every orifice of the human body! One of the main reasons for their survival is that they are extremely adaptable and that their behavior is unpredictable. Globalization has worked for the spread of microbes due to increased international travel both of humans, food, and other products. The most recent example is the emergence of swine flu H1N1 in April 2010 and the chaos it caused on a global level. Despite all the scientific knowledge we had about the influenza virus from the previous pandemic, we were simply unable to predict the behavior of the new H1N1 strain.

Intensive farming to mass produce food, abuse of antimicrobial agents both in medical and veterinary practice, crowded urban populations with lack of safe water and provision of basic sanitation in low resource countries, continuing world conflicts, war, famine, drought, and tsunami have all resulted in massive displacement of people, and climate change has lead to the emergence and re-emergence of new and old infectious diseases. Medical tourism and increase in international travel has contributed to the spread of multi-resistant microorganisms on a global basis. In addition to these changes, during the past two decades, the delivery of health care has seen a substantial change. Innovations in medical sciences, improvement in public health education, and improved socioeconomic conditions have led to longer life expectancy resulting in an increased elderly population who are more prone to infections. Advancement in medical treatment and medical interventions has seen increased survival of immunocompromised patients making the population more susceptible to health care associated infections (HCAIs). As a result of these changes, the prevention and control of HCAIs is now recognized as a major global issue and their prevention is now an integral part of the patient safety and quality improvement programmes of all health care facilities worldwide. HCAIs lengthen patients' hospital stays, increase both morbidity and mortality, and have a profound impact on the delivery of health services. In addition, diagnosing and treating these infections is a costly process and places intense pressure on limited health care resources worldwide.

This new edition of the book, which was previously published as *Manual of Infection Control Procedures*, has been renamed *Manual of Infection Prevention and Control*. This new expanded edition is radically different from previous editions in terms of content as all of the chapters have been extensively revised and rewritten to include the latest knowledge and new evidence which has been published in the past seven years in the field of infection prevention and control. Like previous editions, the main aim of the book remains unchanged—to provide a comprehensive overview and to give practical and easy-to-follow advice on strategies to prevent and control cross-infection in all health care facilities.

I found that revising the third edition of the book as a single author was a daunting task and I am grateful to all my reviewers for their valuable input in their individual area of expertise. I am grateful to Margaret Mullan for the secretarial assistance. The production of the book would not have been possible without the help of Nicola Wilson, Siân Jenkins, Vimal Stephen, and Hema Kustagi of Oxford University Press. I am grateful to my wife Laila for her understanding and willingness to accommodate her life to my chaotic schedules for the past four years during the writing of the book.

Nizam Damani

Acknowledgements

I would like to thank Dr Rajesh Rajendran and Dr Judith Troughton, Consultant Microbiologists, for reading the manuscript and making useful comments, and Michele Gorham, Nurse Consultant at the National Hospital Neurology & Neurosurgery, London, for her input on the section on Prion Disease.

Figures 1.1, 1.2, 1.3, 1.4, 3.2, 3.3, 5.1, 5.2, 6.3, 8.3, 9.3, 9.4, 9.5, 9.6, 11.1, 11.3, 12.1, 12.2, 13.1, and 15.3 were produced with permission from the *Infection Control Manual* published by Craigavon Area Hospital, Portadown, N. Ireland.

Reviewers

Dr Benedetta Allegranzi
MD
Deputy Lead
First Global Patient Safety Challenge
World Health Organization
Geneva, Switzerland

Christina Bradley
BMS, MIBMS
Manager, Hospital Infection Research
Laboratory
Queen Elizabeth Hospital
Birmingham, UK

Peter Hoffman
B.Sc, Hon DipHIC
Consultant Clinical Scientist
Health Protection Agency
London, UK

Dr Conall McCaughey
FRCPath
Consultant Virologist
The Royal Hospital Group
Belfast
N. Ireland, UK

Dr Michael Borg
MD, MSc, DLSHTM, MMCPath, DipHIC
Consultant Hospital Infection Control
Mater Dei Hospital, Msida, Malta

Dr Andrew Ferguson
MEd FRCA, FCARCSI, DIBICM,
FCCP, FJFICMI
Consultant in Anaesthetics and
Intensive Care Medicine
Craigavon Area Hospital, Portadown
Co. Armagh, N. Ireland, UK

Prof. Hilary Humphrey
MD, FRCPath, FRCPI, FFPath, DipHIC
Professor of Microbiology
Royal College of Surgeons &
Beaumont Hospital, Dublin
Republic of Ireland

Dr John Yarnell
MD, FFPHM
Senior Lecturer in Epidemiology and
Public Health, Queen's University
Belfast
N. Ireland, UK

Contents

Abbreviations

AAFB	acid and alcohol fast bacilli		ELISA	enzyme-linked immunosorbent assay
ACDP	Advisory Committee on Dangerous Pathogens, UK		ESBL	extended-spectrum beta-lactamase
AER	automatic endoscope reprocessors		EtO	ethylene oxide
A&E	accident and emergency department		GP	general practitioner
			GRE	glycopeptide-resistant enterococci
AGP	aerosol-generating procedure		HAP	hospital-acquired pneumonia
AIDS	acquired immune deficiency syndrome		HAV	hepatitis A virus
APIC	Association for Professionals in Infection Control & Epidemiology, USA		HBeAg	hepatitis B e antigen
			HBIG	hepatitis B immunoglobulin
			HBsAg	hepatitis B surface antigen
BBV	blood-borne viruses		HBV	hepatitis B virus
BSAC	British Society for Antimicrobial Chemotherapy		HCAI	health care-associated infections
			HCV	hepatitis C virus
BSE	bovine spongiform encephalopathy		HCW	health care worker
CR-BSI	catheter related-blood stream infections		HELICS	Hospital in Europe Link for Infection Control through Surveillance
CA-UTI	catheter associated-urinary tract infections		HEPA	high efficiency particulate air filter
CA-MRSA	community-associated meticillin-resistant *Staphyloccocus aureus*		HICPAC	Health Care Infection Control Practices Advisory Committee, USA
CCDC	consultant in communicable disease control		HIV	Human immunodeficiency virus
CDC	Centers for Disease Control and Prevention, USA		HMSO	Her Majesty's Stationery Office
CDSC	Communicable Disease Surveillance Centre, UK		HPA	Health Protection Agency
			HSE	Health and Safety Executive, UK
CFU	colony forming unit		ICU/ITU	intensive care/therapy unit
CJD	Creutzfeldt–Jakob disease		IDSA	Infectious Diseases Society of America
CMV	cytomegalovirus			
CVC	central venous catheter		IFH	International Scientific Forum for Home Hygiene
DH	Department of Health, UK			
ECDC	European Centre for Disease Prevention and Control		IFIC	International Federation of Infection Control
EIA	enzyme immunoassay		IGT	interferon-gamma test

IHI	Institute of Health Improvement, USA
IP	incubation period
IPC	infection prevention and control
IPS	Infection Prevention Society
IT	information technology
IV	intravenous
JCAHO	Joint Commission on Accreditation of Healthcare Organization
JCR	Joint Commission Resource, USA
MDA	Medical Device Agency, UK
MDRO	multidrug-resistant microorganism
MHRA	Medicines and Healthcare products Regulatory Agency
MRGN	multi-resistant Gram-negative
MRD-TB	multidrug resistant tuberculosis
MRSA	meticillin-resistant *Staphyloccocus aureus*
NaDCC	Sodium dichloroisocyanurate
NDSC	National Disease Surveillance Centre, Ireland
NDM	New Delhi metallo-beta-lactamases
NHSN	National Healthcare Safety Network, USA
NICE	National Institute for Health and Clinical Excellence, UK
NIOSH	National Institute for Occupational Safety & Health
NNU/SCBU	neonatal/special care baby unit
OCC	Outbreak Control Committee
OHD	Occupational Health Department
OSHA	Occupational Safety and Health Administration
PCR	polymerase chain reaction

PEP	post-exposure prophylaxis
PHAC	Public Health Agency of Canada
ppm av Cl2	parts per million of available chlorine
PI	period of infectivity
PICC	peripherally-inserted central (venous) catheter
PPE	personal protective equipment
PVL	Panton–Valentine leucocidin
QAC	quaternary ammonium compound
RCA	root cause analysis
SARS	severe acute respiratory syndrome
SCBU	special care baby unit
SENIC	Study on the Efficacy of Nosocomial Infection Control
SHEA	Society for Healthcare Epidemiology of America
SSD	sterile supply department
SSI	surgical site infection
TSE	transmissible spongiform encephalopathy
TPN	total parenteral nutrition
UTI	urinary tract infection
vCJD	variant Creutzfeldt–Jakob disease
VAP	ventilator-associated pneumonias
VHF	viral haemorrhagic fever
VRE	vancomycin-resistant *Enterococcus*
VZIG	varicella zoster immunoglobulin
VZV	varicella zoster virus
XDR-TB	extra-drug-resistant tuberculosis
ZN	Ziehl–Neelsen
WHO	World Health Organization

Glossary of infection control terms

Additional (transmission based) precautions Infection control precautions required when the standard precautions may not be sufficient to prevent transmission of infection. These are used for patients known or suspected to be infected or colonized with pathogens that can be transmitted by airborne, droplet, or contact routes. Additional precautions are transmission-based precautions and should be used in addition to *standard precautions*.

Airborne transmission Transmission of infectious agents by either airborne nuclei or particles of <5 mm in size. See also *droplet transmission*.

Antimicrobial A chemical agent that, on application to living tissue or by systemic administration, will selectively kill or prevent the growth of susceptible organisms. This definition includes antibacterials, antivirals, antiprotozoals, antifungals, antiseptics, and disinfectants.

Antisepsis The destruction or inhibition of microorganisms on living tissues, having the effect of limiting or preventing the harmful results of infection.

Antiseptic A chemical agent which, when applied to *living tissue*, will destroy or inhibit the reproduction of microorganisms.

Asepsis The prevention of microbial contamination of living tissues or sterile materials by removal, exclusion, or destruction of microorganisms.

Aseptic technique A technique in which the instruments, drapes, and the gloved hands of the health care worker are sterile when performing surgery or invasive procedures.

Asymptomatic infection Infection which does not display any clinical signs/symptoms, but may still be capable of transmitting disease or microorganisms.

Bacteriuria The presence of bacteria in the urine, with or without consequent urinary tract infection.

Carrier A person (host) who harbours a microorganism (agent) but does not necessarily display clinical signs/symptoms of disease. Carriers may shed organisms into the environment intermittently or continuously and therefore act as a potential reservoir or source of infection.

Case A person with symptoms.

Chemoprophylaxis The administration of antimicrobial agents to prevent the development of an infection or the progression of an infection to active manifest disease.

Cleaning The physical removal of foreign material, e.g. dust, soil, organic material such as blood, secretions, excretions, and microorganisms. Cleaning physically removes (rather than inactivates) microorganisms. Cleaning is accomplished with water, detergents, and mechanical action.

Cohort A group of patients infected or colonized with the same microorganism, grouped together in a designated area of a unit or ward.

Colonization The presence of microorganisms at a body site(s) without the presence of symptoms or clinical manifestations of illness or infection. Colonization may be a form of carriage and is a potential method of transmission.

Commensal A microorganism resident in or on a body site without causing clinical infection.

Community-acquired infection This is an infection which was present, or incubating, at the time the patient was admitted to hospital. It is possible that the infection may only become apparent after the patient has been admitted. As a general rule, an infection which appears within 72 hours of admission may be considered to have been 'community-acquired', though more exact criteria will take into account the nature of the infecting organism and the incubation period of the disease.

Contact An exposed individual who might have been infected through transmission from another host or the environment.

Contamination The presence of microorganisms on a surface or in a fluid or material.

Cross-infection An infection transmitted from one patient to another, or from a member of staff, or from the environment, to another patient.

Decontamination A process which removes or destroys contamination and thereby prevents microorganisms or other contaminants from reaching a susceptible site in sufficient quantities to initiate infection or any other harmful response.

Disinfectant A chemical agent which, under defined conditions, is capable of disinfection. A substance that is recommended by its manufacturer for application to an inanimate object to kill a range of microorganisms.

Disinfection The inactivation of non-sporing microorganisms using either thermal (heat alone, or heat and water) or chemical means.

Droplet nuclei Particles produced when aqueous droplets of a suitably small size are dispersed into air. Larger droplets expelled from the nasopharynx can only travel about 1 metre at most before impaction by gravity. Small droplets, or nuclei (after surface evaporation) can travel quite a large distance.

Endemic The usual level or presence of an agent or disease in a defined population during a given period.

Endogenous infection Microorganisms originating from the patient's own body which may cause infection in another body site.

Epidemic An unusual, higher than expected level of infection or disease by a common agent in a defined population in a given period.

Exogenous infection Microorganisms originating from a source or reservoir which are transmitted to a person, i.e. contact, airborne, droplet, ingestion, vertical, sexual, or vector-borne.

Exposure-prone procedures A subset of 'invasive procedures' characterized by the potential for direct contact between the skin (usually finger or thumb) of the health care worker and sharp surgical instruments, needles, or sharp tissues (spicules of bone or teeth) in body cavities or in poorly visualized or confined body sites (including the mouth). In the broader sense, an exposure-prone procedure is considered to be any situation where there is a potentially high risk of transmission of blood-borne disease from the health care worker to patient during medical or dental procedures (UK Department of Health).

Flora (normal) The 'normal' flora (also termed 'commensal' or 'resident' flora) comprises microbes which are found commonly on, or in, humans. In general, the normal flora live, multiply, and die without any adverse effects on their hosts.

Flora (transient) Organisms that are not considered to be part of the normal flora and are not multiplying to any significant extent are termed 'transients'. Transient organisms are normally picked up on the hands of health care workers from contaminated environments or patients with infection. These transient flora usually do not cause the health care worker any harm and sooner or later will die, or be lost, usually by shedding of epithelial layers. Hand washing is the most effective way to remove transient flora picked up from the contaminated environment.

Fomite An inanimate object which can act as an intermediate source of infecting organisms, e.g. equipment that is used for more than one patient and is not decontaminated between uses.

Health care-associated infections The term *health care-associated infections* refers to infections associated with health care delivery in any setting (e.g. hospitals, long-term care facilities, ambulatory settings, home care). This term reflects the uncertainty in always being able to determine where the pathogen is acquired. Patients may be colonized with, or exposed to, potential pathogens outside of the health care setting before receiving health care, or may develop infections caused by those pathogens when exposed to the conditions associated with delivery of health care. Additionally, patients frequently move among the various settings within a health care system.

Health care workers Refers to all health care professionals (including students and trainees) and employees of health care establishments who have clinical contact with patients or with blood or body substances.

High-risk/critical items Items in close contact with a break in the skin or mucous membrane or which have been introduced into a sterile body area (e.g. surgical instruments, dressings, catheters, and prosthetic devices). Items in this category must be sterile before they are used on a patient. The recommended decontamination method is sterilization.

Hospital-acquired infection (nosocomial infection) Infection acquired during hospitalization; not present or incubating at the time of admission to hospital. In general, infections that occur more than 72 hours after admission and within 10 days after hospital discharge are defined as *nosocomial* or *hospital acquired*. The time frame is modified for infections that have incubation periods less than 72 hours (e.g. gastroenteritis caused by Norwalk virus) or longer than 10 days (e.g. hepatitis A). Surgical site infections are considered nosocomial if the infection occurs within 30 days after the operative procedure or within 1 year if a prosthetic device or foreign material is implanted. Also see *health care-associated infections.*

Humectant Ingredient(s) added to hand hygiene products to moisturize the skin.

Immunity The resistance of a host to a specific infectious agent.

Immunocompromised A state of reduced resistance to infection. It can result from malignant disease, drugs, radiation illness, or a congenital defect.

Incidence The number of new cases of a disease (or event) occurring in a specified time.

Incidence rate The ratio of the number of new cases of infection or disease in a defined population in a given period to the number of individuals at risk in the population.

Incubation period The time interval between initial exposure to the infectious agent and the appearance of the first signs or symptoms of the disease in a susceptible host.

Index case The first case to be recognized in a series of transmissions of an infective agent in a host population.

Infection The host reaction to invasion by microorganisms. The damaging of body tissue by microorganisms or by poisonous substances released by the microorganisms.

Intermediate-risk/semi-critical items Items that make direct contact with intact mucous membranes. Semi-critical items need not be sterile when used, although this is desirable; but they do need to be free of the common vegetative microorganisms. The recommended decontamination method is disinfection, preferably by moist heat.

Invasive procedure Any procedure that pierces skin or mucous membranes or enters a body cavity or organ. This includes surgical entry into tissues, cavities, or organs or repair of traumatic injuries. See also *Exposure-prone procedures.*

Lookback investigation The process of identifying, tracing, recalling, counselling, and testing patients or health care workers who may have been exposed to an infection, usually a blood-borne virus.

Low-risk/non-critical items Objects that make contact with intact skin (e.g. chairs, baths, washing bowls, toilets, and bedding). The recommended decontamination method is cleaning and drying. Disinfection is necessary if there is a known infection risk.

Medical device According to the UK Medical Device Agency a medical device is an instrument, apparatus, appliance, material, or other article, whether used alone or in combination, intended by the manufacturer to be used on human beings for the purpose of: diagnosis, prevention, monitoring, treatment, or alleviation of disease, diagnosis, monitoring, treatment, alleviation of or compensation for an injury or handicap, investigation, replacement, or modification of the anatomy or physiological process and control of conception.

Microbiological clearance The reduction of the number of pathogenic microorganisms in a specimen below that detectable by conventional means.

Microorganism (microbe) A microscopic entity capable of replication. These include bacteria, viruses, fungi, and protozoa.

Negative pressure ventilation Used to denote airflow which is negative in relation to surrounding air pressure. It is usually created by mechanical airflow devices (e.g. exhaust fans).

Nosocomial infection See *Hospital-acquired infection* and *Health care associated infection.*

Notifiable disease A disease or condition which is notifiable to the Director of Public Health as required under UK Public Health Order.

Outbreak An outbreak can be defined as two or more epidemiologically-linked cases of infection caused by the same microorganism in place and/or time. However, a more realistic definition of an outbreak would be the occurrence of disease at a rate greater than that expected within a specific geographical area and over a defined period of time.

Pathogen A microorganism capable of producing disease in a susceptible host.

Pathogenicity The power of an infectious agent or microorganism to produce disease in a susceptible host.

Prevalence rate The ratio of the total number of individuals who have a disease at a particular time to the population at risk of having the disease.

Prion A small proteinaceous infectious unit that appears to cause transmissible spongiform encephalopathies.

Protective isolation The physical separation of immunocompromised patients in an attempt to prevent the transmission of infectious agents.

Reservoir Any animate or inanimate focus in the environment in which an infectious agent may survive and multiply and which may act as a potential source of infection.

Re-usable item An item designated or intended by the manufacturer as suitable for reprocessing and re-use.

Seroconversion The development of antibodies not previously present, resulting from a primary infection.

Sharps Any objects capable of inflicting penetrating injury, including needles, scalpel blades, wires, trochors, auto lancets, stitch cutters, etc.

Single-use items Items designated by the manufacturer for single-use only.

Skin antiseptic An antiseptic that is intended for application to intact, healthy skin to prevent the transmission of transient or resident skin bacteria from person-to-person or from a surgical operation site to underlying tissue. Skin disinfectants include antiseptic preparations, antiseptic soaps and hand washes, and antiseptic hand rubs.

Source isolation The physical separation of an infected or colonized host from the remainder of the 'at-risk' population in an attempt to prevent transmission of the specific agent to other individuals and patients.

Sporadic case A single case which has not apparently been associated with other cases, excreters, or carriers in the same period of time.

Standard precautions Work practices required to achieve a basic level of infection control. Standard precautions are recommended for the treatment and care of *all* patients. Standard precautions include good hygiene practices, particularly washing and drying hands before and after patient contact, use of personal protective equipment, careful handling and disposal of sharps and clinical waste, and the use of aseptic techniques.

Sterile Free from all living microorganisms and spores.

Sterilization A process which renders an item sterile or free from all living microorganisms and spores. For practical reasons, a process can be said to sterilize if it can kill or remove 10^6 spores of a type specified to test the process within the time specified.

Surveillance Systematic collection, analysis, and interpretation of data on specific events (infections) and disease, followed by dissemination of that information to those who can improve the outcomes.

Susceptible A person not possessing sufficient resistance (or immunity) to an infectious agent to prevent them from contracting infection when exposed to the agent.

Transmission The method by which any potentially infecting agent is spread to another host, i.e. contact, airborne, droplet, ingestion, vertical, sexual, and vector-borne.

Transmission-based precautions These are additional precautions, used for patients infected or colonized with pathogens that can be transmitted by contact, droplet, or airborne routes.

Virulence The intrinsic ability of a microorganism to infect a host and produce disease.

Window period The period immediately after a person is exposed with an agent, during which the infection is not detected by laboratory tests, although the person may be infectious.

Zoonosis An infection or infectious disease transmissible under natural conditions from vertebrate animals to humans.

Chapter 1

Basic concepts

> For creatures your size I offer
> a free choice of habitat,
> so settle yourselves in the zone
> that suits you best, in the pools
> of my pores or the tropical
> forests of arm-pit and crotch,
> in the deserts of my fore-arms,
> or the cool woods of my scalp.
>
> A New Year Greeting, *W.H. Auden (1907–1973)*

Microbes are ubiquitous. They live inside and outside of our bodies and in the surrounding environment, including water, food, vegetables, animals, etc. The vast majority of microbes are harmless and according to J. Ingraham 'the percentage of disease-causing microorganisms (pathogens) are far, far less than the percentage of humans that commit first-degree murder'.

For a particular anatomical site, there is a normal flora which is part of a synergistic host–microbe relationship. It not only contributes to the maintenance of a healthy host but is also essential for our survival. They also act as a protective barrier in *resisting* the establishment of pathogenic microorganisms—this defence mechanism is called '*colonization resistance*'. The classical example is that when an antibiotic is prescribed to an individual, it kills and disturbs the normal healthy microflora of the gut which acts as a protective 'wall paper', thus allowing *Clostridium difficile* and other enteric pathogens to establish, thus causing diarrhoeal diseases. Figure 1.1 shows the normal flora of humans on various body sites.

Human microflora

Although the microflora of a human being develops over time, initial colonization occurs rapidly after **birth** via passage through the birth canal. For example, the skin of a newborn is colonized within 2 hours at almost all sites, the oral cavity and the rectum are colonized within 72 hours, while the vagina takes up to 4 days after birth to be colonized.

The **skin** is a tough dry exterior that protects the body from the external environment. It has an acidic environment, with a pH of about 5.5, and a temperature range

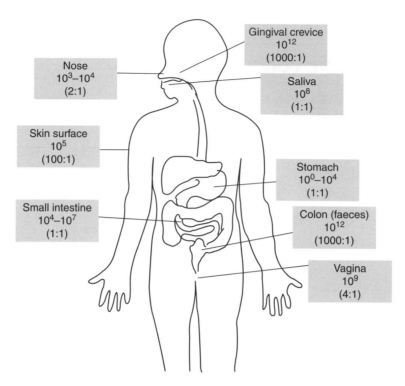

Fig. 1.1 Figure showing numbers of bacteria which colonize different parts of the body with (anaerobic: aerobic) ratio.

from 26°C to 35°C. It provides an environment of low humidity on exposed surfaces and of higher humidity in occluded sites such as the groin, axilla, and toe web. There is plenty of oxygen available on the outermost layers of the surface of the skin (stratum corneum), but none beneath the surface in its hair follicles where bacteria exist as microcolonies. The skin is also rich in protein, exudes oils, and its surface is covered with desquamated cells which are shed on a daily basis. This environment permits microorganisms which are proteolytic (protein eating), lipophilic (utilizing lipids or oils), acidophilic (preferring an acid environment), and versatile enough to live either aerobically or anaerobically (with or without oxygen) to successfully colonize the skin. The microbial species that best fit the environment and are part of skin flora are *Staphylococcus epidermidis*, *Staph. aureus*, 'diphtheroids', and *Propionibacterium* spp.

All surfaces of the **mouth** are constantly washed by saliva, which maintains a relatively neutral pH except when high-sucrose foods are eaten, at which time the oral cavity pH can drop to 4–5. The microflora of the oral cavity consists of over 200 bacterial species. The upper part of the *gastrointestinal tract* (oesophagus, stomach, and upper part of the small intestine) is free from microbes mainly as a result of gut motility. However, the concentration of microorganisms in the contents of the intestinal tract increases from a low level of 10^2 colony-forming units (cfu)/ml in the upper part of the small intestine to 10^{12} cfu/ml (one trillion bacteria per gram) in the lower large intestine.

The multilayered **vagina** lacks hair follicles or glands. The microflora of the vaginal environment is present at a level of 10^8–10^9 organisms/g of secretion. It is mainly comprised of different strains of lactobacilli which are acid producers and which therefore create a protective acid environment (pH 4–6). The characteristics of the vaginal microflora change not only throughout the reproductive life of a woman but also within the menstrual cycle. The concentration of anaerobes remains constant throughout the menstrual cycle, but the total aerobic and facultative organism counts decrease 100-fold during the week preceding menstrual flow. During menstruation, when the blood flows over the acidic mucosal surfaces of the vagina and vulva, the pH of the vagina increases to become more neutral or alkaline. This allows *Escherichia coli* and other normal faecal flora to grow efficiently in large numbers in the vaginal vault. Therefore it is advisable that women who are more prone to recurrent urinary tract infections should avoid sexual intercourse during menstruation.

Types of microbes

Microbes can be divided into three main categories:

Eukaryotic organisms

These organisms have a complex cellular structure, similar to those of humans and animals. Their cells have nuclei and mitochondria and they are largely self-sufficient and capable of independent life. These include **fungi** which exist either in the form of moulds which grow by tubular branching filaments (e.g. *Aspergillus* spp.), or yeasts (e.g. *Candida* spp.) which are oval or spherical and grow by budding, and parasites (e.g. helminthes and protozoans) which are much larger in size from a few millimetres to metres. **Protozoa** are also unicellular organisms, can move about on their own, and are larger than bacteria, e.g. *Entamoeba histolytica*, *Giardia lamblia*.

Prokaryotic organisms

These include bacteria, which are simple and largely self-sufficient unicellular organisms which have no nuclei or internal dividing membranes but are usually capable of independent life. However, some genera, e.g. *Rickettsia* and *Chlamydia*, are not capable of independent life and are therefore named 'atypical bacteria'. The latter group of organisms are obligate intracellular pathogens which require the presence of viable eukaryotic host cells for growth and reproduction.

Bacteria are 0.5–1 μm broad, 0.5–8 μm long, and vary in shape and size and can be seen under light microscopes. Different bacteria have different growth characteristics. Strictly *aerobic* bacteria *need oxygen* to grow; strictly *anaerobic* bacteria *cannot grow* in the presence of oxygen, while facultative anaerobic bacteria can grow in the presence or absence of oxygen. Some bacteria are fastidious and have specific nutritional or other environmental requirements for growth.

The basis of differentiation of bacteria into Gram positive and negative is done by a staining method devised by Hans Christian Gram in 1884. The structural differences between Gram-positive and Gram-negative bacteria is that the cell wall in Gram-positive bacteria is composed of the peptidoglycan layer, while Gram-negative bacteria possess an outer membrane in addition to the peptidoglycan layer.

Viruses are too small to be seen by an ordinary light microscope, but can be seen under an electron microscope. They vary in shape and structure and many species have distinctive morphological characteristics and are usually classified into DNA and RNA viruses. There are some differences between viral and bacterial infections, i.e. all viruses are incapable of independent survival and require host cells for growth and reproduction; they are a much smaller size; provide a relatively high degree of immunity following infection; and may require antiviral agents to treat infections as the antibiotics used to treat bacterial infections are *not* effective.

Prions

Prions are proteinaceous infectious agents composed primarily of protein. Prion disease is caused by accumulation in the brain of an aberrant form of prion protein (PrP^{Sc}). In humans, prion diseases include Kuru, sporadic, familial, iatrogenic and variant Creutzfeldt–Jakob disease (CJD), and in animals includes bovine spongiform encephalopathy (BSE or 'mad cow disease' in cattle), sheep/goat scrapie, etc.

Pathogenesis of infectious diseases

The establishment of an infection in the body is depended on the three main factors:

Number of microbes

Each microorganism has a set infective dose and microorganisms which have low infective doses spread more quickly than microorganisms which have high infective doses. In addition, if the person is immunosuppressed, the infective dose required to cause infection is even lower.

Virulence

This is the capacity for a microbial strain to produce diseases. Each microorganism has a different virulence factor. In addition, microorganisms within the same species have different virulence factors, e.g. Panton–Valentine leucocidin (PVL) toxin-producing *Staph. aureus* are more virulent then non–PVL-producing *Staph. aureus* and the 027 strain of *C. difficile* are more virulent then the non-027 strain.

Immune status of patients

This is also one of the most important factors as patients who are at an extreme age, immunosuppressed, e.g. patients with a transplant, AIDS, and patients on cancer chemotherapy are more susceptible to infection. In addition, patients who are immunized or who have been exposed to certain infectious disease (e.g. chickenpox) are less likely to get the same disease due to lifelong immunity.

$$Infection \ \alpha \ \frac{Number \ of \ microbes \times Virulence \ characteristics}{Immune \ status \ of \ the \ host}$$

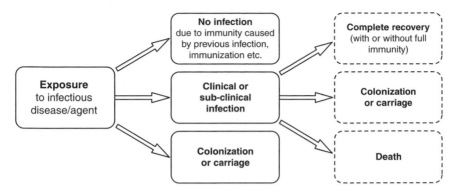

Fig. 1.2 Diagram showing possible outcomes if an individual is exposed to an infectious agent.

It is important to note that exposure to a microorganism *does not always* necessarily lead to infection and Figure 1.2 summarizes the possible outcome. Healthy individuals may be 'colonized' without disease (meticillin-resistant *Staph. aureus* (MRSA), extended-spectrum beta-lactamase (ESBL), vancomycin-resistant *Enterococcus* (VRE), etc.) or carry infectious agents without overt symptoms of infection (HIV, hepatitis B and hepatitis C, *Chlamydia*, etc.). Colonized or asymptomatic patients are often also described as *carriers*. However, the term colonization should be restricted to the presence of a microbe at an *expected site*, e.g. *E. coli* in the large bowel, or *Staph. epidermidis* on the skin, but occasionally it is also used to describe the presence of a potential pathogen in an unexpected site without causing symptomatic infection, e.g. presence of *Staph. aureus* or MRSA in the upper respiratory tract or *E. coli* in the urine of a catheterized patient with *no* symptoms. Therefore, it is essential that the *bacteriology report must be interpreted in the presence of clinical symptoms* and one should treat patient with clinical symptoms and *not* a positive bacteriology report.

Due to underlying illness, immunosuppressive therapy, and invasive procedures, hospitalized patients are more prone to develop infections. They can acquire infection either from an *exogenous route,* where the source microorganisms are acquired from health care environment, equipment and from health care workers or via an *endogenous route* where the source of microorganisms is from the patient's own microflora. Endogenous infections are commonly seen in an immunocompromised host, e.g. neutropenic and transplant patients.

Chain of infection

In order to prevent health care-associated infections (HCAIs), it is essential to understand the six vital links of transmission; the prevention and control strategies of HCAI in health care settings rely on breaking these links in the chain to interrupt transmission.

1. Causative agent

The causative agent for infection is any microorganism capable of producing disease. Microorganisms responsible for infectious diseases include bacteria, viruses, rickettsiae, fungi, protozoa, and helminthes.

2. Reservoir of infection

The reservoir of infection could be an infected person, animal, items/equipment, and/ or the environment on which microorganisms can survive and, in some cases, multiply. Animals and human beings can all serve as reservoirs, providing the essential requirements for a microorganism to survive at specific stages in its life cycle. In some inanimate environments, some microorganisms not only survive but also multiply (e.g. *Pseudomonas* spp. in wet environment), while in others the microorganisms survive but do not multiply on the surface (e.g. hepatitis B virus).

Infectious reservoirs abound in health care settings, and may include everything from patients, visitors, and staff members to furniture, medical equipment, food, water, and blood. A human reservoir may be either an infected case or a carrier. A case is a patient with an acute clinical infection while a carrier is a person who is colonized with a specific pathogenic microorganism but shows no signs or symptoms of infection (e.g. MRSA).

Carriers fall into four categories: an *incubatory carrier* is one who has acquired the infection and has been incubating the illness but does not yet show symptoms. Incubation periods vary from one infectious disease to other (see Appendix 7.2, page 131). A *convalescent carrier* is in the recovery stage of an illness but continues to shed the pathogenic microorganism for an indefinite period, e.g. a patient who has had a *Salmonella* infection commonly sheds the organism in their faeces even after symptoms disappear. An *intermittent carrier* occasionally sheds the pathogenic microorganism from time to time, e.g. some people are intermittent carriers of *Staph. aureus*. A *chronic carrier* always has the infectious organism in their system, e.g. chronic carriers of hepatitis B and C virus. Asymptomatic carriers may present a risk of cross-infection in health care facilities because their illnesses go unrecognized and therefore adherence to standard infection control prevention is essential at all the time.

3. Portal of exit

The portal of exit is the path by which an infectious agent leaves its reservoir. Usually, this portal is the site where the microorganism also grows. Common portals of exit associated with human reservoirs include the respiratory, genitourinary, and gastrointestinal tracts, the skin, and mucous membranes.

4. Mode of transmission

The microorganism can be acquired via various routes. However it is important to remember that some microorganisms use more than one transmission route to get from the reservoir to a new host.

Contact transmission: contact is the most frequent mode of transmission of HCAIs. It occurs when microorganisms are transferred from one infected person to another person. This can occur either as:

Direct contact: direct contact occurs when there is physical contact with a patient, e.g. during activities such as bathing, dressing changes, insertion and maintenance of invasive devices, etc. Diseases that spread by direct contact include scabies and herpes simplex (if direct contact with infected lesions or secretions occurs on mucous membrane). Hand washing is the *most effective way* to prevent transmission by the contact route.

Indirect contact: indirect contact transmission occurs when an infectious agent is transmitted through a contaminated intermediate object (items and equipments) or person. In health care settings, effective cleaning, disinfections and sterilization of items/equipment is essential to prevent transmission through this route. Effective environmental cleaning is necessary to reduce the bioburden of microorganisms. Use of personal protective equipment is used as an additional barrier to prevent contamination of clothing, e.g. uniforms when nursing infected/colonized individuals. Hands are contaminated not only after touching infected/colonized patients but also by touching contaminated items/equipment and environment and therefore hand hygiene is key in preventing this mode of transmission.

Droplet transmission: droplet transmission occurs when microorganisms come into contact with the mucous membranes of a person's nose, mouth, eyes, etc. such as when an infected person coughs, sneezes, or talks. Droplet transmission is considered to be a form of contact transmission, as microbes in droplet nuclei (mucus droplets >5 μm in size) can travel only up to about 1 metre (~3 feet) and therefore cause also cause very heavy contamination of the surrounding environment. Droplet transmission differs from airborne transmission in that the droplets are heavy and therefore do not remain suspended in the air for a long time and settle on surfaces very quickly due to gravity—therefore special air handling and provision of negative pressure ventilation is not necessary. In order to prevent transmission via this route, it is recommended to wear a surgical mask when within *1.8–3 metres (6–10 feet)* of the patient or upon entry into the patient's room. In addition, it is essential that overcrowding of patients in the ward should be avoided and adequate bed spacing between patients should be kept. UK Health Estates recommend 3.6 metres (~12 feet) between the canters of adjacent beds.

Examples of diseases spread by droplets include influenza, whooping cough, etc. Although *Staph. aureus* is mainly transmitted by a contact route, if colonized individuals suffer from an upper respiratory tract infection caused by a virus, they can disperse *Staph. aureus* into the air for a distance of about 1.2 metres (4 feet). These individuals are called as the *'cloud baby*/adult' and have been responsible for causing outbreaks.

Airborne transmission: transmission via airborne route occurs when pathogens are transmitted to a susceptible person though inhalation of small droplet nuclei of particle size (<5 μm). Such particles are very light in nature and therefore can disperse well beyond 1 metre (3 feet) and remain airborne for long periods. Because these particles are very light in nature, on inhalation they can reach the alveoli by passing the bronchial tree to cause infection. Therefore, health care workers (HCWs) should wear a respirator when entering the room. Ideally these patients should be nursed in an isolation room with negative pressure ventilation (6–12 changes/hour) to dilute and remove the infective microorganisms safely. Microorganisms for which airborne precautions are necessary include *Mycobacterium tuberculosis*, varicella-zoster virus (chickenpox), and rubeola virus (measles). If possible, a non-susceptible person should replace a HCW who is susceptible to measles or chickenpox. Figure 1.3 shows host defence mechanisms in the respiratory tract.

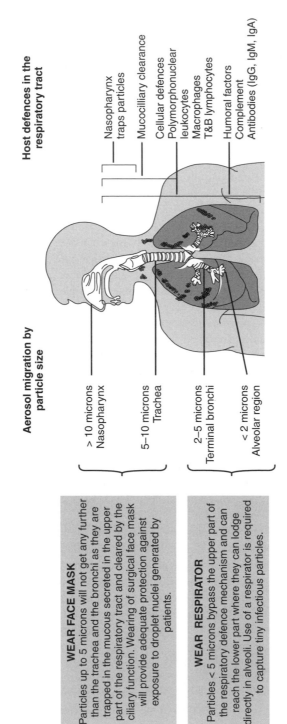

Fig. 1.3 Figure showing host defence mechanisms in the respiratory tract and use of appropriate personal protection equipment to protect against infection spread by droplet and air-borne routes.

5. Portal of entry

The portal of entry is the path by which an infectious agent invades a susceptible host and this is usually the same as the portal of exit.

6. Susceptible host

The final and most important link in the chain of infection is the susceptible host (see Table 1.1). The human body has many defence mechanisms for resisting the entry and multiplication of pathogens. When these mechanisms function normally, infection does not occur. However, in immunocompromised patients, where the body defences are weakened, infectious agents are more likely to invade the body and cause an infection. In addition, the very young and the very old are at higher risk for infection because in the very young the immune system does not fully develop until about 6 months of age, while old age is associated with declining immune system function as well as with chronic diseases which also weaken host defences.

The body's defence mechanisms

First line of defence

External and mechanical barriers such as the skin, other body organs, and secretions serve as the body's first line of defence. Intact skin, mucous membranes, certain chemical substances, specialized structures such as cilia, and normal flora can stop pathogens from establishing themselves in the body. The gag and cough reflexes and gastrointestinal tract peristalsis work to remove pathogens before they can establish a foothold. Chemical substances that help prevent infection or inhibit microbial growth include secretions such as saliva, perspiration, and gastrointestinal and vaginal secretions as well as interferon (a naturally occurring glycoprotein with antiviral properties). Normal microbial flora controls the growth of potential pathogens through a mechanism called *microbial antagonism*—microbial flora use nutrients that pathogens need for growth, compete with pathogens for sites on tissue receptors, and secrete naturally occurring antibiotics to kill the pathogens. When microbial antagonism is disturbed, such as by prolonged antibiotic therapy, an infection may develop; for example, antibiotic therapy may destroy the normal flora of the mouth, leading to overgrowth of *Candida albicans* and consequent thrush.

Second line of defence

If a microorganism gets past the first line of defence by entering the body through a break in the skin, white blood cells and the inflammatory response come into play. Because these components respond to any type of injury, their response is termed non-specific. The main function of the inflammatory response is to bring phagocytic cells (neutrophils and monocytes) to the inflamed area to destroy microorganisms. If a pathogen gets past non-specific defences, it confronts specific immune responses, cell-mediated immunity or humoral immunity. Cell-mediated immunity involves T cells. Some T cells synthesize and secrete lymphokines and orchestrate the cell-mediated immunity, these are the CD4 subsets of the T lymphocytes also known as helper T cells. Others become killer (cytotoxic) cells, predominantly the CD8 subsets of the

Table 1.1 Innate host first-line defence mechanisms

Mechanism	Examples	Examples of disturbances in first-line defences
Physical barriers	Skin	Skin abrasion/laceration
		Burns
		Skin condition, e.g. psoriasis
		Inoculation injuries
		Trauma to the skin
		Surgical site/wound infections
		Insertion of intravenous line
		T-tube biliary drain tubes
		Insertion of urinary catheter
		Insertion of nasogastric tube
		Insertion of endotracheal tube
	Interference with mucociliary clearance mechanism	Smoking
		Respiratory viral infections
		Sticky nature of mucus in the respiratory tract
		Drying airway secretions due to dehydration or tracheostomy
Mechanical barriers	Washing action of secretions/excretions and dilution factor of fluids: urine, tears, bile, etc.	Insertion of urinary catheter
	Coughing, sneezing gag, effective swallow etc.	Impaired conscious state
		General anaesthesia
		Endotracheal intubation and tracheostomy
		Surgery procedures that restrict coughing esp. on abdomen and chest
		Post-traumatic/postoperative pain
Chemicals antimicrobial	Hydrochloric acid in stomach	H_2 antagonists and proton pump inhibitors
		Previous gastric surgery
	pH and chemical barriers: stomach acid, skin fats, vaginal pH	Enteral tubes feeding
		Achlorhydria
	Antibiotic therapy	Diabetes mellitus (altered skin fats)
		Disturbance of normal flora which may leads to colonization by hospital microflora

T lymphocytes, setting out to track down infected body cells. Once the infection is under control, suppresser T cells bring the immune response to a close. Humoral immunity, mediated by antibodies, involves the action of B lymphocytes in conjunction with helper T cells. Antibodies produced in response to the infectious agent help fight the infection. In response to the effects of suppressor T-cell activity, antibody production then wanes. Impaired host defences make patients more susceptible to infection. Conditions that may weaken a person's defences include malnutrition, extremes of age, AIDS, chronic disease, immunosuppressive therapy, surgery, and inadequate immunization.

Strategies to control and prevent health care-associated infections

Figure 1.4 summarizes the five pillars of infection prevention and control. Surveillance (process and outcome) and audits should be carried out to monitor the compliance with the recommended practice. In recent years, various strategies to control and prevent HCAIs have been applied successfully and these interventions have been very successful in reducing HCAIs substantially and they are discussed briefly in this chapter.

Concept of zero tolerance

Some health care facilities have introduced the *concept of zero tolerance*. This concept originates on the premise that no *preventable* HCAI is considered tolerable and no

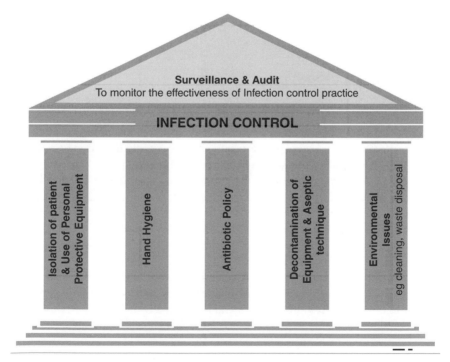

Fig. 1.4 Five pillars of infection prevention and control.

benchmark or mean is good enough unless it is zero. Clinical teams should be accountable for performing at the highest level in the interest of patient safety and quality. For various factors, we fully recognize that *not all HCAIs are preventable* and for certain types of infections, it may not be possible to achieve zero infection rates. However, it is important that clinical teams *must focus on doing everything under their control* to prevent patients getting HCAIs and reduce their rate to 'irreducible minimum'. They should create a culture of *zero tolerance* to poor infection control practice which puts patients at risk.

Root cause analysis

In the UK, root cause analysis (RCA) has been effectively used to control MRSA bacteraemia and *C. difficile* infection and tools are available from http://hcai.dh.gov. uk/website. RCA is a reactive method with the aim of identifying the *root causes* of preventable HCAIs and is based on the concept that problems are best solved by attempting to address and take corrective action to eliminate the *root causes* rather than merely addressing the immediately obvious issues which have resulted in infections. Information gathered by the RCA over a long period may make it useful as a *proactive method* and if effectively carried out it can be used to *forecast* or predict probable events even *before* they occur. It is recognized that complete prevention of recurrence by one corrective action is not always possible and for this tool to be effective, corrective action must be taken at an appropriate time and all the recommendations to prevent its recurrence must be followed and implemented both by clinical and non-clinical staff to close the loop. Thus, RCA is often considered to be an iterative process, and is frequently viewed as a tool of *continuous improvement.*

Care bundle approach

The concept of a 'care bundle' in the health care setting was introduced by Dr Donald Berwick, the CEO of the Institute for Healthcare Improvement (IHI) who gave a speech on 14 December, 2004 to a room full of hospital administrators at a large industry convention and said 'Here is what I think we should do. I think we should save 100,000 lives. And I think we should do that by 14th June 2006—18 months from today. Some is not a number; soon is not a time. Here's the number: 100,000. Here's the time: 14th June 2006—9 am'. Eighteen months later he announced that the hospitals enrolled in the *100,000 Lives Campaign* had collectively prevented an estimated 122,300 avoidable deaths. The campaign has been extremely successful and has been re-named *Protecting 5 Million Lives from Harm* and the concept has now been adapted by many hospitals in developed countries.

The concept of care bundles has emerged from the acknowledgement that health care delivery is too dependent on individual clinicians' knowledge, motivation, and skills, with the result that most of the patients do not receive *all the recommended care all the time* due to variation in practices. *Care bundle* is defined as a 'group of evidence-based interventions that, when implemented together, result in better outcomes than when implemented individually'. As the IHI has pointed out, the strength of a bundle comes from the simplicity, consistency, and evidence behind each of its components.

Care elements / Observation	Care element 1	Care element 2	Care element 3	Care element 4	All elements performed
1	✔		✔	✔	
2	✔	✔		✔	
3	✔	✔	✔	✔	✔
4	✔	✔	✔		
5	✔	✔	✔	✔	✔
Total number of times an individual element was performed	5	4	4	4	2
% when element of care was given	100%	80%	80%	80%	40%

Fig. 1.5 This example of a care bundle shows that while most care elements were performed, on only two occasions were all elements performed correctly. Overall compliance with all elements was only 40% and as a result the risk of infection was significantly increased. With permission from UK Department of Health (2007).

To make it simple, a bundle should consist of three to six elements of well-established/evidence-based practices which should be packaged together into a 'care bundle' that should be delivered by a health care team at one point in time to *every patient* meeting the bundle criteria. Trying to add additional components, although well intentioned, may be associated with lower rates of adherence and, thus, worse outcomes. The point in time for implementation varies according to the type of bundle, as some care bundles may be completed once, while other care bundles should be repeated daily for the same patient. For its success, it is essential that *all the elements* of the care bundle must be implemented on *all the patients* and compliance with the bundle should be monitored (see Figure 1.5).

Care bundles for various interventions are summarized in the relevant chapters of this book. Further information and various implementation tools and resources to reduce HCAIs are available from the Institute of Healthcare Improvement website (http://www.ihi.org/) and the UK Department of Health (High Impact Interventions) website (http://hcai.dh.gov.uk/).

Risk management in infection control

Risk is defined as the possibility of incurring misfortune and loss. Risk management is a *proactive approach* and its aim is to prevent or minimize harm. The implementation of a formal risk management process will identify potential problems and the potential for harm to patients. Once the risks are identified, actions are then planned to reduce the likelihood of the problem arising or to limit the harm caused. In infection control the risks can be biological agents that have the potential to cause infection or a mechanism that allows the transmission of an infectious agent to occur. The risk management process can be divided into four key stages.

1. Risk identification
2. Risk analysis

3. Risk control

4. Risk monitoring.

Risk identification

The process of risk management starts with risk identification and involves identifying:

- Activities and tasks that put patients, HCWs, and visitors at risk
- Infectious agent involved, and
- Mode of transmission.

The aim is to identify common problems/practices that have an impact on a large number of patients or rarer problems which can cause severe infection or death. Once a problem is identified, it is essential to obtain evidence which usually requires the expert knowledge of the Infection Prevention and Control (IPC) team and can be achieved by observational or experimental studies.

Risk analysis

Once the risk has been identified, the likely consequences to patients must be estimated. This can be achieved by analysing four key questions:

- *Why* are infections happening?
- How *frequently* are they happening?
- What are the likely *consequences* if the appropriate action is not taken?
- How much is it going to *cost* to prevent it?

Why are infections happening? A range of system failures can result in patients acquiring HCAIs and it is important to analyse these failures in detail.

- *Type I error*: these occur due to an act of omission, e.g. failure to comply with current professionally accepted practice. The basic cause of a Type I error is lack of knowledge and it is typically common in health care institutions where there is inadequate provision of education, training, and supervision. In a low-resource setting, a scarcity of goods can also contribute to this type of error. Regular education and competence based training, good communication and availability, and regular supplies of goods are necessary to address this issue.
- *Type II error*: these occur due to an act of commission, i.e. an act should not have been committed. These are due to lack of commitment or consideration for others. This type of error is more complex and amongst other things may also require management reinforcement.
- *Type III error*: these mainly occur due to a failure to understand the true nature of the problem. Real solutions are adopted to deal with the wrong problems, rather than incorrect solutions to real problems. This is often due to lack of communication, or misinterpretation of information as a result of inadequate research or information.

How frequently are they happening? This information is quantitative and can be obtained by ongoing surveillance data (if available) or by performing a point prevalence study. The information can be gathered from other sources, e.g. as a part of outbreak investigation, local prevalence data, data published in the literature, or clinical evidence. Frequency can be measured as the percentage or rate of persons who developed infection following either a clinical procedure or exposure to a pathogen. If surveillance data are not available, probability can be used instead. Severity can be measured in terms of morbidity (disability or increased length of stay in hospital) or mortality experienced by persons who had the procedure or exposure.

How much is it going to cost to prevent it? It is also important to estimate the cost of prevention of each risk. Estimated costs are acceptable, as the exact cost may be difficult to obtain. The cost of prevention of infections is important because it helps IPC practitioners to target resources where they will deliver the greatest advantage in terms of preventing harm to patients.

Risk control

Once the risk analysis has been completed, review the possible solutions. Ideally, the risk should be completely eliminated; if this is impossible then the risk should be reduced to a minimum/acceptable level. In some situations, it may be more cost-effective to transfer the risk to a third party, such as a private contractor. For example, if there is a problem with the supply of sterile goods it may be more cost-effective to purchase these items from another source.

If resources are severely constrained, then it may be possible to accept the risk in both the short and possibly long term. Willingness to tolerate known risks in a health care institution is different in different parts of the world and is based mainly on the availability of resources and the fear/level of litigation.

Risk monitoring

Once appropriate measures are in place to reduce the risk, it is essential to monitor their effectiveness. Depending on the availability of resources, this can be achieved by regular audit, process monitoring and outcome, and surveillance of HCAIs. Timely feedback must be given to front-line HCWs and senior management.

Audit in infection control

The aim of infection control audit is to carry out systematic review (or audit) of recommended policies and procedures in infection prevention and control and is based on the evidence-based/best practice to ensure that what *should* be done is *being* done. The audit process will identify the 'gap in the practice' and this process should continue until the recommended best practice is achieved by implementing change to improve quality in health care delivery. The key elements to the success of this process are communication, consultation, and timely feedback of information to all the key stakeholders and making sure that the audit loop is closed. However, the main barriers to audit can be lack of resources, lack of expertise or advice in audit process and analysis, lack of an overall plan for audit, fear of litigation, and hierarchical and territorial suspicions.

Key references and further reading

Bialachowski A et al. The Audit Process: Part I : Pre-preparation, Part II : Setting the audit criteria and Part III : Closing the Loop. *Canadian Journal of Infection Control*, 2010; Spring issue: 68–70; Summer issue:109–111 and Fall issue: 161–165.

CDC. *Hospital Infection Control Practice Advisory Committee. Guidelines for Isolation Precautions in Hospitals. Preventing Transmission of Infectious Agents in Healthcare Settings 2007*. Atlanta, GA: Centers for Disease Control and Prevention, 2007.

Damani NN. Risk management. In: Friedman C, Newsom W (eds). *Basic Concepts of Infection Control*, pp. 179–85. Portadown: International Federation in Infection Control.

Heymann DL. *Control of communicable disease manual*, 19th edn Washington, DC: American Public Health Association, 2008.

Ingraham J. *March of the microbes: sighting the unseen*. Cambridge: The Belknap Press of Harvard University Press, 2010.

Nolan T, Berwick DM. All-or-none measurement raises the bar on performance raises. *Journal of the American Medical Association* 2006; **295**:1168–70.

Roberts G. Risk management in healthcare. 2nd ed. London: Witherby & Co., 2002.

UK Department of Health. *Using high impact interventions: Using care bundles to reduce healthcare associated infection by increasing reliability and safety*. London: Department of Health, 2007. Available at: http://hcai.dh.gov.uk/.

Chapter 2

Administrative arrangement

If you think you're too small to make a difference,
try sleeping in a closed room with a mosquito.

Anonymous

It has been estimated that in developed countries up to 10% of hospitalized patients develop infections every year. The risk of HCAIs in developing countries is much higher than in developed countries (Allegranzi et al., 2011). In the UK, approximately 100,000 patients develop HCAIs which are responsible for over 10,000 deaths per annum and cost the UK National Health Service in excess of one billion pounds per year (UK National Audit Office, 2000). Similarly, in the USA it has been estimated that approximately two million patients suffer HCAIs and nearly 90,000 patients die each year (Scott, 2009). The overall annual direct medical costs of HCAI to US hospitals ranges from $28.4 to $33.8 billion. The European Commission estimates that approximately four million patients acquire HCAIs each year in the European Union, which are responsible for 37,000 deaths, and cost 5.5 billion Euros a year (European Centre for Disease Prevention and Control, 2008).

Impact of health care-associated infections

It is important to bear in mind that in addition to the financial burden to the health care facility, HCAIs also have a profound impact on the delivery of health services which includes:

- Increased length of stay due to HCAI and a number of readmissions to hospital leading to the loss of available bed days to treat other patients. This has a direct impact on patient throughput in the hospital and in an outbreak situation, cancellation of surgical operating lists.
- Private hospitals may lose revenue due to lack of throughput of patients.
- Under 'Pay for Performance', some HCAIs in the USA are now classified as preventable events. Hospitals will no longer be paid for eight conditions presented by the Centers for Medicare and Medicaid Services. Three of the eight conditions are HCAIs: catheter-associated urinary tract infection, vascular catheter-associated infection, and surgical site infection/mediastinitis after coronary artery bypass graft.

Some other profound impacts on the delivery of health services include:

◆ Additional cost of surveillance, isolation measures, and environmental cleaning.

◆ Additional laboratory, radiological, and other investigation costs related to diagnosing and managing HCAIs.

◆ Use of expensive antimicrobials to treat multi-resistant microorganisms.

◆ Lack of adequate isolation facilities may increase the risk of cross infection to other patients, staff, and visitors.

◆ Additional resources are needed to deal with patient's complaints and with the added cost of litigation and public enquiries.

◆ Adverse publicity and loss of confidence of patients in delivery of a quality service.

It is important to bear in mind that the cost of HCAIs to individuals and families should not be underestimated. For example, if a patient is employed, and has to stay in hospital or at home, s/he loses time and/or salary due to being off work. In addition, it also adds an indirect cost to family members in terms of time lost from work in caring for the affected individual. The illness also causes increased suffering to the patient and may have psychological effects not only of 'isolation' in a single room but in certain cultures, the concepts of pestilence and contagion are still inextricably intertwined with beliefs that such diseases are divine punishments for sinners and for those who live dissolute lives.

Responsibilities of health care facilities

HCAIs are now recognized as a major cause of morbidity and mortality worldwide. Therefore, provision of an effective infection prevention and control (IPC) programme is essential for all health care facilities and should be part of the *patient safety* and *quality improvement programme* of the organization. Since the hospital's chief executive/ administrator are managerially responsible for provision of such a service, it is essential that they provide adequate resources, support, and managerial back-up to the IPC team so that agreed infection prevention programmes are implemented *effectively*. The World Health Organization (WHO) has published a core component for provision of an effective infection prevention and control in health care facilities (WHO, 2009).

All *employers* have a legal obligation to ensure that all their employees are appropri- ately trained and proficient in the procedures necessary for working safely. They must be given adequate education and training on all issues relating to IPC and provide a safe work environment, resources, and material to carry out their tasks effectively. In addition, every *employee* also has equal responsibility to ensure that they take all rea- sonable steps while at work to ensure their own health and safety, and that of others who may be affected by their acts and omissions at work. It is the responsibility of each individual employee to be aware of their own role in IPC and to incorporate good practices into *their daily activity* to ensure that they do not jeopardize the health and safety of themselves or any other person.

Managers of all health care establishments must ensure that all HCWs are made aware of the importance and principles of IPC. They should also emphasize the importance of continuing education and training for all HCWs. New employees should be offered an orientation and induction programme to increase their awareness and to assist in their understanding of the institutional policies and programmes for IPC. Education and training programmes should be flexible enough to encourage participation.

Policies and procedures manual

It is essential that each health care establishment should develop a manual of policies and procedures and this manual should establish standards for performance in all aspects of IPC. The recommendations in the manual must be based on the relevant national guidelines. They should be practical, workable, and sufficiently flexible to ensure their implementation. Policies and procedures should identify IPC indicators and desired outcomes. They should also include some basis for the risk assessment of each procedure. A comprehensive procedures manual should include policies and procedures on:

* Isolation of patients.
* Hand hygiene and appropriate use of personal protective equipment.
* Cleaning, decontamination, and sterilization of items and equipment.
* Environmental cleaning and decontamination.
* Management of spills or accidents with infectious substances.
* Safe handling and transport of pathology specimens.
* Handling and cleaning/disinfection of contaminated linen.
* Handling and safe disposal of clinical and related waste.
* Handling and safe disposal of sharps.
* Management of sharps injuries and other exposure of HCWs to infectious diseases.
* Policies and procedures for insertion and maintenance of all indwelling devices, e.g. intravenous and urinary catheters.

The IPC manual must be updated on a regular basis and issue and review dates must be clearly stated. Staff should be informed of changes to current policies and procedures, as well as the introduction of new ones. New policies should be carefully monitored by regular audit and should include feedback to the clinical team. The manual should be easily accessible to all HCWs and availability of the manual on the intranet should be considered, if possible.

Reduction of health care-associated infections

In 1985, the SENIC Project (Study on the Efficacy of Nosocomial Infection Control) study provided evidence that a well-organized infection control programme is not only effective in reducing nosocomial infections, but provision of such a programme in every hospital is also cost-effective. The study also highlighted that 6% of infections can be prevented by using minimal infection control efforts, and 32% could be prevented by a well-organized and highly effective IPC programme (Haley et al., 1985).

However, recent data suggest that if evidence-based infection control practices are implemented, HCAIs can be reduced even further. Based on the published data, it has been estimated that if various evidence-based infection control interventions are successfully implemented, the risk of developing HCAIs can be substantially reduced.

It has been estimated that up to a 70% reduction in HCAIs can be achieved for IV catheter-associated bloodstream infections and infections associated with the use of urinary catheters. Similar interventions can reduce ventilated-associated pneumonias and surgical sites infections by 55%. However, due to the complexity of various factors, it is not possible to achieve a 100% reduction in HCAIs (Umscheid et al., 2011).

Public reporting of health care-associated infection data

Although public reporting of HCAI data is controversial it has also had some success as 'naming and shaming' has put pressure on the hospital management and clinicians to take HCAI reduction more seriously. In the UK, HCAIs public reporting and targets were introduced to reduce MRSA bacteraemias and *Clostridium difficile* infections by the Department of Health due to pressure both from the media and the public. Introduction of HCAI targets has been extremely successful as the political commitment was matched with additional resources and the chief executives were made responsible for achieving these targets. This strategy clearly demonstrated that substantial and sustained reduction of HCAIs can be achieved provided there is clear commitment from the senior management. In addition, there was also a fundamental shift in the approach to prevent HCAIs in the UK by making infection prevention and control *everybody's responsibility*.

Organization of an infection prevention and control programme

Although the organization of an IPC programme varies from country to country depending on the available resources, in the majority of countries the IPC programme is delivered through an IPC team who is not only responsible for the day-to-day running of the IPC programme but is also responsible for setting priorities, applying evidence-based practice, and advising hospital administrators on issues relating to IPC. The IPC team usually comprises the IPC doctor(s) and nurse(s).

Infection prevention and control doctor

The IPC doctor/officer must be a registered medical practitioner. In the majority of countries, the role is performed either by a medical microbiologist, hospital epidemiologist, or consultant in infectious diseases. Irrespective of their professional background, the IPC doctor should have knowledge and experience in medical microbiology and infectious disease, hospital epidemiology and surveillance, asepsis, disinfection, and sterilization. It is recommended that at least one IPC doctor is required for every 1000 beds. However, this may vary greatly depending on their role and responsibility in the organization and type of health care facility.

The role and responsibilities of the IPC doctor/officer are summarized as follows:

- Serves as a specialist advisor and takes a leading role in the effective functioning of the IPC team.
- Should be an active member of the hospital IPC committee and may act as its chairperson.

◆ Assists the hospital IPC committee in drawing up annual plans, policies, and long-term programmes for the prevention of HCAIs.

◆ Advises the chief executive/hospital administrator directly on all aspects of HCAIs and on the implementation of agreed policies.

◆ Participates in the preparation of tender documents for the support services and advises on IPC aspects.

◆ Is involved in setting of quality standards, surveillance, and monitoring of HCAIs.

In order to increase the profile of IPC, in 2003, the post of Director of Infection Prevention and Control (DIPC) was created in the UK to lead the IPC programme. Every hospital is required to appoint a DIPC at board level with direct reporting to the chief executive. Roles, responsibilities, and competencies of the DIPC are available at the UK Department of Health website: http://www.dh.gov.uk.

Infection prevention and control nurse

An IPC nurse/practitioner is a registered nurse with an additional academic education and practical training which enables him or her to act as a specialist advisor. A recognized qualification in IPC should be held which will allow recognition of the nurse as a specialist practitioner. The role and responsibilities of the IPC nurse are summarized as follows:

◆ Serves as a specialist advisor and take a leading day-to-day role in the effective functioning of the IPC team.

◆ Should be an active member of the hospital IPC committee.

◆ Assists the health care facility IPC committee in drawing up annual plans and policies.

◆ Provides specialist nursing input in surveillance, prevention, monitoring, and control of HCAIs.

◆ Identifies, investigates, and takes timely action on all hazardous practice and procedures relating to IPC.

◆ Advises the contracting departments, participating in the preparation of documents relating to service specifications and quality standards.

◆ Ongoing contribution to the development and implementation of IPC policies and procedures, participating in audit, and monitoring tools related to IPC and infectious diseases.

◆ Presentation of educational programmes and membership of relevant committees where IPC input is required.

It is essential that the IPC nurse should have an expert knowledge of both general and specialist nursing practice and must also have an understanding not only of the functioning of clinical areas but also operational areas and services. S/he must also be able to communicate effectively with all grades of staff, negotiate and effect change, and influence practice.

In order to perform the job effectively, IPC practitioners *must* possess a higher level of knowledge in clinical and diagnostic microbiology, epidemiolog,y and infection prevention and control. In addition, they must possess essential skills and understanding of their role and responsibilities. In the UK, the Infection Prevention Society has developed a competency-based framework that will assist IPC nurses to continually expand on their existing knowledge, understanding, and skills to help IPC staff to address the challenges that HCAI presents in our ever changing health care environment (Burnett, 2011).

Infection prevention and control team

The team is comprised of an IPC doctor and IPC nurse(s). The team is responsible for the day-to-day running of the IPC programme. It is important that all acute hospitals should have an IPC team, although smaller health care providers may not find this a feasible option. In cases where the provision of an IPC team is not possible, arrangements for the provision of and access to the IPC service should be arranged with a nearby acute hospital. The role of the IPC team can be summarized as follows:

- Production of an annual IPC programme with clearly defined objectives.
- Production of written policies and procedures on IPC, including regular evaluation and update.
- Education of all grades of staff in IPC policy, practice, and procedures relevant to their own area of practice.
- Surveillance of infection to detect outbreaks at the earliest opportunity and provide data that should be evaluated to allow for any change in practice or allocation of resources to prevent HCAIs.
- Provide advice to all grades of staff on all matters in relation to IPC on a day-to-day basis.
- Participate in the audit activity.

For an effective working of the IPC team, it is essential that:

- All IPC practitioners should be resourced appropriately to meet the goals and objectives of the health care facility in surveillance, detection, and management of an outbreak, provision of education and training to the staff, etc.
- They must be trained and educated in all aspects of IPC, clinical microbiology, and infectious diseases, and should attend conference and educational meetings on an ongoing basis to keep them abreast of the current knowledge and evidence-based practice.
- They must have access to the Internet and most up-to-date textbooks, current journals, and standards and/or guidelines in IPC.
- Adequate office space and secretarial support with computers must be provided so that they can function effectively.
- They should have access to expert resources, e.g. medical microbiologist, infectious disease physician, epidemiologist, consultant in communicable disease control, microbiology, and virology laboratory.

The role of the IPC team is to ensure that an effective IPC programme is implemented and its impact is monitored and evaluated. Whilst they will actively participate in most of these areas, some aspects of the IPC programme may fall under the remit of others. In such cases the IPC team will provide advice and direction, ultimately ensuring that all tasks reach completion. It is important to ensure that there is provision made for 24-hour access to the IPC team for advice.

The number of IPC nurses/practitioners required to run an effective programme depends on various factors—number of beds, number of health care facilities, and the distance, types of acute care settings with specialized units, tertiary care centre, etc. It is recommended that three full-time equivalents are required per 500 beds in acute care hospitals and one full-time equivalent IPC nurse/practitioner is required per 150–250 beds in long-term care facilities (Public Health Agency of Canada, 2010). The results of the USA Delphi project recommended a ratio of 0.8–1.0 IPC nurse for every 100 occupied acute care beds (O'Boyle et al., 2002).

Infection prevention and control committee

The IPC committee is charged with the responsibility for the planning, evaluation of evidence-based practice and implementation, prioritization, and resource allocation of all matters relating to IPC. The membership of the hospital IPC committee should reflect the spectrum of clinical services and administrative arrangements of the health care establishment so that policy decisions take account of implementation issues. As a minimum, the committee should include:

- IPC doctor or hospital epidemiologist who may act as a chairperson.
- IPC nurse/practitioner(s).
- Medical microbiologist.
- Infectious disease physician (if available).
- Chief executive or hospital administrator or his or her nominated representative.
- Director of nursing or his/her representative.
- Occupational health physician or a representative.
- Representative from the major clinical specialties—medical, surgical, obstetrics and gynaecology, paediatrics, etc.
- Representative from the community health sector, e.g. consultant in communicable disease control for UK.

Additionally, representatives of any other department may be invited as necessary.

Large institutions, or those operating on multiple sites, may need to enlarge this membership to ensure that all aspects of clinical service are adequately represented. The IPC committee should meet regularly according to local need. A minimum of three planned meetings a year is recommended.

The function of the local IPC committee is that of supporting the development of an effective IPC programme. The committee should discuss surveillance (outcome and compliance monitoring) reports, outbreaks of HCAIs, needle stick injury incidents,

HCW immunization and education, purchasing of equipment, etc. In addition, it is important that the members of the committee voice areas of concern including any problems relating to either IPC practice or policy, in particular highlighting areas which have not been addressed within their own sphere of responsibility.

Infection prevention and control link nurse

One effective way of developing infection control education and operational support can be through the development of a link system. It has been shown that competent infection control link nurses can motivate ward staff by enabling more effective practice. Success and effectiveness of the link nurses programme is reliant on the ongoing support and backing of senior management. However, high staff turnover, lack of adequate training time, lack of recognition of their role, and the requirement for the IPC team to monitor the link programmes are all resource pressures which are important for the effectiveness of this programme.

Key references and further reading

Allegranzi B, Bagheri Nejad S, Combescure C, *et al*. Burden of endemic health-care-associated infection in developing countries: systematic review and meta-analysis. *Lancet* 2011; **377**: 228–41.

Burnett E. Infection Prevention Society and Competency Steering Group. Outcome of competences for practitioners in infection prevention and control. *Journal of Infection Prevention* 2011; **12**(2):67–90.

European Centre for Disease Prevention and Control. *Annual Epidemiological Report on Communicable Diseases in Europe 2008*. Stockholm: European Centre for Disease Prevention and Control, 2008. Available at: http://www.ecdc.europa.eu/.

Haley RW, Culver DH, White JW, *et al*. The efficacy of infection surveillance and control programs in preventing nosocomial infections in US hospitals. *American Journal Epidemiology* 1985; **121**:182–205.

HICPAC Guidance on Public Reporting of Healthcare-associated infections: Recommendations of the Health care Infection Control Practices Advisory Committee. *Infection Control Hospital Epidemiology* 2005; **26**(6):580–7.

O'Boyle C, Jackson M, Henly SJ. Staffing requirements for infection control programs in US health care facilities: Delphi project. *American Journal of Infection Control* 2002; **30**(6):321–33.

Public Health Agency of Canada. *Essential resources for effective infection prevention and control programs: A matter of patient safety: A discussion paper*. Ottawa: Public Health Agency of Canada, 2010.

Scott RD. *The Direct Medical costs of Healthcare-Associated Infections in U.S. Hospitals and the Benefits of Prevention*. Atlanta: Centers for Disease Control and Prevention, 2009.

UK National Audit Office. *The management and control of hospital acquired infection in acute NHS Trusts in England*. London: The Stationery Office, 2000.

Umscheid CA, Mitchell MD, Doshi JA, *et al*. Estimating the proportion of healthcare-associated infections that are reasonably preventable and the related mortality and costs. *Infection Control and Hospital Epidemiology* 2011; **32**(2):101–14.

WHO. *Core components for infection prevention and control*. Geneva: World Health Organization, 2009.

Chapter 3

Surveillance

There may be infection control without surveillance, but those who practice without measurement will be like the crew of an orbiting ship travelling through space without instruments, unable to identify their current bearings, the probability of hazards, their direction or their rate of travel.

Richard Wenzel

Surveillance has been described as systematic collection, analysis, and interpretation of data on specific events/infections and disease, followed by dissemination of that information to those who can improve the outcomes. Surveillance of HCAIs is the foundation for organizing, implementing, and maintaining an effective IPC programme in the health care facility; as Lord Kelvin has said: 'If you don't measure it, you cannot improve it'.

Objectives of surveillance

The ultimate aim of surveillance is to *reduce* HCAIs. The process of surveillance must incorporate four key stages, i.e. data must be *collected*, *validated*, *analysed*, and *interpreted*. The most vital component of surveillance is ensuring that the information obtained is conveyed in a *timely manner* to those who may influence practice, implement change, and provide financial resources and managerial back-up which are necessary to improve the outcomes. This means that the information must be provided not only to the clinical team but also to the relevant senior health service managers. Collecting and recording data is a futile exercise if no further action is taken. The main objectives of surveillance can be summarized as follows:

- Establish endemic/baseline rate of infections as part of benchmarking exercise.
- Compare HCAI rates within/between health care facilities.
- Convince the clinical team to adopt best practices.
- Reduce HCAIs rates within health care facilities by introducing evidence-based and cost-effective interventions.
- Identify and control outbreaks.

◆ Evaluate success of IPC interventions using both outcome and process monitoring tools.

In addition, information obtained from surveillance data is a useful tool for the IPC team and committee to identify areas of priority so that resources are allocated accordingly. Therefore it is essential that each health care establishment has their own surveillance systems based on the local priorities and institutional objectives.

In some countries, HCAI rates between hospitals are published and such comparisons are a contentious issue which needs careful consideration and sensitive handling. This is mainly because the surveillance data may not be comparable, and the range of institutions involved will introduce confounding factors inherent in all surveillance systems. Problems of data interpretation can be overcome when surveillance systems are set up with clearly defined surveillance objectives included in the expected outputs of surveillance. Unfortunately, at this time, surveillance objectives rarely underpin surveillance methods.

Surveillance methods should be flexible enough to accommodate technological changes within health care facilities, shortening lengths of stay and the necessity to provide post-discharge surveillance, including surveillance of procedures carried out in the community. Irrespective of the methods used, it is essential that data generated from the surveillance is appropriately *risk-adjusted* for the generation of meaningful infection rates, especially when the information is released beyond the institution.

Incidence of various health care-associated infections

Incidence of various HCAIs in US intensive care units is summarized in Figure 3.1. The four most common HCAIs are: 1) urinary tract infections which are mostly associated with the use of indwelling urinary catheters, 2) lower respiratory tract infections which are mainly associated with ventilated patients in the ICU, 3) surgical site infections, and 4) bloodstream infections mainly associated with the use of intravascular devices.

Data from the USA indicate that the estimated increase in length of stays due to the four most common HCAIs were: 1–4 days' extra stay for a urinary tract infection, 7–8 days for a surgical site infection, 7–21 days for a bloodstream infection, and 7–30 days for pneumonia.

Definitions of health care-associated infections

During the past decade, delivery of health care has seen substantial changes. The changes are not only due to innovations in medical sciences, but also due to ever increasing pressure on managers to provide health services which are both efficient and cost-effective. In addition, improvement in public health education and improved socioeconomic conditions (especially in developed countries) have led to increasing survival of the elderly population. Advancement in medical treatment and medical interventions has seen an increased survival of immunocompromised patients making the population more susceptible to HCAIs. Advancement in surgical practices has resulted in higher throughput of surgical patients and provision of treatment and care in non-acute care settings. As a result of these changes, the term *health care associated infection* (HCAI) is used instead of *hospital-acquired* or *nosocomial infection*. The new

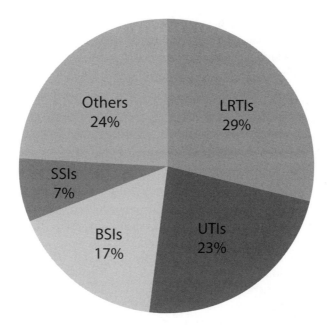

Fig. 3.1 The four major infection sites in US intensive care units. Adapted from National Nosocomial Infections Surveillance System (NNIS) hospitals, 1990–1998. BSI, bloodstream infection; LRTI, lower respiratory tract infection; SSI, surgical site infection; UTI, urinary tract infection.

term HCAI refers to infections associated with health care delivery in *any setting* (e.g. hospitals, long-term care, and ambulatory settings). This term reflects the uncertainty that some patients are going through the 'revolving doors' amongst various health care facilities and it is not always possible to establish with certainly the primary source of infection in these patients.

An infection is classified as HCAI if it was not present or incubating at the time the patient was admitted to the health care facility. Infections should be considered as HCAIs if they are related to procedures, treatments, or other events. Most HCAIs appear *before* the patient is discharged, although some are incubating at discharge and do not become apparent until later. Thus, an infection is not considered a HCAI if it represents a complication or extension of an infectious process present on admission. In general, infections that occur more than 48–72 hours after admission and within 10 days after discharge from the health care facility are defined as HCAIs. The time frame is modified for infections that have incubation periods less than 48–72 hours (e.g. gastroenteritis caused by Norwalk virus) or longer (e.g. viral hepatitis B and C). Surgical site infections are considered as HCAI if the infection occurs within 30 days after the operative procedure or within 1 year if a device or foreign material is implanted.

Although definitions of HCAIs have been developed by various countries and organizations, the definition developed by the Centers for Disease Control and Prevention/ National Healthcare Safety Network (CDC/NHSN, 2008) and Hospital in Europe for Link Infection Control through Surveillance (HELICS) (http://www.ecdc.europa.eu)

has been most commonly used in the USA and in Europe respectively. However these definitions are complex and require training of individuals for its interpretation in the clinical setting. In addition, it also requires good laboratory support and input from a clinical microbiologist/epidemiologist. Therefore, adaptation of these definitions are not suitable for all health care facilities, especially in countries and/or hospitals with limited resources where availability of trained IPC personnel, laboratory support, and clinical microbiologist/epidemiologist input is not readily available.

Data collection for surveillance

A minimum data set for surveillance should include: details of the infected individual, i.e. name or other unique identifier, date of birth, sex, hospital record number, ward or unit in the hospital, name of the consultant, unit involved, date of admission, date of onset of infection and date of discharge or death, site of infection/colonization, organism isolated with antibiotic sensitivities. This minimum data set should also include information on medical treatment/procedures at the time of infection and any other information relevant to why the infection may have occurred, including the patient's underlying medical risk factors, clinical outcome, and an assessment of whether the incident was preventable. It is vital that *both* numerator and denominator data should be collected in all situations for the calculation of rates of infection. For surveillance purposes, the analysis of numerator data alone is meaningless.

Methods of surveillance

Different methods of surveillance exist and their advantages and disadvantages are summarized in Tables 3.1 and 3.2. The type of surveillance method depends on the local factors, i.e. the type and size of hospital, case mix, availability of resources, etc.

Surveillance is an expensive and time-consuming business. Therefore it is essential that the objectives must be set at the very outset. They must be targeted at the preventable health care infections in the high-risk area/unit. Incidence surveillance is ideal but is time-consuming and expensive; prevalence surveillance can be done once or twice a year, which can give you a snapshot of the situation (Figure 3.2).

Targeted surveillance aimed at high-risk areas (e.g. Intensive Care Unit and Neonatal Units), type of infections (e.g. bloodstream and surgical site infections), or procedure directed (e.g. infections associated with central venous or urinary catheters) are the most cost-effective and manageable, and should be used in health care facilities.

On a day-to-day basis *laboratory-based ward liaison surveillance* is the most commonly used surveillance by the IPC team. This is carried out with a daily visit of the IPC nurse to the wards and other clinical areas so that information is collected on *alert conditions* (see Box 3.1) on all new admissions with suspected infections, as laboratory investigation may take time to confirm a diagnosis or the laboratory may not have the facilities to establish a diagnosis. This type of surveillance must be used in conjunction with a search for positive reports from the microbiology laboratory for *alert organisms* (see Box 3.2), which may result in a case review of patients or a search for other carriers/infected patients by ward visits. It is the responsibility of the ward staff to notify the IPC team of all the suspected cases of infection, either during the ward

Table 3.1 Various methods of surveillance used in infection control

Methods	Sources of data	Comments
Continuing surveillance of all patients	Medical, nursing, laboratory records including temperature charts, x-ray and antibiotic treatment reports	Time-consuming and not cost-effective Infection rates are low in some specialties
Ward liaison	Twice-weekly visits to wards Discuss all patients with staff and review records	Less comprehensive than *continuing surveillance*, with similar disadvantages
Laboratory-based	Laboratory records only	Depends on samples taken and information on request forms
Laboratory-based ward surveillance	Follow up of *laboratory-based* in wards	Disadvantages of *laboratory-based*, but more accurate
Laboratory-based ward surveillance and selected continuing surveillance	As for *laboratory-based ward surveillance* and reporting of outbreaks by ward staff and *continuing surveillance* in special units (e.g. ICU) or infections (e.g. wounds)	As for *laboratory-based ward surveillance*, but early detection of outbreaks and incidence in studies in selected areas of infection
Laboratory-based ward liaison	Combination of *laboratory-based* and laboratory-based ward surveillance	Time-consuming but most sensitive after *continuing surveillance*

With permission from Glenister HM, Taylor LJ, Bartlett CLR, *et al.* An evaluation of surveillance methods for detecting infections in hospital inpatients. *Journal of Hospital Infections* 1993; **23**:229–42.

Table 3.2 Advantages and disadvantages of various surveillance strategies

Strategy	Advantages	Disadvantages
Hospital-wide surveillance		
Incidence	Provides data on infections due to all organisms, on all infection sites, and on all units Identifies clusters Establishes baseline infection rates Allows outbreaks to be recognized early Identifies risk factors	Expensive and labour intensive Large amounts of data are collected, and there is little time to analyse it No defined prevention objectives; it is difficult to develop interventions Not all infections are preventable
Prevalence	Inexpensive Uses time efficiently; can be done periodically	Over or underestimates infection rates and does not capture data on important differences Has limited value in small institutions

(continued)

Table 3.2 (*continued*) Advantages and disadvantages of various surveillance strategies

Strategy	Advantages	Disadvantages
Targeted surveillance		
Site specific	Flexible and can be combined with other strategies	No defined prevention strategies or objectives
	Can include a post-discharge component	May miss clusters
		Denominator data may be inadequate
	Identifies risk factors	No baseline rates in other units
	Easily adapted to interventions	
Unit specific	Focuses on patients at greater risk	May miss clusters
		Denominator data may be inadequate
	Requires fewer personnel	
	Simplifies surveillance effort	
Rotating	Less expensive	May miss clusters, or underestimate or overestimate rates
	Less time-consuming and labour intensive	Includes all hospital areas
		Risk stratification may be difficult
		Baseline infection rates may be unreliable
Outbreak	Valuable when used with other strategies	Thresholds are institution-specific types of surveillance
	Does not provide baseline infection rate	Baseline infection rates not available
Limited periodic	Decreases possibility of missing a significant problem	May miss clusters
	Liberates infection preventionist for other activities, including interventions	Baseline infection rates may be unreliable
	Increases the efficiency of surveillance	
Objective or priority based	Can be adaptable to institutions with special populations and resources	Baseline infection rates not available
	Focuses on specific issues at the institution	May miss clusters or outbreaks
	Identifies risk factors	
	Easily adapted to interventions	
	Can include a post-discharge component	

Table 3.2 (*continued*) Advantages and disadvantages of various surveillance strategies

Strategy	Advantages	Disadvantages
Syndromic	Can identify events that may be missed by traditional surveillance systems	Non-specific and not sensitive
		Not validated in most types of settings
	May facilitate early recognition of an outbreak or event	Validation is very time-consuming
		Baseline infection rates not available
	Uses data from administrative systems; less resource intensive	
	Automated	

With permission from Perl TM, Chaiwarith R. Surveillance: An overview. *Practical Healthcare Epidemiology*, 3rd edn, pp. 111–142.Chicago, IL: University of Chicago Press, 2010.

visit or by telephone to the IPC team. Alert conditions and alert microorganisms outlined in this chapter provide a guide and each hospital/country should modify this list based on their epidemiology of communicable diseases.

Types of surveillance

All types of surveillance are resource intensive, expensive, and time-consuming. It requires trained IPC personnel, IT support (both hardware and software), administrative and clerical staff for input of data, statisticians, and good microbiology laboratory support. In addition, the clinical team responsible for collecting the data

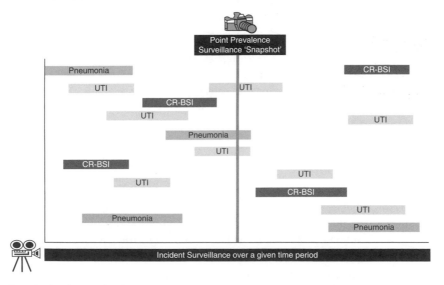

Fig. 3.2 The data in the figure shows routine incidence surveillance of eight cases of nosocomial urinary tract infection (UTI), four cases of catheter related-bloodstream infection (CR-BSI), and four cases of hospital-acquired pneumonia. Prevalence surveillance at a given point identifies two hospital-acquired UTIs and one hospital-acquired pneumonia.

Box 3.1 Alert infectious conditions

- Surgical site infections
- Diarrhoea and/or vomiting
- Diarrhoea with blood (dysentery or colitis)
- Severe cellulitis e.g. necrotizing fasciitis
- Tuberculosis
- Exanthemata
- Chickenpox or shingles
- Mumps, measles, rubella, parvovirus
- Whooping cough
- Poliomyelitis
- Diphtheria
- Scabies
- Meningitis
- Viral hepatitis
- Ophthalmia neonatorum
- Pyrexia of unknown origin
- Typhoid and paratyphoid fevers
- Viral haemorrhagic fever

needs to be trained in the interpretation of HCAI definitions and all the data collected must be validated for accuracy. Therefore, before embarking on any surveillance, it is essential that definitions of surveillance must be agreed with the clinical team and resources must be identified, taking into consideration the availability of trained personnel, laboratory facilities, and patient workload. Personnel involved in surveillance must be trained and once the definitions are agreed, they should not be altered once the surveillance has started.

Outcome surveillance

The aim of outcome surveillance is to *count* the number of HCAIs. Outcome surveillance will inform you about the magnitude of the problem but will not provide you with information regarding what factors might be contributing to the problem. It is important to bear in mind that outcome surveillance is inherently fraught with the following problems:

- There are no internationally agreed definitions on surveillance. The most commonly used definitions were developed by the CDC/NHSN in the USA and ECDC in Europe. Worldwide, CDC/NHSN definitions with/without modification have been used. Both definitions assume availability of good diagnostic laboratory support which is a major issue especially in countries/hospitals with limited resources.

Box 3.2 Alert organisms

Bacteria

◆ MRSA, other resistant *Staph. aureus*, and Panton–Valentine leucocidin (PVL)

◆ *Streptococcus pyogenes* (Group A *Streptococcus*)

◆ *Streptococcus agalactiae* (Group B *Streptococcus*)

◆ Penicillin-resistant *Streptococcus pneumoniae* (PRP)

◆ Influenza virus

◆ *Legionella* spp.

◆ Glycopeptide/vancomycin-resistant enterococci (GRE/VRE)

◆ Pathogenic *Neisseria* spp.

◆ *Clostridium* spp., e.g. *C. difficile*

◆ *Salmonella* or *Shigella* spp.

◆ *Escherichia coli* 0157

◆ Multi-resistant Gram-negative bacilli, e.g. ESBL, NDM beta-lactamase

◆ Any unusual bacteria e.g. *Legionella*

Viruses

◆ Rotavirus

◆ Norovirus and other small round structured virus

◆ Respiratory syncytial virus

◆ Chickenpox/varicella zoster

◆ Measles

◆ Mumps

◆ Rubella

◆ Parvovirus

◆ To ensure consistency and accurate interpretation, the clinical team responsible for surveillance *must be trained* in the interpretation of HCAIs definitions.

◆ Surveillance data must be *validated* and must be *fed back* to the clinical team in a *timely manner*. For surgical site infections (SSIs) surveillance, the data must be *risk adjusted* and this is essential for inter- and intrahospital comparisons.

◆ Infections acquired in health care settings can be grossly underestimated, especially if the throughput of patients is high and there is no follow-up of patients in the community after discharge. It has been estimated that up to 70% of SSIs are missed as a result of failure to follow-up these patients in the community.

◆ Published data cite examples where feedback of outcome surveillance to the clinical team has resulted in reduction of HCAIs, but these reductions are modest and some are due to reinterpretations of surveillance definitions in the post-surveillance period to create an illusion of success.

Process surveillance

A *process* is series of steps taken that lead to an outcome. If all the steps in the process occur correctly, then the desired outcome will prevent the adverse incident, i.e. infection (Figure 3.3). Therefore monitoring of compliance to evidence-based and/or best

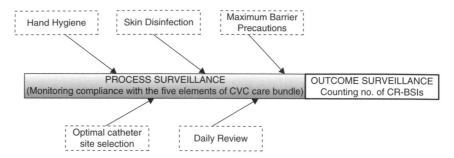

Fig. 3.3 Diagram to show the difference between the process surveillance which requires monitoring of compliance with the five elements of the CVC care bundle to prevent catheter related-blood stream infections (CR-BSIs) and outcome surveillance which provides information on the number of CR-BSIs.

practice is a key to its success. If the best practice is implemented and the infection rate is still high, monitoring of compliance will determine any deviations in adherence to the best practices so that appropriate steps are taken to improve compliance. Since process surveillance is also resource intensive, it is essential to prioritize which processes/steps will be monitored.

Issues with monitoring of compliance *only* includes problems with the reliability of data as some health care facilities collect data based on review of a few selected patients for each care bundle. In addition, the hospital may have good compliance with all the elements of the care bundle but this type of surveillance will not provide you with the information of whether the task was performed *effectively* or not. In addition, collection data by the clinical team on the process monitoring who are part of the ward/unit may introduce bias. Therefore, it is essential to emphasize that process surveillance *must* be linked to reduce HCAIs (outcome surveillance) and not just monitoring of compliance with the processes which may not always be accurate and/or effective.

Learning from the airline industry

In the past, unlike the airline industry, IPC teams and epidemiologists worldwide invested substantial amounts of resources on outcome surveillance (*counting*) and minimal resources in process surveillance (*controlling*). In recent years, with the introduction of various HCAI 'care bundles' (see 'Care bundle approach', Chapter 1, p. 12.) and with the emphasis on monitoring of compliance, health care facilities have achieved a significant reduction in HCAIs. In summary, for substantial and sustained reduction of HCAIs, a combination of *both outcome and process surveillance* is essential to assess the problem and monitor the effectiveness of interventions. It can be argued that if we *control the process* (which must be monitored and carried out *effectively* on all the patients all the time) then we can *control the outcome* (Damani, 2007).

Key references and further reading

Damani NN. Surveillance in countries with limited resources. *International Journal of Infection Control* 2008; **4:**1 doi:10.3396/ijic.V4i1.003.08. www.theific.org.

Damani NN. Simple measures save lives: an approach to infection control in countries with limited resources. *Journal of Hospital Infection* 2007; **65**(S1):151–4.

Glenister HM, Taylor LJ, Bartlett CLR, *et al.* An evaluation of surveillance methods for detecting infections in hospital inpatients. *Journal of Hospital Infection* 1993; **23**:229–42.

Haley RW, Culver DH, White JW, *et al.* The efficacy of infection surveillance and control programs in preventing nosocomial infection in US hospitals. (SENIC study). *American Journal of Epidemiology* 1985; **121**(2):182–205.

HELICS. Surveillance of nosocomial infections in Intensive Care units. Hospital in Europe for Link Infection Control through Surveillance: September, 2004. Available at: http://www.ecdc.europa.eu.

HICPAC guidance on public reporting of healthcare-associated infections: Recommendations of the Health care Infection Control Practices Advisory Committee. *Infection Control Hospital Epidemiology* 2005; **26**(6):580–7.

Horan TC, Andrus M, Dudeck, MA. CDC/NHSN surveillance definition of health care-associated infection and criteria for specific types of infections in the acute care setting. *American Journal of Infection Control* 2008; **36**:309–32.

Lee TB, Montgomery OG, Marx J, *et al.* Recommended practices for surveillance: Association for Professionals in Infection Control and Epidemiology (APIC), Inc. *American Journal of Infection Control* 2007; **35**(7):427–40.

Perl TM, Chaiwarith R. Surveillance: An overview. In: *Practical Healthcare Epidemiology*, 3rd edn, pp.111–42. Chicago, IL: University of Chicago Press, 2010.

Chapter 4

Outbreak management

First, get the cow out of the ditch. Second,
find out how the cow got into the ditch.
Third, make sure you do whatever it takes so the
cow doesn't go into the ditch again.

Anne Mulchay

An outbreak of infection or food-borne illness may be defined as two or more linked cases of the same illness or the situation where the observed number of cases exceeds the expected number, or a single case of disease caused by a significant pathogen (e.g. diphtheria or viral haemorrhagic fever). It is can also be defined as the occurrence of disease at a rate greater than that expected within a specific geographical area and over a defined period of time (Beck-Sague et al., 1997). Outbreaks may be confined to some of the members of one family or may be more widespread and involve cases either locally, nationally, or internationally.

The rapid recognition of outbreaks is one of the most important objectives of the routine surveillance performed by the IPC team and effective surveillance systems should facilitate the early detection of outbreaks. In some instances, the occurrence of an outbreak may be obvious, such as in an episode of food poisoning that affects both HCWs and patients, while in other instances the onset may not be immediately apparent for various reasons. Some outbreaks may arise more insidiously and reach considerable proportions before they become apparent. These outbreaks are detected by the laboratory, but under some circumstances may be identified only through the vigilance of clinical staff based on clinical presentations.

Major outbreaks of transmissible infection in both the hospital and community require appropriate planning to ensure effective management of such episodes. Therefore it is important that the health care facilities must draw up detailed outbreak control plans appropriate to local situations. These plans should be discussed and endorsed by the hospital IPC committee and should include the criteria and method for convening the outbreak control committee. The plan should also clearly address the areas of individual responsibilities, and action plans for all involved. Those who are or may be involved in the management of a major outbreak must be aware of such a plan and their individual role. The plan must be reviewed and updated on 1- to 2-yearly bases and urgently if there is change in the health care facility management structure

> ## Box 4.1 Advice to clinical team if outbreak is suspected
>
> ◆ **Inform** IPC team if you suspect an outbreak. In the community setting, all suspected outbreaks should be reported to the appropriate medical officers (CCDC in the UK).
>
> ◆ **Isolate** all the suspected cases as soon as possible and record information on all cases with date of admission, time of onset of symptoms, clinical diagnosis, etc. Relevant specimens for investigation should be sent to the laboratory *after* consultation with the member of the IPC team and medical microbiologist. Restrict movement of staff and patients.
>
> ◆ **Implement** appropriate infection control measures based on the most likely mode of transmission of pathogens as per local infection control guidelines.

to ensure that lines of communication, responsibility, and accountability are clear. A clinical team who suspect an outbreak must take immediate action (see Box 4.1).

Case definitions

Case definitions in an outbreak situation can be divided into three categories: 1) *confirmed case* when the patients have clinical signs and symptoms of the disease and the diagnosis is confirmed by laboratory analysis of the appropriate specimen(s), 2) *probable case* when the patients have clinical signs and symptoms of the disease or are epidemiologically linked (been exposed to a confirmed case, eaten the same food, stayed in the same hotel, etc.) to a confirmed case, and 3) *possible case* when the patients have clinical signs and symptoms without being a confirmed or probable case.

Role of microbiology laboratory

Effective outbreak investigation requires adequate laboratory support and therefore it is essential that the IPC team liaise with the microbiology laboratory as soon as possible for both hospital and community outbreaks. This liaison is essential as the laboratory may require additional resources in term of staffing, consumables, and reagents to deal with the additional specimens and may have to arrange transport to send specimens to other laboratories. A request should be made to the laboratory to ensure that outbreak isolates are stored for further investigation. This is because many of the infectious agents that cause outbreaks in health care facilities are endemic microorganisms, and it may be necessary to use appropriate typing methods to evaluate which isolates are part of any putative outbreak. Although simple antimicrobial susceptibility testing may be enough to distinguish some isolates, against a background of increasing resistance, other molecular methods of typing may be necessary which are usually available from a reference laboratory. In other outbreaks, storage of blood and other specimens is also necessary to make a diagnosis. Depending on the nature and type of an outbreak, food and other environmental samples may be collected and investigated at the request of the outbreak team in consultation with a medical microbiologist. The role of a microbiology laboratory in the investigation and management of an outbreak can be summarized as followed:

♦ Actively collaborate in epidemic investigations.

♦ Give advice to the IPC on the appropriate collection of specimens.

♦ Give diagnosis as soon as possible by use of new methods—polymerase chain reaction (PCR) for *Mycobacterium tuberculosis, Clostridium difficile* 027 strains, MRSA, and detection of *Legionella* by urinary antigen EIA, etc.

♦ Grow and detect microbial pathogens and carry out appropriate test.

♦ Accurately identify the causative organisms to species level.

♦ Accurately determine the antimicrobial susceptibilities.

♦ Send the microorganisms to reference laboratories for appropriate typing to establish an epidemiological link.

♦ Store microorganisms and/or acute serum sample for further investigations as appropriate depending on the type of outbreak.

♦ Carry out internal quality control on a regular basis and participate in the external quality control programme.

♦ Constantly review and update its laboratory methodology to keep pace with the advances in diagnosis of microbial diseases and to improve early detection and diagnosis by use of molecular and non-molecular methods.

♦ Before introduction of a new test or a method, it must access evidence both for sensitivity and specificity of the test and ensure its cost-effectiveness.

Is it really an outbreak?

The confirmation of an outbreak by the IPC team requires not only clinical experience but also expertise and knowledge in microbiology, epidemiology, and behaviours of various microorganisms. Therefore, it is essential that the infection control practitioner *must* have good understanding of the microbiology and diagnostic methods used to diagnosis infectious diseases. This knowledge can be gained by spending time in the local microbiology laboratory to understand the methods employed in identifying microbes and microbial diseases and to understand the strengths and limitations in the diagnosis of microbial disease both local and regionally.

Before launching into a full-scale outbreak investigation, the IPC team must gather all the relevant information by visiting the ward(s) or facility and line list all the essential clinical and laboratory information and establish the local endemic rate. Once this information is available, they should pause and reflect and pose a question: it is really an outbreak? It is important to note that pseudo-outbreaks are not uncommon and can take a considerable amount of time to identify. One of the reasons is that the human body contain normal microflora (see 'Human microflora', Chapter 1) and specimens from non-sterile sites can grow bacteria *without* clinical symptoms, therefore a positive culture may represent colonization rather than infection so it is essential that a positive bacteriology report should correlate with the clinical condition of the patient.

Cause of pseudo-outbreaks

Laboratory factors

+ Introduction of new test which was previously unavailable locally.

+ Improved laboratory techniques for identification.

+ Introduction of new laboratory test with poor specificity and/or sensitivity.

+ Contamination during processing in the laboratory, e.g. due to contamination of media or cross contamination of specimen during processing.

Ward level

+ Incorrect diagnosis of clinical entity.

+ Mislabelling of specimens. Remember, if in doubt ask for a repeat specimen!

+ Contamination during collection if the correct procedure for collection of specimens is not followed. Please refer to local guidelines for collection of specimens.

+ Failure to distinguish community-versus hospital-acquired infection.

Environmental factors

+ Use of water of poor microbiological quality in the washer disinfectors used for decontamination has been responsible for pseudo-outbreaks. Misdiagnosis of tuberculosis has been reported due to contamination of the endoscope with environmental mycobacteria (e.g. *Mycobacterium chelonae*) from the rinse water which subsequently contaminated bronchial washings sent for culture.

+ Tap water contains microbes including *Mycobacterium* spp. If tap water is used by the microbiology laboratory to perform a Ziehl–Neelsen (ZN) stain, it can give a false positive diagnosis for tuberculosis.

The epidemic curve

An epidemic curve is a graph (histogram) in which the cases of a disease that occurred during an outbreak/epidemic are plotted by date of onset of illness and this information is gathered from line listing of all the cases during an outbreak. This curve depicts the number of cases/patients on the vertical (y) axis, and time on the horizontal (x) axis. The shape of the curve can provide data on the mode of transmission and help us to:

+ Determine whether the source of infection was common or continuous or both.

+ Identity the probable time of exposure of the cases to the source(s) of infection.

+ Identity the probable incubation period.

+ Determine if the problem is ongoing or not.

   Point source: in a *point source* outbreak all cases have the same origin, i.e. index case/same person or a single vehicle which has been identified as the primary reservoir or means of transmission. For example, if there is an abrupt increase in the number of cases over a short time period, the curve suggests single exposure to a point source of contamination. With a common source outbreak, the epidemic curve approximates a normal distribution curve if there are a sufficient number of cases and if cases are limited to a short exposure with maximum incubation of a few days or

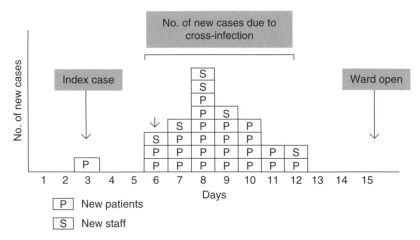

Fig. 4.1 Epidemic curve showing a *point source* outbreak with a bell-shaped curve. A patient is admitted with norovirus gastroenteritis and subsequently infected both patients and staff (secondary and tertiary cases). After implementation of infection control measures, the number of cases was decreased and ward was opened to new admission after 72 hours of the last symptomatic case as the incubation of norovirus is between 24–72 hours.

less (Figure 4.1). It is important to note that in an outbreak situation, sometimes it may be possible that when an extended case finding is carried out, an index case may not be the primary case but the case who has been either not noticed or not reported initially or has been discharged from the health care facility.

Continuous source: in a *continuous source* outbreak, the infections are transmitted from a reservoir and cases occur over a longer period (Figure 4.2). Epidemics can occur due to person-to-person transmission, from the environment, or from contaminated food or water. To determine the probable period of exposure of cases in a *continuous source* outbreak it is necessary to know the specific disease involved, dates of onset of cases, and either mean or median, or minimum and maximum, incubation period(s) for the specific disease. It is important to note that exposure may be continuous or intermittent; if the exposure is intermittent then the curve will have irregularly spaced peaks.

Outbreak control measures

Hospital setting

Preliminary control measures should be introduced as soon as possible by the clinical team and must be based on mode of spread of microorganisms (see Box 4.1). In hospital settings, initial investigation and management of an outbreak will be the responsibility of the IPC team who will investigate to determine whether or not there is an outbreak and decide on further action. If the outbreak is confirmed, the IPC team will liaise with the appropriate personnel as per local outbreak policy and procedures. It may be necessary to close the ward for new admissions as part of an outbreak control measure. If the closure of the ward is considered necessary, the IPC team *must* discuss this

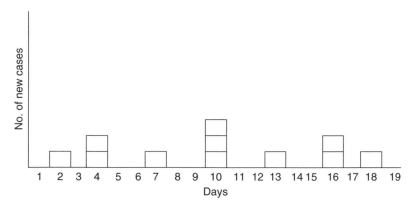

Fig. 4.2 Epidemic curve showing a *continuous source* outbreak in which the epidemic cure is relatively flat as the numbers of cases are spread over long periods due to intermittent exposure of microorganisms.

recommendation with the senior managers and clinicians as this can have a profound impact on the delivery of services.

Depending on the type of outbreak, visiting should be restricted and movement of staff and patients from the outbreak ward may also be restricted to a minimum until the outbreak is over. Patients can be discharged home, if considered fit by the clinical team. Nursing staff (permanent, student, and agency) should remain dedicated to the ward, if possible. The summary for investigation of an outbreak is outlined in Table 4.1.

Management of an outbreak

Most minor outbreaks in hospital are successfully dealt with by the members of the IPC team; however, in certain cases, e.g. if the outbreak is large or serious or if the microorganism is unusual, an Outbreak Control Committee (OCC) should be convened as per local outbreak plan. Where there is a major incident, e.g. a substantial outbreak of food poisoning or a case of an unusual communicable disease, the OCC should seek advice from experts at both regional and national levels. A special incident room must be set up to coordinate the outbreak which amongst other things must have a computer with Internet connection, dedicated telephone line, and faxing facilities. The membership of the committee varies depending upon the type of health care facility. The aims of the OCC are to:

♦ Facilitate the investigation of the outbreak.

♦ Implement necessary control measures to contain the outbreak as soon as possible.

♦ Monitor the effectiveness of the control measures.

♦ Oversee communication to all relevant groups.

♦ Facilitate the medical care of patients with the involvement of relevant clinical team.

The control measures may include:

♦ Full implementation of infection control measures as recommended by the IPC.

♦ Special nursing procedures including isolation of cases.

Table 4.1 Summary for investigation of an outbreak

Confirm the existence of an outbreak	◆ Ascertaining the reliability of both clinical and laboratory information ◆ Beware aware of pseudo-outbreaks (see 'Is it really an outbreak?') ◆ Look at changes that may have affected the rate of infection—new staff, new procedures, new laboratory tests, staff:patient ratio, etc. ◆ If, after investigation, an outbreak is not confirmed then the IPC team must inform the clinical team who have reported the outbreak and provide reassurance
Confirm the diagnosis	◆ Do a full investigation to confirm an outbreak based on the clinical presentation of the disease, incubation period, etc. ◆ Seek advice from the medical microbiologist so that appropriate specimens are collected to confirm and/or exclude the diagnosis ◆ Consider rapid diagnostic tests, e.g. PCR for diagnosis of tuberculosis, *C. difficile* 027 and urinary antigen for *Legionella* ◆ For bacterial infection, take specimens *before* the start of antibiotic therapy ◆ For virology take swab for culture/PCR and blood sample for base-line serology
Create a case definition	◆ At the start of an outbreak, use a broad case definition and then narrow the case definition down at a later date when more information is available from the clinical and laboratory investigation
Develop line listings	◆ Create a line listing which contain information on the date of admission, date of onset of clinical symptoms, risk factors, location of the patients in contact with the index cases, etc.
Construct an epidemic curve	◆ Identify and count cases or exposures both in patients and staff ◆ Construct an epidemic curve (Figures 4.1 and 4.2) to determine the source of the outbreak ◆ Describe the data in terms of time, place, and person ◆ Remember that cases may have been discharged from the hospital so alert GPs and appropriate medical officer in the community (CCDC in the UK)
Develop and test the hypothesis	◆ In larger outbreaks, a case–control method may be the most efficient way of testing a hypothesis ◆ If a single hospital ward is affected, a retrospective cohort study should be done
Implement control measures	◆ Take action and implement infection control measures without delay ◆ Isolate patients with appropriate infection control measures depending on the mode of transfer of pathogens ◆ Determine patients/staff at risk of becoming ill and offer appropriate treatment, e.g. antimicrobial agents, active and/or passive immunization ◆ Depending on the type of pathogen, incubation period, and susceptibility, consider isolation of patients, staff, and visitors and initiate contact tracing, as appropriate

Table 4.1 (*continued*) Summary for investigation of an outbreak

Communicate	◆ Communicate information to the patients and their families ◆ Inform relevant personnel e.g. GPs, A&E department, local/national health authority, as appropriate ◆ Develop strategy for dealing with the media and nominate a person who can answer quires from the media
Screen personnel and environment	◆ Screen personnel and environment as indicated after consultation with the members of the IPC team, medical microbiologist, and CCDC in the UK ◆ Involve environmental health officer for an outbreak of food poisoning
Write an outbreak report	◆ Write preliminary and final confidential outbreak reports ◆ The report must summarize full investigations, lessons learnt, and recommendations to prevent a recurrence in the future ◆ The report must be sent to the senior management and other appropriate personnel/authorities for action

- ◆ Closure of health care facilities, if necessary.
- ◆ Special cleaning and disinfection procedures.
- ◆ Closure of catering facilities, if considered appropriate.

Communication

In an outbreak situation, communication to relevant staff is important and this is best done by the Occupational Health Department (OHD). The IPC team will liaise with the OHD to provide further information as and when required.

It is also essential that worried patients and patients' relative must be kept informed by the clinical team. In order to avoid confusion, this information must be *consistent and accurate* and if the clinical team need more information then they must discuss this with a member of IPC team.

It is also essential that members of staff *must not* communicate directly with the media. All queries related to the outbreak/incident must be referred to the Public Relations Officer or a person designated by the health care facilities management. The designated person must have formal training in dealing with media. The spokesperson must be attending the OCC meetings on a daily basis and if this is not possible s/he must be kept informed of all the developments by the chairperson of the OCC on daily basis.

End of outbreak

At the end of an outbreak, the OCC will call the final meeting to:

- ◆ Review the experience of all participants involved in the management of the outbreak.
- ◆ Identify any shortfalls and particular difficulties that were encountered.

- Revise the outbreak control plan in view of the current experience.
- Recommend, if necessary, structural or procedural improvements which would reduce the chances of recurrence.
- Write the final outbreak report with recommendations outlining action needed to be taken with timeline to prevent it recurrence.

It is important to note that all outbreaks provide the opportunity to educate HCWs about infection prevention and control measures. It is essential that all outbreaks, however minor, must be thoroughly investigated and the outcomes of such investigations and recommended actions taken must be documented by the IPC team and others for legal purposes.

Look-back investigations

Look-back investigations refer to the process of identifying, tracing, recalling, counselling, and testing patients or HCWs who may have been exposed to an infection. An example is the case of a HCW who has undertaken exposure-prone procedures on surgical patients and is later found to be positive for a blood-borne virus (e.g. HIV, hepatitis B or C virus) or a HCW who has been diagnosed with open pulmonary tuberculosis and has been working in the health care facility in a clinical area especially with susceptible patients.

A similar process may be needed if there is a breakdown and failure in the normal processes of disinfection or sterilization of instruments (e.g. failure to adequately disinfect/sterilize endoscopes or items/equipment which may have put patients at risk from infection). The summary of recommended actions and follow-up for exposure investigation after a failure of disinfection and sterilization procedures is summarized in Box 4.2.

All types of look-back investigations have the potential to generate a great deal of publicity and can take up a great deal of time and resources and therefore they must be handled carefully. It can also cause a great deal of unnecessary anxiety in patients treated at the health care facility who have not been exposed to infection, as well as anger and distress among patients who were put at risk of infection.

The senior management of the health care facility must establish an incident team (see 'Management of an outbreak') as soon as possible with members who have expertise in infection prevention and control, infectious disease, microbiology, the discipline involved, public relations, and representatives of the health authority. Legal and indemnity issues should also be considered. At the very outset, the senior management must clearly set procedures to be undertaken and how these are presented to at-risk patients and the public. These procedures should also clearly set out protocols for tracing, counselling, and referral of at-risk patients in a timely manner. Test results should be available with minimal delay, and the incident team should ensure that the all the tasks are completed and a final report produced as soon as possible.

Box 4.2 Summary of protocol for exposure investigation after a failure of disinfection and sterilization procedures

◆ Confirm disinfection or sterilization reprocessing failure.

◆ Impound any improperly disinfected/sterilized items.

◆ Do not use the questionable disinfection/sterilization unit (e.g. sterilizer, automated endoscope reprocessor) until proper functioning can be assured.

◆ Inform key stakeholders.

◆ Conduct a complete and thorough evaluation of the cause of the disinfection/sterilization failure.

◆ Prepare a line listing of potentially exposed patients.

◆ Assess whether disinfection/sterilization failure increases patient risk for infection.

◆ Inform expanded list of stakeholders of the reprocessing issue.

◆ Develop a hypothesis for the disinfection/sterilization failure and initiate corrective action.

◆ Develop a method to assess potential adverse patient events.

◆ Consider notification of local and national authorities.

◆ Consider patient notification.

◆ Develop long-term follow-up plan.

◆ Perform after-action report.

With permission from Rutala WA, Weber DJ. *Infection Control Hospital Epidemiology* 2007; **28**:146–55.

Key references and further reading

Arias KM. *Outbreak Investigation, Prevention, and Control in Health Care Settings: Critical Issues in Patient Safety*, 2nd edn. Sudbury, MA: John Bartlett Publishers, 2009.

Beck-Sague C, Jarvis W, Martone W. Outbreak investigations. *Infection Control Hospital Epidemiology* 1997; **18**:138–45.

Department of Health. *Management of outbreaks of Food borne illness.* London: Department of Health, 1994.

Rutala WA, Weber DJ. How to assess risk of disease transmission to patients when there is a failure to follow recommended disinfection and sterilization guidelines. *Infection Control Hospital Epidemiology* 2007; **28**:146–55.

WHO. *Communicable Disease Control in emergencies: A field manual.* Geneva: World Health Organization, 2005.

Chapter 5

Epidemiology and biostatistics

There are three kinds of lies: lies, damned lies, and statistics.

Mark Twain

Epidemiology

The word epidemiology is derived from the Greek *epi*, upon + *demos*, people—which literally means tracking what is on people. Epidemiology is defined as 'the study of the distribution and determinants of health-related states, conditions, or events in specified populations and the application of the results of this study to the control of health problems' (Last, 2001). The first scientific explanation and description of how a disease spreads from person to person, and from place to place, was given by a Danish physician, Peter Ludwig Panum, when he submitted his report to the Danish government in 1847 on the epidemic of measles in the Faeroe Islands.

There are two major categories of epidemiological studies, i.e. experimental and observational. In *experimental studies*, the investigator controls the exposures to specific factors and then follows the subjects to determine the effect of the exposure, e.g. a clinical trial of a new drug. In *observational studies*, the group being compared is already defined and the investigator merely observes what happens. These observations are used to analyse outbreaks because the investigator is observing the outcomes to prior exposures over which the investigator has no control. Case–control, cross-sectional, and cohort are types of observational studies that typically consider features of the past, present, and future respectively, to try to identify differences between the groups.

Case–control studies

Case–control studies are analytical epidemiological studies whose aim is to investigate the association between disease and suspected causes and are usually cross-sectional or retrospective in nature (Figure 5.1).

In case–control studies, people with an outcome (an infection or a disease) are identified and their medical and social history examined retrospectively in an attempt to identify exposure to potential infectious agent or risk factors. A matched control group free from the disease or infection is also identified and data collected from them in an identical fashion. The two sets of data are compared to determine whether the disease group was exposed in significantly higher numbers to the suspected risk factors than the control group.

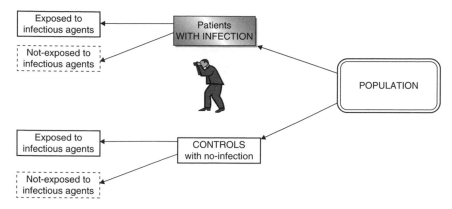

Fig. 5.1 The structure of a case–control study.

A case–control study must contain a sufficiently large number of study subjects in order to be able to detect an association, if one exists, between an exposure and a disease. As the number of study subjects increases, the power to detect a statistically significant association increases.

When designing a case–control study, it is important to tightly define what constitutes a 'case'. However, in the initial stages of an outbreak, a case definition may be broad in order to identify all potential cases. The case definition may be refined as the investigation progresses and potential risk factors are identified. If the number of cases is small, it is possible to include all of them in a case–control study. In a large outbreak, however, it may not be practical, or possible, to identify and include all of the cases. In this instance, cases are selected from those who are ill. Care must be taken to ensure that the cases selected are representative of the entire population with disease so that the study findings can be extrapolated to the whole population. Controls must come from the same environment where the cases' exposures occurred, i.e. they must be from the same population at risk for exposure and must be at the same risk of acquiring the disease. Controls should be similar to the cases in many respects except for the presence of the disease being studied. Ideally, controls should be randomly selected from the population at risk to avoid selection bias.

Advantages of a case–control study:

◆ These studies are relatively quick and cheap to perform.

◆ Case–control studies are useful for investigating rare diseases.

◆ Case–control studies can be used to evaluate interventions.

Disadvantages of a case–control study:

◆ It is not possible to calculate the true incidence and relative risk. The results should be expressed as odds ratios.

◆ The study design inevitably means that data are collected retrospectively and hence the information may not be available or may be of poor quality.

Case–control or cohort studies can be used in outbreak investigations to compare rates of infection in various populations in order to determine which exposures or risk factors are most likely responsible for the infection. A case–control study differs from a cohort study in that the subjects are enrolled into a case–control study based on whether or not they have a *disease*. In a cohort study, subjects are included in the study based on their *exposure* and are then followed for the development of disease. Case–control study is the method most commonly used to investigate outbreaks because it is relatively inexpensive to conduct, is usually of short duration, and requires relatively few study subjects.

Cohort studies

Cohort studies are observational studies usually carried out over a number of years, and designed to investigate the aetiology of diseases or outcomes. The aim of such studies is to investigate the link between a hypothetical cause and a defined outcome. Prior to undertaking a cohort study, investigators should seek statistical advice regarding the number of subjects needed in each group.

Cohort studies originate with a hypothesis that the outcome (an infection or a disease) is caused by exposure to an infectious agent or event (risk factor). Subjects exposed to the suspected risk factor (cases) and similar groups that have not been exposed (control) are identified (Figure 5.2). Often, a complete population sample (cohort) is followed prospectively over a period of time (usually a number of years) to identify the incidence of the outcome in both groups. These results are then analysed to determine if the group exposed to the risk factor has a higher incidence of disease than those not exposed. Cohort studies are usually prospective but they can be performed retrospectively if there is a clearly documented point of first exposure.

Advantages of cohort studies:

◆ The prospective design of the 'standard' cohort study provides an opportunity for accurate data collection that is not normally available from retrospective studies.

◆ The incidence, relative risk, and attributable risk can be calculated from the results.

◆ An estimate of the time from exposure to disease development is possible.

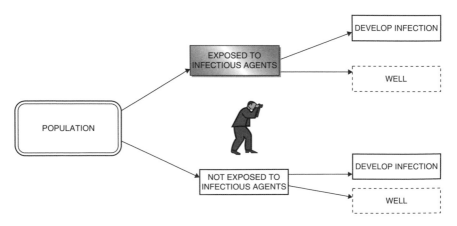

Fig. 5.2 The structure of a cohort study.

- ◆ Occasionally, cohort studies can be performed retrospectively and can thus be cheaper and less time-consuming.

  Disadvantages of cohort studies:
- ◆ Time-consuming and costly (unless the outcome has a high incidence and short latent period).
- ◆ Long studies inevitably increase the drop-out rates.
- ◆ Cohort studies are not useful investigations for rare diseases as large numbers of subjects are required.

Cross-sectional (prevalence) surveys

Cross-sectional studies are descriptive studies in which a sample population's status is determined for the presence or absence of exposure and disease at the same time. These surveys take a 'snapshot' of the population and thus detect the presence of disease at a point in time (prevalence) as opposed to the frequency of onset of the disease (incidence).

The cases in a specified population can either be calculated during a given period of time (period prevalence) or at a given point in time (point prevalence).

Measures of disease frequency

Rates describe the *frequency with which events occur*. In other words, a rate measures the occurrence of an event in a defined population over time. Rates are used to track trends, such as the occurrence of nosocomial infections over time. The rates most frequently used are incidence, prevalence, and attack rates. When an increase in a disease or other health-related event is suspected, rates can be calculated and used to determine if there is a change in the occurrence of disease from one period of time to the next.

Basic formula for all type of rates:

$$\text{Rate} = \frac{\text{Numerator}}{\text{Denominator}} \times \text{Constant (k)}$$

where k = 100 for discharges and 1000 for device-days e.g. IV lines.

Incidence rates

Incidence rates are used to measure and compare the frequency of new cases or events in a population.

$$\text{Incidence rate} = \frac{\text{Number of new cases that occur in a defined period}}{\text{Population at risk during the same period}} \times k$$

where k = 100 for discharges and 1000 for device-days e.g. IV lines.

Prevalence rate

A prevalence rate is used to describe the *current status* of active disease. It is a measure of the number of active (new and old) disease at any one time as the numerator and the exposed population at that point as the denominator. The cases in a specified population can either be calculated during a given period of time (period prevalence) or at a given point in time (point prevalence).

It is sometimes helpful to review the incidence and prevalence simultaneously.

Prevalence rate =

$$\frac{\text{Number of all (new and existing) cases of a disease at specified period or point in time}}{\text{Population at risk during the same time period}} \times k$$

Attack rate

Attack rate is another type of incidence rate that is expressed as cases per 100 population (or as a percentage). It is used to describe the new and recurrent cases of disease that have been observed in a particular group during a limited time period in special circumstances, such as during an epidemic.

Attack rate =

$$\frac{\text{Number of new and recurrent cases that occur in a population in a specified time period}}{\text{Population at risk for same time period}} \times 100$$

Measures of association

Measures of association are used during outbreak investigations to evaluate the relationship between exposed and unexposed populations. These statistical measures can express the strength of association between a risk factor (exposure) and an outcome (disease).

Risks

Risk represents chance—usually the chance of an unwanted event. There are several ways to express risk, such as the relative risk, the odds ratio, the relative risk reduction, or the absolute risk reduction. The measures of association used for outbreak investigations are the risk ratio (or relative risk) and the odds ratio.

Risk ratio

The *risk ratio* is the ratio of the attack rate (or risk of disease) in the exposed population to the attack rate (or risk of disease) in the unexposed population. If the value of the risk ratio (relative risk) is equal to 1, the risk is the same in the two groups and there is no evidence of association between the exposure and outcome. If the risk ratio is greater than 1, the risk is higher for the exposed group and exposure may be associated with the outcome. If the risk ratio is less than 1, the risk is lower for the exposed group and the exposure may possibly protect against the outcome.

Relative risk, absolute risk, and individual risk

Relative risk provides an estimate of the chances of an exposed individual to develop an illness, complication, or response to therapy in comparison with a non-exposed individual.

The *absolute risk* is the risk in the exposed and the non-exposed group as a whole and the individual risk computes the risk according to the levels of exposure. However, one should remember that these chances have been calculated from observations on large groups of patients and the result of the group as a whole may not automatically apply to the patient that is presently sitting in front of you.

Risk ratio (relative risk) =

$$\left(\frac{a/(a+b)}{a/(c+d)} \right) \text{ (risk of disease in exposed compared to that in unexposed)}$$

$$\text{Relative risk} = \frac{\text{Incidence rate among exposed}}{\text{Incidence rate among unexposed}}$$

Odds ratio

The *odds ratio* is similar to the risk ratio except that the odds, instead of the risk (attack rates), are used in the calculation. It is the ratio of the probability of having a risk factor if the disease is present to the probability of having the risk factor if the disease is absent. If the odds ratio is equal to 1, the odds of disease are the same if the exposure is present (i.e. there is no evidence of association between the exposure and disease). If the odds ratio is greater than 1, the odds of disease are higher for the exposed group and the exposure is probably associated with the disease.

Odds ratio =

$$\frac{\text{Number of diseased persons exposed }(a) \times \text{number without disease and not exposed }(d)}{\text{Number of well persons exposed }(b) \times \text{number with disease but not exposed }(c)}$$

Bias and confounders

Bias

Bias refers to errors in study design and execution, and to interpretation and implementation of its results, which systematically influence the eventual outcome for the patient. Bias occurs in both quantitative and qualitative research and it can occur at any stage from conception of a study through to marketing and implementation of its results. Bias can be deliberate or unintentional.

The perfect study is one that is both accurate and precise without bias. An accurate study may be imprecise but not biased. A biased study can be precise but still be inaccurate.

The following are the most common and important biases occur in study design:

Selection bias can occur when the cases selected for study do not represent the entire population at risk. This can occur if a non-random method is used to select study subjects (e.g. the selection is unconsciously or consciously influenced in some way) or if some of the study subjects are unavailable (e.g. they refuse to participate, their records are missing, their disease is mild and they do not seek medical care and are therefore not detected, and their disease is undiagnosed or misdiagnosed).

Information bias can occur if the information collected is incorrect because of inaccurate recall or because it is inconsistently collected (observer bias). Observer bias occurs when collection or interpretation of data about exposures is systematically different for persons who have the disease than those who do not or when data about outcomes are systematically different for persons who are exposed than for persons who are not exposed.

Bias can result from misuse of statistical tests. The most common types of bias are:

◆ Using the wrong test for the data.

◆ Inferring that there is no difference between treatments when the study is under-powered.

◆ Multiple testing.

Confounders

Confounders are factors extraneous to the research question that are determinants of the outcome of the study. If they are unevenly distributed between the groups they can influence the outcome. A confounder need not be causal; it might be just a correlate of a causal factor. For example, age is associated with a host of disease processes but it is only a marker for underlying biological processes that are causally responsible for these diseases. Similarly, the water pump disconnected by John Snow in Limehouse was not the cause of the cholera, just the conduit that delivered the causal agent.

Procedures for dealing with confounders prior to a study include exclusion, stratified sampling, pairwise matching and randomization. After a study, corrections can be made by using standardization techniques, stratified analysis or multivariate analysis. Prior randomization, whenever possible, is the preferred method of eliminating the effect of confounders.

Biostatistics

It is important that those responsible for implementing infection prevention and control and quality management programmes are familiar with statistical measures. Basic statistical methods can be used to organize, summarize, and analyse data to determine if there are trends or associations in observations. Numerous computer databases and statistical programs are available and these have virtually eliminated the need to calculate complicated mathematical formulas by hand or by using a hand-held calculator. However, the investigator still needs to understand which statistical methods to use and when to use them. There are several computer software programs that can be used to store, manage, and analyse epidemiological data. *Epi Info* is a software program that was developed by the CDC to manage and analyse data collected during an epidemiological investigation and can be downloaded from the CDC website (http://www.cdc.gov) free of cost.

Measures of central tendency

A set of data, which comprises a number of individual results for a particular single variable, is said to make up a distribution in the group as a whole. Measures of central tendency describe the values around the middle of a set of data. The mean, median, and mode are the principal measures of central tendency.

Mean: the mean is an arithmetic *average of a group* of numbers. The value of the mean is affected by extreme values in the data set. When extreme values appear in a data set, the distribution of the data becomes skewed and the mean does not give a representative picture of the data.

Median: the median is *the middle number* or point in an ordered group of numbers—the value at which half of the measurements lie below the value and half above the value. The median is useful when there are extreme values in a data set, i.e. the data are skewed.

Mode: the mode is the *most frequently occurring value* in a set of observations. Mode is not often used as a measure of central tendency, particularly in small data sets.

In a normal (symmetric) distribution, the mean, median, and mode have the same values. A curve of a histogram that is not symmetrical is referred to as skewed or asymmetrical. A curve that is said to be negatively skewed has a tail off to the left and most of the values are above the mean. The mean is less than the median, which is less than the mode. In contrast, a positively skewed curve value would depict a mirror image of this and the mean will be greater than the median, which will be greater than the mode.

Measures of dispersion

Measures of dispersion describe the distribution of values in a data set around the mean. The most commonly used measures of dispersion are range, deviation, variance, and standard deviation. The difference between the highest and lowest values in a data set is termed the *range*. The *deviation* is the difference between an individual measurement in a data set and the mean value for the set. A measurement may have no deviation (equal to the mean), or a positive deviation (greater than the mean). The *variance* measures the deviation around the mean of a distribution. The *standard deviation*, which may be represented as *s* or SD, is a measure of dispersion that reflects the distribution of values around the mean. A normal distribution represents the natural distribution of values around the mean with progressively fewer observations toward the extremes of the range of values. A normal distribution plotted on a graph shows a bell-shaped curve, in which 68.3% of the values fall within one standard deviation of the mean, 95.5% of the values fall within two standard deviations of the mean, and 99.7% of the values fall within three standard deviations of the mean (Figure 5.3).

Hypothesis testing

The traditional method of determining whether one set of data is different from another is hypothesis testing. By convention, the investigator will usually assume the null hypothesis, which predicts that the two sets of data are from the same population and therefore not different. The probability that the null hypothesis is correct is then determined. This probability is referred to as the *P* value. A *P* value of 0.10 tells us that there is a 0.10 probability or 10% chance that the null hypothesis (that there is no difference) is correct. An arbitrary cut-off of 0.05 or 5% has been chosen to indicate that the null hypothesis can be reasonably rejected. If the *P* value falls below this level, the observed difference is regarded as a true difference or a statistically significant difference. Of course, there is a 5% chance that this inference is incorrect.

Error of hypothesis testing

An investigator's inference about an association can be wrong if the findings are due to bias or confounding factors in the study or to chance alone.

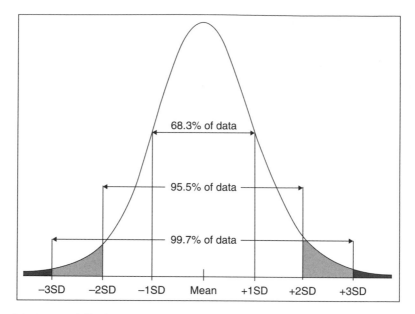

Fig. 5.3 A normal distribution curve that lies between one, two, and three standard deviations on either side of the mean.

Type I (alpha) error: a type I (alpha) error occurs when an investigator states that there is an association when in fact there is no association, i.e. the investigator rejects a true null hypothesis.

Type II (beta) error: a type II (beta) error occurs when the investigator states that there is no association when in fact there is an association, i.e. the investigator fails to reject a null hypothesis that is actually false. Although these errors are not always avoidable, the likelihood of making a type II error can be minimized by using a larger sample size. By choosing the statistical cut-off level, the investigator decides before beginning the study what probability of committing a type I error can be accepted (usually 5%).

Tests of statistical significance

Chi-square test

The chi-square test is commonly used in outbreak investigations to evaluate the probability that observed differences between two populations, such as cases and controls, could have occurred by chance alone if an exposure is not truly associated with disease. It is calculated by using two-by-two contingency tables (Table 5.1). Because it takes a lot of patience to calculate chi-squares by hand, most investigators opt to use a computer with a statistical software package. The chi-square test can be used if the number of subjects in a study is approximately 30 or more. For smaller populations, or if the value of any of the cells in a two-by two table is less than 5, the Fisher exact test should be used.

Table 5.1 Two-by-two table

	Disease	**No disease**	
Exposed	a	b	a = b
	number of individuals with exposure and disease	number of individuals with exposure and *no* disease	
Unexposed	c	d	c = d
	number of individuals with no exposure and disease	number of individuals with *no* exposure and *no* disease	
Total	a + c	c + d	N

a + b = total number with exposure; a + c = total number with disease; b + d = total number with no disease; c + d = total number with no exposure; N = a + b + c + d = total population in the study.

Fisher exact test

The Fisher exact test is used for evaluating two-by-two contingency tables, and is a variant of the chi-square test. The Fisher exact test is the preferred test for studies with few subjects. The formula for the Fisher exact test calculates the P value directly, so a table of chi-squares is not needed. However, in order to calculate the P value for the study, one must calculate the P value for the observations in the study and then add this P value to the P values of all possible combinations that have lower P values. This calculation should be done with the aid of a computer.

The P value

In the results of most research reports and scientific articles the P value seems to play a pivotal role. A P value less or greater than 0.05 conventionally indicates whether the findings are statistically, 'significant' or 'not significant' respectively.

This level of P value certainly means that there is statistical significance but does *not* necessarily mean that the results are clinically significant. Sometimes, a statistically significant difference may be clinically irrelevant.

Pitfalls of the P value As has been mentioned earlier, the absence of a P value of 0.05 does not mean that there is no difference between the groups. The P value does not convey any information about the magnitude of differences between groups. Furthermore, the P value is equally influenced by the precision of the study results. Hence, a small (but consistent) difference may be highly statistically significant and a very large difference may lack statistical significance due to a variability of the test result. The P value can only be considered as an instrument to express the statistical certainty of a detected difference.

Alternatives to the use of the P value Many researchers and biomedical journals prefer the use of 95% confidence intervals (CIs) to the use of the P value. Briefly, a 95% CI reflects the range of differentiation that may be encountered in 95% of the cases if the experiment were repeated endlessly.

Confidence intervals

CIs are estimates of where 'true' answers are most likely found. Whereas P values denote statistical significance, CI indicates clinical significance. The CI (sometimes referred to as the margin of error) of a study with a stated probability (usually 95%) indicates that the true value of a variable, such as the mean, proportion, or rate, falls within the interval. In other words, a person using a 95% CI can be confident that if a study were repeated many times, the observed value would fall within the CI in 95 out of 100 studies. Unlike the P value, which provides information on statistical significance only, the CI expresses the statistical precision of a point estimate and the strength of an association. The statistical precision is measured by the size (range) of the CI: the narrower the computed interval, the more precise the estimate. The strength of the association is measured by the magnitude of the difference in the measured outcomes between the two groups, e.g. the higher the numerical value of the risk ratio, the more likely the exposure is related to the outcome.

CIs provide an alternative to hypothesis testing when ratios of risk or rates are being compared. A 95% CI provides information on whether or not an observation is statistically significant with a P value less than or equal to 0.05. As noted previously, an odds (or risk) ratio of 1.0 means that the odds (or risk) of disease are the same between the comparison groups whether or not the exposure occurs. If the value of a risk ratio is greater than one, the risk of disease in the exposed population is greater than the risk of disease in the unexposed population. If a ratio of 95% CI does not include 1.0, then statistical significance is implied ($P = 0.05$). If the CI for an odds or risk ratio includes 1.0, then the findings are not statistically significant.

For example, if the odds ratio (the point estimate) for an exposure is said to be 8.1 with a 95% CI of 6.3–10.7, this means:

- Persons with the disease were 8.1 times more likely to have been exposed to the risk factor than those without the disease, *and*

- One can be 95% confident (probability of 0.95) that the odds ratio in the population is between the confidence limits of 6.3 and 10.7 (i.e. it may be as low as 6.3 or as high as 10.7).

Although P values alone have traditionally been used to show the statistically significance between disease and risk factors in outbreaks, odds ratios/risk ratios and 95% CI are now frequently reported.

The calculation of a CI depends on a representative sample from a normally distributed population. The width of the interval is determined by the degree of confidence desired (i.e. 90%, 95%, or 99%), the variability of the data (standard error), and the number of observations (n). Larger numbers of observations result in narrower intervals.

Sensitivity and specificity

Sensitivity and specificity are terms that provide information about the accuracy of a diagnostic test. A diagnostic test is usually performed to establish the presence or absence of a disease. However, diagnostic tests are rarely 100% accurate and may give false-positive (i.e. the test indicates there is a disease, while this is in fact not true) or false-negative (i.e. the test falsely overlooks the presence of the disease) results.

The *sensitivity* of a test reflects the proportion of patients with the disease that have a positive test result, from the total number of patients with the disease. The *specificity* of a test reflects the proportion of healthy patients that have a negative test result, from the total number of patients that do not have the disease.

Test result: disease present, disease absent

Positive: true-positive (TP), false-positive (FP)

Negative: false-negative (FN), true-negative (TN)

Sensitivity = Percentage of cases with the disease who are detected by the test:

$$\frac{TP}{TP + FN} \times 100\%$$

Specificity = Percentage of people without the disease who were correctly labelled by the test as not diseased:

$$\frac{TN}{TN + FP} \times 100\%$$

Positive predictive value = Percentage of all test-positives who are truly positive (e.g. diseased):

$$\frac{TP}{TP + FP} \times 100\%$$

Negative predictive value = Percentage of all test-negatives who are truly negative (e.g. not diseased):

$$\frac{TN}{TN + FN} \times 100\%$$

Statistical process control

Statistical process control (SPC) charts are used to measure processes or parameters (i.e. infection rate) over time. They allow us to evaluate trends to ensure that the process/parameter is being maintained within acceptable statistical bounds. SPC charts assume that the process, e.g. infection rate, will be largely similar over time. Previous data can be used to calculate a mean rate upon which SPC limits can be set. To ensure the mean rate is reflective of the process it is recommended that the SPC charts are based on 10–12 data points. Warning limits are set at two standard deviations above/below the mean with action limits set at three standard deviations above/below (see Figure 5.4). A process within these statistical bounds is said to be in control. If the process exceeds the action limit during one data point this is deemed statistically significant variation which cannot be explained by chance alone. Other also rules exist for the warning limits.

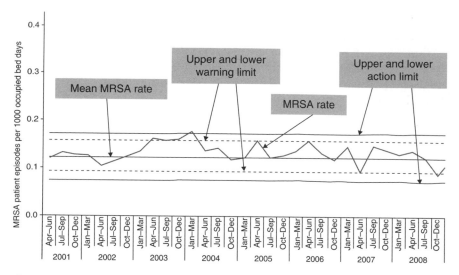

Fig. 5.4 Statistical process control for quarterly MRSA bacteraemia.

Key references and further reading

Abramson JH. Making sense of data: *A self-instruction manual on the interpretation of epidemiology data*, 2nd edn. New York: Oxford University Press, 1994.

Birnbaum D, Sheps S. The merits of confidence intervals relative to hypothesis testing. *Infection Control and Hospital Epidemiology* 1992; **13**:553–5.

Centers for Disease Control and Prevention. *Principles of Epidemiology: An Introduction to Applied Epidemiology and Biostatistics*, 2nd edn. Atlanta, GA: US Dept of Health and Human Services, 1992.

Freeman J, Hitchison GB. Prevalence, incidence and duration. *American Journal of Epidemiology* 1980; **112**:707–23.

Gardner MJ, Aftman DG. Confidence intervals rather than *P* values: estimation rather than hypothesis testing. *British Medical Journal* 1986; **292**:746–50.

Giesecke J. *Modern Infectious Disease Epidemiology*, 2nd edn. London: Arnold, 2002.

Last JM. *A Dictionary of Epidemiology*, 4th edn. New York, Oxford University Press, 2001.

Chapter 6

Disinfection and sterilization

The dream of a bacterium is to become two bacteria.

F. Jacob

Basic concepts

Contaminated medical and surgical devices may serve as vehicles for the transmission of infection to susceptible hosts. Therefore, it is important that all health care facilities have a comprehensive disinfection policy to ensure that re-usable medical items and equipment are adequately cleaned, disinfected, and/or sterilized before use on patients as per manufacturers' instructions and in accordance with the local policy and/national guidelines.

Where applicable, items of reusable medical devices or equipment will have a record kept of the decontamination procedures used and a list of the patients on whom the item was used so that if there is a failure in the decontamination process, the patients can be recalled. Please refer to (see Chapter 4, Box 4.2) which summarizes the protocol for exposure investigation after failure of disinfection and sterilization procedures.

- Every health care facility should have a nominated Decontamination Lead who should have clear line management responsibility to the senior management. S/he should ensure that the roles and responsibilities of all personnel who may be involved in the use, installation, and maintenance of decontamination equipment are clearly defined. S/he should be responsible for the implementation, monitoring, and all the operational issues and policy for decontamination.

- Staff who are responsible for the decontamination of medical devices and equipment must have training and be deemed competent in the relevant decontamination procedures. The training must be update on a regular basis and when new equipment is purchased. Records of training must be kept in the Department.

- Before purchase of any equipment, it is essential to ensure that the equipment may be adequately decontaminated. New items of equipment should have a written procedure that complies with the manufacturer's recommendations on decontamination of equipment.

- Equipment used for sterilization or disinfection must be commissioned on installation, regularly serviced, maintained, and tested in accordance with the manufacturer's instructions and current advice from the Department of Health. The equipment performance must be monitored to ensure that accepted standards of safety are achieved as per guidance and a written record must be kept by the head of department.

◆ Where applicable, equipment must be adequately decontaminated prior to service, inspection, or repair.

Medical devices and degree of risks of infection

Earle Spaulding (1968) devised a classification of medical devices and equipment based on the degree of risk infection from these items. These classifications have been used as the benchmark when assessing risk and selecting the decontamination processes. Spaulding classified items into three categories:

◆ Critical items or high-risk items.

◆ Semi-critical items or intermediate-risk items.

◆ Non-critical items or low-risk items.

Later, an additional category of 'minimal risk items' was added to Spaulding's original classification for items and environmental surfaces that do not come into close contact with the patient. Please refer to Appendix 6.1 for disinfection procedures for individual items and equipments.

Critical or high-risk items

Critical or high-risk items are those which come into contact with a break in the skin or mucous membrane or are introduced into a sterile body area. Such items must be rendered free from contamination by any microorganism, including bacterial spores. This category includes surgical instruments and implants, invasive devices such as cardiac catheters, urinary catheters, and intravascular devices. Sterilization is the recommended process for items in this category. In the health care setting, many of these items are available as single-use sterile items. Heat-labile items may be treated with low-temperature steam and formaldehyde, ethylene oxide, or by irradiation. Liquid chemical 'sterilant' should be used only if other methods are unsuitable.

Semi-critical or intermediate-risk items

Semi-critical or intermediate-risk items are those which come into contact with non-intact skin or mucous membranes. Such items should be rendered free from all microorganisms, although small numbers of bacterial spores may be present. This category includes respiratory therapy and anaesthetic equipment, endoscopes, laryngoscope blades, oesophageal probes, and other non-invasive items.

High-level disinfection is the recommended process for items in this category. As disinfection using chemicals is not always reliable; heat sterilization should be used, if possible. If the item is heat labile, it may be treated using chemical disinfection.

Non-critical or low-risk items

Non-critical or low-risk items are those which come into contact with intact skin. This category includes patient-care equipment such as blood pressure cuffs. Cleaning is the recommended process for items in this category, although in some cases, disinfection may be required.

Minimal risk items

Minimal risk items do not come into close contact with the patient or their immediate surroundings. Items in this category are either unlikely to be contaminated with significant numbers of potential pathogens, or transfer to a susceptible site on the patient is unlikely, e.g. items or environmental surface e.g. flower vases, walls, floors, ceilings, sinks and drains. Cleaning with detergent and drying of these items is adequate.

Methods of decontamination

The choice of method of disinfection or sterilization depends mainly on the:

- Type of material to be disinfected.
- Level of decontamination required for the procedure.
- Microorganisms involved. It is important to have a clear understanding of the following terms used in this context.

Cleaning

Cleaning of instruments *before* decontamination is an essential procedure as it allows physical removal of microorganisms which not only prevents inactivation of the disinfectant by organic matter, but also allows complete surface contact during further decontamination procedures. Therefore thorough cleaning of items is a prerequisite before disinfection and sterilization is commenced.

Cleaning should be carried out by trained staff in the sterile supply department (SSD). Machine washing is the preferred option; however, some instruments may require washing by hand. Staff performing these procedures must be trained in safe systems of work and wear appropriate PPE. During cleaning, care should be taken not to produce splashes, high pressure sprays, or aerosols.

Disinfection

Disinfection by either heat or chemicals will destroy microorganisms but not bacterial spores. Chemical disinfection does not necessarily kill all microorganisms present but reduces them to a level not harmful to health. Chemical disinfection should only be used if heat treatment is impractical or may cause damage to the equipment. 'High-level' disinfection refers to a process using an agent which is normally used for disinfection purposes, but under specific circumstances, when used in sufficient concentrations and with suitable extended exposure times, is capable of destroying bacterial spores. Sometimes this process is referred to as 'chemical sterilization' and the agent as a 'chemical sterilant, however use of this term should be avoided. The outcome of a disinfection procedure is affected by the

- Presence of organic load (bioburden) on the item.
- Type and level of microbial contaminant prior to cleaning of the object.
- Concentration of disinfectant.
- Exposure time.
- Physical structure of the object.
- Temperature and pH of the disinfection process.

Besides effective *cleaning* of items or equipments, the *concentration* and *contact time* are critical factors that determine the effectiveness of disinfection process.

Sterilization

Sterilization is a process which achieves the complete destruction or removal of all microorganisms, including bacterial spores. Equipment and materials used in procedures involving a break in the skin or mucous membranes should be sterilized in an accredited SSD.

It is essential that all the instruments must be thoroughly clean prior to sterilization and stored in a clean and dry place before use (see Box 6.1 on guidance of storage of sterile items). Figure 6.1 shows the symbols used on medical devices and their packaging. Sterilization can be achieved by:

+ **Dry heat sterilization:** dry heat sterilization requires higher temperatures for much longer exposure periods than moist heat sterilization to kill all microorganisms.

Box 6.1 Storage of sterile products

+ The storage area for sterile products *must be separated* from dirty linen, dirty utility/sluice area, and must be away from storage of clinical waste. In addition, the sterile material should be far from sources of moisture.

+ The storage area should be large enough for the amount of material that needs to be stored, should have an adequate level of lighting, and the walls should be smooth and easy to clean. Access to the area should have restricted.

+ They storage shelves should be located at a minimum distance of 30 cm from the floor, 45 cm from the ceiling, and 5 cm from the wall and should be maintained at the temperature between 15–28°C and humidity between 30–50%. Recommended air exchange in the storage room should be 10 changes per hour for a theatre sterile pack store.

+ Shelving or cabinets should be selected based on the rotation of the materials and of personnel access to the area and must always be kept in optimal conditions in terms of order and cleanliness.

+ Packages should be placed on shelves or in cabinets. If they are small packages, they should be placed in drawers or baskets. It is recommended that the storage containers should *not* be wooden.

+ The material should be placed in a position that makes it simple to see the label and visualize the expiry date indicated on the container.

+ When accessing the materials needed, don't touch the other material when removing the one that is needed.

+ Before use, it should be inspected in order to verify that it meets the requirements of a sterile product.

Adapted from Pan American Health Organization. *Sterilization manual for health centres.* Washington, DC: Pan American Health Organization, 2009.

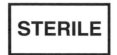

2002-06-30

CE marking indicates that the manufacturer has declared that the item complies with the requirements of the Directive(s) relevant to that device.

DO NOT REUSE. Synonyms for this are Single-use or Use only once.

STERILE Item.

USE BY DATE: The symbol is intended to indicate that the device should not be used after the end of the month or day shown.

Fig. 6.1 Symbols used on medical devices and their packaging.

Exposure in an oven for 2 hours at 170°C (328°F) is generally used for the dry heat sterilization of glassware and other items.

◆ **Moist heat sterilization:** moist heat is far more penetrating than dry heat and, hence, more effective for killing microorganisms. Steam under pressure is frequently used in sterilization procedures which can be achieved in an autoclave or sterilizer. A sterilizer is basically a chamber that can withstand pressures of greater than two atmospheres. Refer to Figure 6.2 which shows the basic features of a sterilizer or autoclave. The materials to be sterilized are placed in the chamber, which is then sealed. Steam is introduced under pressure into the chamber and held in there for the necessary time and then vented from the chamber. Sterilizers have pressure gauges and thermometers that monitor the sterilization process. In addition to these, sterilizers are also monitored using chemical and biological indicators. The cycles most frequently used for sterilization are 134–138°C for 3 min, 121–124°C for 15min, or 115°C for 30 min.

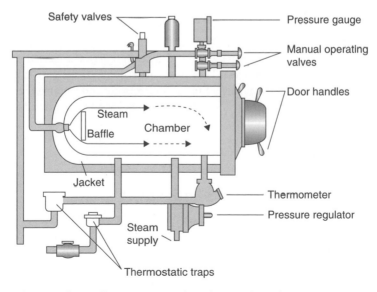

Fig. 6.2 Diagram of a sterilizer or an autoclave showing basic features.

If sterilization is not carried out in the hospital SSD then it is vital that sterilization procedures outside a central processing department promote the same level of safety and efficiency. Requirements include routine biological, mechanical, and chemical monitoring to ensure that all parameters of sterilization are met before using the instrument on patients.

- ◆ **Ethylene oxide (EtO):** EtO has several applications as a sterilizing agent. The ethylene portion of the molecule reacts with proteins and nucleic acids. EtO kills all microorganisms and endospores. It is toxic and explosive in its pure form, so it is usually mixed with a non-flammable gas such as carbon dioxide or nitrogen. A special autoclave-type sterilizer is used for EtO sterilization. Because of their ability to sterilize without heat, gases like EtO are also widely used on medical supplies and equipment that cannot withstand steam sterilization. Examples include disposable sterile plastic-ware such as syringes and Petri plates, linens, sutures, lensed instruments, artificial heart valves, heart-lung machines, and mattresses. Once the item is sterilized, it requires aeration time to remove EtO residue as is toxic and a carcinogen. The sterilizing cycle is lengthy. EtO cartridges should be stored in flammable liquid storage cabinet.

Benchtop sterilizers

Gravity displacement benchtop sterilizers

Traditional or gravity displacement benchtop sterilizers are those which displace air *passively* from the chamber and load by steam generated within the sterilizer chamber or in a separate chamber within the sterilizer's casing. Only *unwrapped* instruments without crevices or lumens may be processed in these machines.

Vacuum benchtop sterilizers

Vacuum benchtop sterilizers are those which have a pump or some other *active* method of removing air from the chamber and load. 'Porous loads', i.e. instruments which are hollow, tubular or have crevices or are wrapped, can only be processed in these machines. Vacuum benchtop sterilizers are much more complicated machines than traditional benchtop sterilizers. They therefore require greater care in their use and maintenance to ensure that they function effectively and require regular and rigorous testing. Benchtop sterilizers should only be used as an alternative if the items cannot be decontaminated in the SSD. If benchtop sterilizers are used in health care facilities then it is essential that they are properly used, adequately maintained, and monitored according to manufacturer's instruction (see Box 6.2).

Chemical disinfectants and antiseptics

A *disinfectant* is a chemical agent which, under defined conditions, is capable of disinfection. It is a substance that is recommended for application to inanimate surfaces to kill a range of microorganisms. The equivalent agent, which kills microorganisms present on skin, mucous membrane, is called an **antiseptic**. Two factors must be evaluated in determining the effectiveness of antiseptics, i.e. the agents must have effective antimicrobial activity and must not be toxic to living tissues.

Box 6.2 Maintenance of benchtop sterilizers

Commissioning, validation, and maintenance: before use, all benchtop steam sterilizers must be installed and validated in line with the manufacturer's recommendations. An authorized person should provide advice on the validation process and commissioning tests according to the manufacturer's recommendations. Details of this process must be recorded in the logbook, which must be retained with the sterilizers. It is essential to ensure that all persons who will use the machine are *properly trained* and deemed *competent* to use it.

Periodic testing: a schedule for periodic testing must be drawn up at the time of validation and the owner/user of the benchtop sterilizer must ensure that these tests are performed according to schedule as outlined in the relevant documents.

Maintenance: maintenance should be performed routinely as recommended by the manufacturer. The test schedule should be carried out on daily, weekly, quarterly, and yearly intervals as specified in the documents. These tests are always preceded by safety checks to ensure that the sterilizer is safe to use.

Routine monitoring: In addition to the periodic testing, routine monitoring of the process is necessary to ensure that sterile loads are consistently being produced. For each production cycle:

- Note any fault or malfunction of the sterilizer.
- Note whether the sterilizer's controller has indicated a passed or failed cycle.
- Note the actions taken, if a failed cycle was indicated.
- Examine printouts from the sterilizer's record to ensure that they are within the prescribed limits.
- Keep printed records of every cycle which must be retained with the sterilizer logbook.

Record keeping: all records of testing should be kept according to the guidance provided by the manufactures. The following results must be logged on the production cycle.

- Date and cycle number.
- Type of load, e.g. porous load, solid instrument, hollow instrument, or a mixture.
- Sterilization cycle selected.
- Whether the cycle was a pass or fail and the chart record for the cycle.
- Identity of the operator.

The results of the daily test must be recorded in the logbook, dated, and signed by the user. Stream penetration indicator test sheets marked with the result of the test must be signed and dated by the operator and stored as recommended by the manufacturer for a period of at least 6 months. Chemical indicators should meet the requirements as specified in EN 867 and must only be used for the process specified by the manufacturer. The use of an inappropriate indicator may give misleading results. Biological indicators should meet the requirements of EN 866. These are of limited value in steam sterilization.

Various chemical agents are used to disinfect items or equipment in a health care setting. Ideally, a disinfectant should have high germicidal activity. They should rapidly kill a wide range of microorganisms, including spores. The agent should be chemically stable and effective in the presence of organic compounds and metals. The ability to penetrate into crevices is desirable. It is essential that a disinfectant should not damage the materials to which it is applied. Furthermore, it should be inexpensive and aesthetically acceptable.

Microorganisms vary in their sensitivity to particular disinfectants and antiseptics (see Tables 6.1 and 6.2). Generally, growing microorganisms are more sensitive than microorganisms in dormant stages, such as spores. Figure 6.3 shows the descending order of resistance to germicidal activity of chemical disinfectants against various microorganisms.

Chemical disinfectants are hazardous substances and may cause damage on contact with skin, eyes, or mucous membranes, by inhalation of vapours, or by absorption through the skin. Some individuals may be allergic to individual disinfectants, or more sensitive to them than other people. This may take the form of skin rashes, contact dermatitis, or, in rare cases, difficulty in breathing. Therefore it is important that relevant safety precautions are observed when using chemical disinfectants (see Box 6.3). Concentrated disinfectants should always be stored and handled with care and appropriate protective equipment must be worn. For certain chemical disinfectants (e.g. glutaraldehyde) proper ventilation is required.

The following points should be kept in mind when using chemical disinfectants:

- The efficacy of chemical disinfection is often uncertain and, wherever possible, disinfection by heat is preferable to chemical methods.

- All chemical disinfectants must be clearly labelled and used within the expiry date. They should be freshly prepared. They must be used at the correct concentration and stored in an appropriate container. Chemical disinfectant solutions must not be mixed or detergents added unless they are compatible.

- Disinfectant or detergent solutions must not be prepared and stored in multi-use containers for occasional use. Solutions prepared and stored in this manner may easily become contaminated with microorganisms; using such solutions will therefore readily contaminate a surface rather than clean it.

- Disinfectants can be corrosive and may damage fabrics, metals, and plastics. Manufacturers' instructions must be consulted on compatibility of materials with the method of sterilization or disinfection.

Alcohol

The name alcohol is taken from the Arabic *Al Kohl*, which was used for refined antimony sulfide used by ancient Egyptians as a remedy against eye infections, in combination with a blue dye, as a cosmetic.

An important feature for their usability in antisepsis is the miscibility of alcohols with water. Only short-chained alcohols, such as methanol, ethanol, and the propanols, are completely miscible. Of the large chemical group of alcohol substances, three are mainly used in disinfection and antisepsis: ethanol, iso-propanol (or 2-propanol), and n-propanol (or 1-propanol).

Table 6.1 Antimicrobial activity of antiseptic agents

Group	Gram-positive bacteria	Gram-negative bacteria	Mycobacteria	Fungi	Viruses	Speed of action
Alcohols	+++	+++	+++	+++	+++	Fast
Chlorhexidine (2% and 4% aqueous)	+++	+++	+	+	+++	Intermediate
Hexachlorophane (3% aqueous)	+++	++	+	+	+	Intermediate
Iodine compounds	+++	+++	+++	++	+++	Intermediate
Iodophors	+++	+++	+	++	++	Intermediate
Phenol derivatives	+++	+	+	+	+	Intermediate
Triclosan	+++	++	+	−	+++	Intermediate
Quaternary ammonium compounds	+	++	−	−	+	Slow

Activity: +++ = Good; ++ = Moderate; + = Poor; − = no activity or insufficient activity.

Table 6.2 Antimicrobial activity and summary of properties of disinfectants

Disinfectant	Antimicrobial activity					Other properties			
	Bacteria	Mycobacteria	Spores	Viruses		Stability	Inactivation by organic matter	Corrosive/ damaging	Irritant/ sensitizing
				Enveloped	Non enveloped				
Alcohol 60–70% (ethanol or isopropanol)	+++	+++	–	++	++	Yes (in closed container)	Yes (fixative)	Slight (lens cements)	No
Chlorine releasing agents (0.5–1% available chlorine)	+++	+++	+++	+++	+++	No (<1 day)	Yes	Yes	Yes
Clear soluble phenolics (1–2%)	+++	++	–	++	+	Yes	No	Slight	Yes
Glutaraldehyde (2%)	+++	+++	+++	+++	+++	Moderately (14–28 days)	No (fixative)	No	Yes
Peracetic acid (0.2–0.35%)	+++	+++	+++	+++	+++	No (<1 day)	No	Slight	Slight
Peroxygen compounds* (3–6%)	+++	±	±	+++	±	Moderately (7 days)	Yes	Slight	No

Activity: +++ = Good; ++ = Moderate; ± = Variable; – = no activity or insufficient activity. *Activity varies with concentration.

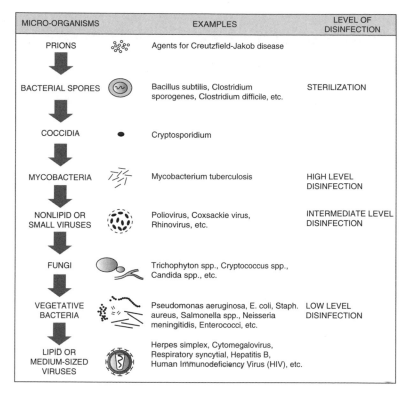

MICRO-ORGANISMS	EXAMPLES	LEVEL OF DISINFECTION
PRIONS	Agents for Creutzfield-Jakob disease	
BACTERIAL SPORES	Bacillus subtilis, Clostridium sporogenes, Clostridium difficile, etc.	STERILIZATION
COCCIDIA	Cryptosporidium	
MYCOBACTERIA	Mycobacterium tuberculosis	HIGH LEVEL DISINFECTION
NONLIPID OR SMALL VIRUSES	Poliovirus, Coxsackie virus, Rhinovirus, etc.	INTERMEDIATE LEVEL DISINFECTION
FUNGI	Trichophyton spp., Cryptococcus spp., Candida spp., etc.	
VEGETATIVE BACTERIA	Pseudomonas aeruginosa, E. coli, Staph. aureus, Salmonella spp., Neisseria meningitidis, Enterococci, etc.	LOW LEVEL DISINFECTION
LIPID OR MEDIUM-SIZED VIRUSES	Herpes simplex, Cytomegalovirus, Respiratory syncytial, Hepatitis B, Human Immunodeficiency Virus (HIV), etc.	

Fig. 6.3 Descending order of resistance to germicidal activity of chemical disinfectants against various microorganisms.

Alcohol does not penetrate well into organic (especially protein-based) matter, and should therefore be used to disinfect only physically cleaned hard surfaces *or* equipment. Alcohol-impregnated wipes are used for disinfection of skin prior to injection. It can be used as a base for other antiseptics, e.g. chlorhexidine and iodine for preoperative skin disinfection.

Alcohol should be stored in a cool place. Alcohol–alcohol mixtures are flammable. Do not allow contact with hot surfaces, flames, electrical equipment or other sources of ignition. If an alcohol preparation is used to disinfect preoperative skin, caution must be exercised whilst using diathermy as it may ignite, causing skin burns if incorrectly used. Therefore all spirit-based skin cleaning and preparation fluids must have a cautionary statement, e.g. 'This preparation contains spirit. When use is to be followed by surgical diathermy, do not allow pooling of the fluid to occur and ensure that the skin and surrounding areas are dry'.

Do not leave uncapped bottles of alcohol as it releases vapours and irritate mucous membranes, especially in an enclosed space. It may cause eye and skin irritation if used in a large quantity in an enclosed space, therefore its use should be avoided in a poorly ventilated area. If inhaled in large quantities, it may cause headache and drowsiness.

Box 6.3 Use of chemical disinfectants

Safety of health care workers

The employer has a duty to *inform*, *instruct*, and *train* employees and non-employees on their premises in relevant safety matters; this includes the use of chemical disinfectants. Disinfectants are chemical agents and may be harmful, irritant, or corrosive and may cause damage by contact with eyes or mucous membranes, by inhalation of vapours, or by absorption through the skin. In addition, environmental disinfectants can damage fabrics, metals, and plastics.

Concentrated disinfectants should always be stored and handled with care and appropriate protective clothing and equipment such as gloves, aprons, respiratory, and eye protection should be used where appropriate. Disinfection should, whenever possible, be carried out in a closed container. Storage containers should never be left open to the atmosphere for longer than absolutely necessary. Work should be carried out in an area with easy access to running water and eye-wash bottle.

Some individuals may be more sensitive or allergic to disinfectants and may develop skin rashes, contact dermatitis, or in rare cases, difficulty in breathing. These individual must inform their line manager who should refer them to Occupational Health Department for assessment and appropriate action.

Therefore it is essential that when disinfectants are selected in health care facilities, risk assessment must be carried out. Their use must follow the manufacturer's instruction and where necessary, the exposure of employees and others who may be exposed should be monitored as per recommended guidelines. In the UK, COSHH (Control of Substance Hazardous to Health) regulations must be followed.

If concentrations are given in fractions of 100 ('per cent'), they must be clearly defined as percentage by weight (g/g or w/w) or by volume (ml/ml or v/v). The transformation of percentage by volume into percentage by weight is not possible by merely multiplying volume per cent by the specific weight of the alcohol, since, in *mixtures with water*, a *volume contraction of the alcohol occurs* that is greatest when mixing equal parts of alcohol and water. The best way to avoid difficulties in preparation of alcohol solutions is to work with concentrations by weight, rather than by volume.

Chlorine-based disinfectants

Hypochlorites are the most widely used of the chlorine disinfectants and are available as Chloros®, Domestos®, Milton®, Actichlor®, etc. Product containing abrasive hypochlorite powders is available as Ajax®, Vim®, etc. They are available as a liquid (sodium hypochlorite 'bleach'), or as a solid (calcium hypochlorite or sodium dichloroisocyanurate [NaDCC]). NaDCC tablets are stable and the antimicrobial activity of a solution prepared from NaDCC tablets may be greater than that of sodium hypochlorite solutions containing the same total available chlorine. Aqueous solutions of sodium hypochlorite are widely used as household bleach. They work on microbes by inhibition of enzymatic reactions, denaturation of proteins and inactivation of nucleic acids.

They are fast acting, low-cost, have a broad spectrum of antimicrobial activity, do not leave toxic residues, and are not affected by water hardness. They are very active against viruses and are the disinfectant of choice for environmental decontamination following blood spillage from a patient with known or suspected blood-borne viral infection. The minimum concentration to eliminate mycobacteria is 1000 ppm for 10 min. Hypochlorites are also incorporated into some cleansing agents which are used for environmental disinfection on hard surfaces such as baths or sinks. It is used in water treatment and in food preparation areas and milk kitchens (see Table 6.3). However, it is important to remember that the following factors affect the stability of chlorine:

- Presence of heavy metal ions.
- Incompatible with cationic detergents.
- Its efficiency diminishes with an increase in pH of the solution.
- Temperature of the solution.
- Presence of biofilms.
- Presence of organic matter (particularly if used in low concentrations).
- Ultraviolet radiation.

Therefore it is important that diluted hypochlorite solutions should be freshly prepared daily. It should be kept in an opaque container as it is degraded by sun rays.

Table 6.3 Uses of hypochlorite and strengths of solution

Uses	Available chlorine mg/L (ppm)*
Blood spills from patients with blood-borne viral infection, e.g. HIV, hepatitis B & C virus	10,000
Laboratory discard jars	2500
General environmental disinfection	1000
Disinfection of clean instruments	500
Infant feeding g bottles and teats	125
Food-preparation areas and catering equipment	125
Eradication of *Legionella* from water supply system, depending on exposure time	5–50
Hydrotherapy pools:	
Routine	1.5–3
If contaminated	6–10
Routine water treatment	0.5–1

*Undiluted commercial products tend to vary between 10% and 0.1% hypochlorite (100,000 and 10,000 ppm av Cl).

With permission from Fraise AD, Bradley C. *Ayliffe's control of Healthcare-Associated Infection. A practical handbook*, 5th edn. London, Hodder Arnold, 2009.

Decomposition is accelerated by light, heat, and heavy metal. They are also corrosive to metal, damaged plastic, rubber, and similar components on prolonged contact (>30 min), or if used at an incorrect concentration. They also bleach fabrics, carpets, or soft furnishings. Hypochlorites can cause irritation to the mucous membranes of the skin, eyes, and lungs if used frequently in a poorly ventilated area. Appropriate protective equipment must be worn when hypochlorite is handled, whether in liquid or powdered/granulated form. Sodium hypochlorite should not be mixed with ammonia or acid or acidic body fluids (e.g. urine), as it release toxic chlorine gas especially in a confined space. They should not be used in the presence of formaldehyde as some of the reaction products are carcinogenic.

Phenolic disinfectants

Phenolic disinfectants (carbolic acid) are probably the oldest recognized disinfectants. Its use as a germicide in operating rooms was introduced by Joseph Lister in 1867. They are usually supplied in combination with a detergent to aid the cleaning process. They also retain their activity in the presence of organic material. They are incompatible with cationic detergents and absorbed by rubber and plastics. Cresols, which are phenolic derivatives of coal tars, are good disinfectants. The active ingredient in Lysol®, a commonly used household disinfectant, is the cresol *o*-phenylphenol. The distinctive aroma of these phenolics gives many hospitals their characteristic smell.

In high concentrations, phenols break the cell wall, penetrate the cell, and precipitate the cytoplasmic proteins. In low concentrations, they cause the death of microorganisms by inactivating the enzymes in the cell wall.

Phenolic disinfectants can be absorbed by porous materials such as plastic, leaving waste that produces irritation in the mucous membranes. It causes respiratory irritation if used at concentrations above those listed in the disinfection policy. Appropriate protective clothing must be worn when handling phenolic disinfectants. Skin and eyes must be protected while 'making up' or discarding a phenolics solution. Phenolic disinfectants can be absorbed through the skin therefore skin must be protected during its use. Use latex gloves for intermittent use; medium weight washing-up gloves are appropriate for more prolonged contact.

Phenolic disinfectants are used for environmental disinfection. Routine-use dilution for the commonly used clear soluble phenolics is 1% v/v for 'clean' (low organic soiling) and 2% v/v for 'dirty' (high organic soiling) conditions. They are the agents of choice for mycobacteria including *M. tuberculosis* in the environment. Clear soluble (2%) phenolics (Stericol ®, Hycolin®, Clearsol®, etc) can be used in laboratory discard jars in bacteriology.

Phenolic disinfectants should *not* be used to clean infant bassinets and incubators because of the occurrence of hyperbilirubinaemia in infants. Phenol must *not* be used on items and equipments that may come into contact with skin or mucous membranes. Phenolic disinfectants may taint food and should not be used on food preparation surfaces.

Chlorhexidine

Chlorhexidine was first synthesized in 1954 in the laboratories of ICI England and is a relatively non-toxic compound. It is available as Hibiscrub®, Hibiclens®, etc.

The chlorhexidine molecule possesses strongly cationic groups and, therefore, binds to surfactants, detergents, and other excipients, reducing the availability of the free compound to exert its antimicrobial effect, therefore it is inactivated by soap, organic matter, and anionic detergents. It also stains fabrics brown in the presence of chlorine-based disinfectants. In addition, if chlorhexidine is used for oral hygiene, brown stains will development on teeth in some users as chlorhexidine reacts with dietary chromogens.

Chlorhexidine is used exclusively as an antiseptic where contact with skin and mucous membranes are involved. The chlorhexidine is combined with alcohol and is used as the antiseptic of choice to disinfect preoperative skin preparation and to disinfect skin before insertion of central venous catheters. It is used as part of MRSA decolonization therapy (see 'Meticillin-resistant *Staphylococcus aureus*', Chapter 10). They are combined with detergent preparations and are used for surgical hand-disinfection. Chlorhexidine gluconate is significantly more effective than povidone-iodine in both the presence and absence of blood and unlike povidone-iodine it has residual activity on the skin after application. It *must not* be allowed to come into contact with the brain, meninges, eye, or middle ear.

Iodine and iodophor

This group includes aqueous iodine in potassium iodide solution and tincture of iodine. It is inactivated by organic matter and may corrode metals. An iodophor is a preparation containing iodine complex with a solubilizing agent, such as a surfactant or polyvinylpyrrolidone ('povidone'). They are available as Betadine®, Disadine®, Videne®, etc). The result is a water-soluble material that releases free iodine when in solution. Unlike iodine, iodophors do not stain skin and are non-irritant.

Alcoholic preparations containing iodine and iodophors are suitable for preoperative skin preparation. Povidone iodine detergent preparations are used for surgical hand-disinfection. An alcoholic iodophor is less irritant than an alcohol/iodine mixture. Tincture of iodine and aqueous iodine solutions can cause skin reactions in some individuals; therefore iodophor solution is preferred. Gloves are required for prolonged handling of iodine/iodophor preparation.

Quaternary ammonium compounds

Quaternary ammonium cations (QACs), also known as 'quats', are positively compounds and they kill microbes by inactivation of energy-producing enzymes, denaturation of cellular proteins, and rupture of the cellular membrane.

QACs at low concentrations inhibit the growth of bacteria (bacteriostatic) but do not kill them. Gram-negative bacilli (e.g. *Pseudomonas* spp.) may cause contamination and grow in diluted or inactivated solution. Therefore, any unused solutions should be discarded immediately after use. Decanting from one container and topping-up should be avoided. This can result in contamination and promote growth of Gram-negative bacilli which may then colonize the wound. Therefore their use in the operating theatre, unless in sterile single-use format, should be avoided because of the danger that they will permit growth of *Pseudomonas* spp. which can cause infection in surgical wounds. To avoid the problem of contamination, the correct strength of solution should be obtained from the pharmacy. Single-use sachets should be used, if possible. Liquid should be stored in closed bottles until immediately before use.

They are good cleaning agents and these compounds are relatively non-irritating to human tissues at concentrations that are inhibitory to microorganisms. However, benzalkonium chloride is one of the leading allergens amongst health care personnel.

Several quaternary ammonium cationic detergents are used as antiseptic agents. The concentrations for use vary according to the combination of each QAC commercial formulation. They are used as antiseptics for cleaning dirty wounds. They act slowly and are *inactivated* by soaps, anionic detergents, and organic matter. Their antimicrobial activity is lowered if they are absorbed by porous or fibrous materials such as cotton or gauze bandages. Hard water containing calcium or magnesium ions interferes with their action. Their use as an environmental disinfectant is usually *not* recommended.

Hexachlorophane

Hexachlorophane is a chlorinated bisphenol and one of the most useful of the phenol derivatives. Unlike most phenolic compounds, hexachlorophane has no irritating odour and has a high residual action. Hexachlorophane is not fast acting and its rate of killing is classified as slow to intermediate. The major advantage of hexachlorophane is its residual effect after application of the product. Soaps and other organic materials have little effect. Hexachlorophane is more effective against Gram-positive than against Gram-negative bacilli. Hexachlorophane (0.33%) powder has good residual effect on the skin and can be used as an anti-staphylococcal agent. However, it should *not* be applied on neonates because it can cause neurological damage. Its use on broken skin or mucous membranes or for routine total body bathing is also contraindicated and currently use of hexachlorophene has been banned worldwide because of its high rate of dermal absorption and subsequent toxic effects.

Triclosan

Triclosan (Irgasan®) is a diphenyl ether and has been used since 1972, and it is present in household antibacterial soaps, deodorants, shaving creams, mouth washes, etc. It has a similar range of antimicrobial activity as hexachlorophane but exhibits no documented toxicity in neonates. It can be absorbed through intact skin but appears to be non-allergenic and non-mutagenic with short-term use. Its activity is only minimally affected by organic matter. Its speed of killing is intermediate but it has excellent persistent (residual) activity on skin. It is used as part of MRSA decolonization therapy (see 'Meticillin-resistant *Staphylococcus aureus*', Chapter 10). Since triclosan shows a lower to immediate reduction and triclosan-containing products are mainly bacteriostatic and are *inactive* against *P. aeruginosa*, its use in operating rooms for surgical scrub is no longer recommended.

Aldehydes

Glutaraldehyde

Glutaraldehyde is available as aqueous, acidic, and alkaline solutions. Its acts on microorganisms by causing alkylation of cellular components that alters the protein synthesis of DNA and RNA. Acidic solutions are stable and do not require activation, but slower in activity than alkaline buffered solutions. Since acidic solutions are not sporicidal, they require alkalinizing agent as activators to make it sporicidal. Once activated, they remain active for 14 days. Most preparations of glutaraldehyde are non-corrosive to metals and other materials and inactivation by organic matter is very low.

Advantages and disadvantages: 2% glutaraldehyde is used to disinfect heat-sensitive items such as endoscopes. Glutaraldehyde may be irritant to the eyes and nasal pathway and may cause respiratory illness (asthma) and allergic dermatitis. Glutaraldehyde should not be used in an area with little or no ventilation, as exposure is likely to be at or above the current occupational exposure standards. The threshold limit value (TLV/exposure value) of glutaraldehyde is 0.02 ppm. (parts per million) to 0.05 ppm in 8 work hours.

Eye protection, a plastic apron, and gloves must be worn when glutaraldehyde liquid is made up, disposed of, or when immersing instruments. Latex gloves may be worn and discarded after use if the duration of contact with glutaraldehyde is brief, i.e. less than 5 min. For longer duration, nitrile gloves must be worn. It should be stored away from heat sources and in containers with close-fitting lids.

Formaldehyde

Formaldehyde (formalin is a stabilized 40% solution of formaldehyde) is an aqueous solution with a penetrating odour. Formaldehyde is used mainly as a gaseous fumigant to disinfect safety cabinets in the laboratory or to disinfect room with highly dangerous pathogens, e.g. VHF. These uses may only be carried out by fully trained persons.

Formaldehyde is a potent eye and nasal irritant and may cause respiratory distress and allergic dermatitis. It is considered potentially carcinogenic. Gloves, goggles, and aprons should be worn when preparing and disposing of formaldehyde solutions. Occupational exposure monitoring is required as per local guidelines.

Peracetic acid

Peracetic acid is an oxidant agent that acts similarly to hydrogen peroxide. It is characterized by a very rapid action against microorganisms (including spores) and act by the denaturation of proteins and altering the permeability of the cell wall.

The greatest advantage is that it does not produce toxic waste and does not require activation. It remains effective in the presence of organic matter and is sporicidal even at low temperatures and does not coagulate blood or fix tissues to surfaces.

An automated machine using peracetic acid chemically sterilizes medical, surgical, and dental instruments including endoscopes and arthroscopes. It is more effective than glutaraldehyde at penetrating organic matter such as biofilms. It is used as a cold 'sterilant' to disinfect endoscopes. The solution is activated to provide the appropriate in-use strength. Once prepared, the current manufacturer's recommendation is that it should be used within 24 hours. Biological indicators may not be suitable for routine monitoring. Peracetic acid can corrode copper, brass, bronze, plain steel, and galvanized iron but these effects can be reduced by additives and pH modifications. It is considered unstable, particularly when diluted. It produces can produces serious eye and skin damage (especially concentrated solution) and cause irritation of the mucous membranes.

Hydrogen peroxide

Hydrogen peroxide kills microorganism by the production of destructive hydroxyl free radicals that can attack membrane lipids, DNA, and other essential cell components. Hydrogen peroxide is active against a wide range of microorganisms including cryptosporidium. Under normal conditions hydrogen peroxide is extremely stable when properly stored (e.g. in dark containers). Hydrogen peroxide and peroxygen compounds have low toxicity and irritancy. No activation is required and it removes organic matter. It does not coagulate blood or fix tissues to surfaces. It has no odour and does not cause irritation or require special disposal.

Commercially available 3% hydrogen peroxide (e.g. Virkon®) is a stable and effective disinfectant when used on inanimate surfaces. It has been used in concentrations from 3–6% for the disinfection of soft contact lenses, tonometer, biprisms, ventilators, and endoscopes.

A chemical irritation resembling pseudomembranous colitis has been reported in a gastrointestinal endoscopy unit with use of 3% hydrogen peroxide. As with other chemical sterilants, dilution of hydrogen peroxide must be monitored by regularly testing the minimum effective concentration (i.e. 7.5–6.0%).

Hydrogen peroxide has not been widely used for endoscope disinfection because of concerns that its oxidizing properties may be harmful to some components of the endoscope. It has compatibility concerns with brass, zinc copper, and nickel/silver plating therefore manufacturer's approval should be obtained before using on equipment where corrosion may present problems, such as endoscopes or centrifuges. It can cause serious eye damage with contact.

Ortho-phthaladehyde

Ortho-phthaladehyde (OPA) (Cidex OPA®) is a chemical agent which is used for high-level disinfection. It corresponds to the group of inorganic aldehydes and contains benzenecarboxaldehyde. It has an excellent antimicrobial activity and its kill microorganisms by alkylation of cellular components and acts directly on nucleic acids.

OPA has several potential advantages compared to glutaraldehyde. The principal advantage is that it has excellent stability in a broad range of pH (3–9) and as a result does not require activation. It is fast acting and has excellent material compatibility and does not coagulate blood or fix tissues to surfaces. Like glutaraldehyde it also has excellent compatibility with any type of material or article and has chemical indicators. It is not a known irritant to the eyes and nasal passages, does not require exposure monitoring, has a barely perceptible odour, and requires no activation. It is not carcinogenic, but it is recommendable to use this compound in ventilated areas since it still has not been determined if it can produce irritation in the eyes and nostrils.

However, it is expensive than glutaraldehyde and has slow sporicidal activity. In addition, it has potential disadvantages as it causes eye irritation with contact and stains proteins grey (including unprotected skin, mucous membranes, clothing, and environmental surfaces) and therefore caution must be exercised when handling the solution and use of PPE, e.g. gloves, eye and mouth protection, fluid-resistant gowns is essential. In addition, equipment must be thoroughly rinsed to prevent discoloration of a patient's skin or mucous membrane. Disposal must be undertaken in accordance with local regulations; OPA solution may require neutralization before disposal to the sanitary sewer system.

The time required for high-level disinfection varies according to the following standards and manufacturers e.g. USA FDA standard 10–12 min at 20 °C, Canadian standard is 10 min and Standard in Europe is 5 min. A concentration of 0.55% is recommended. The solution can be reused for 14 days and has a shelf life of 2 years.

Chlorine dioxide

Chlorine dioxide disinfects by oxidation; however, it does not chlorinate. Chlorine dioxide was first used at a spa in Ostend, Belgium as a water disinfectant. Since the 1950s, it has been used to disinfect drinking water, for the treatment of waste water, and for slime control. In past few years, it has been available (e.g. Tristel®) to disinfect heat-sensitive instrument, e.g. flexible endoscopes.

Chlorine dioxide is a highly effective compound as it is rapidly bactericidal and is active against mycobacteria, viruses, and bacterial spores. It is stable in dilute solution in a closed container in the absence of light. High-level disinfection can be achieved in 5 min; however, 10 min is required for sporicidal activity. Before it is used on any items (flexible endoscopes etc.), user acceptance and instrument and processor compatibility must be established.

Decontamination of endoscopes

The number of endoscopic procedures used on patients for diagnostic and therapeutic reasons is increasing each year. Although the overall incidence of infection following endoscopy is very low, it can only be avoided by maintaining the highest standards of decontamination after each use. Endoscopes are either rigid (e.g. arthroscopes, cystoscopes, laparoscopes) which are relatively easy to clean and mainly heat tolerant, or flexible endoscopes (e.g. bronchoscopes, gastrointestinal endoscopes) which are complex, heat sensitive, and difficult to clean, disinfect, and sterilize. Therefore, effective decontamination of endoscopes requires input from an instrument's manufacturer who is familiar with the design and function of the item and its compatibility with heat and chemical disinfectants. When purchasing, ensure compatibility with the existing hospital decontamination processes, including compatibility with the washer disinfector.

Major problems which occur leading to inadequate decontamination include *inadequate cleaning* which may lead to failure to remove deposits of blood, faeces, tissue, mucous, microorganisms, or slime. These may result in infection, misdiagnosis, or instrument malfunction. In addition if an automated endoscope reprocessor is used, a number of factors have been associated with contamination of machines:

- Inadequate cleaning and maintenance of the machine which may result in the formation of biofilm within the machine.
- Inadequate cleaning of the endoscope resulting in adequate decontamination.

◆ Use of static water within pipe work or tank.

◆ Use of poor microbiological quality of water and/or use of hard water.

General considerations

Endoscopic unit

Facilities where endoscopes are used and disinfected should be designed to provide a safe environment for HCWs and patients. Air-exchange equipment (e.g. ventilation system, exhaust hoods) should be used to minimize the exposure of all persons to potentially toxic vapour of disinfectants. The vapour concentration of the chemical disinfectant used should not exceed allowable limits.

Record keeping

A log must be maintained for each procedure and details of the patient's name and medical record number, the endoscopist who has perform the procedure, and the serial number or identifier of the endoscope used. The log should also include proof of the decontamination procedure and the equipment/method used. This is essential for look-back exercises (see 'Look-back investigations', Chapter 4, Box 4.2).

Education and training

Personnel responsible for the reprocessing of endoscopes must receive training in the reprocessing of equipment to ensure proper cleaning and high-level disinfection or sterilization is carried out according to written instructions based on the manufacturer's instruction. *Competency testing* of personnel should be done on commencement of employment and then at least on an annual basis or if there is change in either endoscopes or introduction of new disinfectants or reprocessors. All personnel working in an endoscopy unit must be educated about the biological, chemical, and environmental hazards. A record of the training received should be retained.

Staff health

Staff should also be immunized against hepatitis B virus. They should wear gloves and a disposable waterproof apron. Gloves should be used for short contact time (15–20 min); nitrile gloves should be worn for longer contact times. Gloves should be removed and the hands washed between tasks. Eye protection should be used to prevent conjunctival irritation and protect the wearer from splashes. An approved vapour respirator should be available in case of spillage or other emergencies. It should be stored away from disinfectants as the charcoal will absorb any fumes.

Cleaning

Thorough *manual cleaning* of the instrument and its internal channels with detergent is the *most important* part of the disinfection procedure. Without this, dry residual organic material such as blood or mucous may lead to channel blockages and also prevent penetration of the disinfectant. It also ensures better contact between the disinfectant (or 'sterilant') and removal of any remaining microorganisms in subsequent stages of decontamination. Cleaning with warm water and a neutral or enzymatic detergent is recommended, though advice on suitable cleaning agents should be sought from the endoscope's manufacturer. The detergent should be changed after each use as per manufacturer's recommendations to prevent its contamination with organic matter. Ultrasonic washers may be used for most rigid endoscope components and accessories with the exception of the telescope. All lumens should be irrigated after ultrasonic cleansing to remove dislodged organic matter. Irrigation pumps are available for flushing instrument lumens and components. Channel cleaning brushes or a similar device should be used in accessible channels prior to flushing with detergent. The brush should be a suitable length and diameter for the channel being brushed.

Automatic endoscope reprocessor

There are many automatic endoscope reprocessors (AERs) available that are capable of cleaning as well as disinfecting endoscopes. However, it is essential that *initial manual cleaning* at the point of use is performed to ensure the effectiveness of subsequent processing and prevent the machine and the disinfectant becoming contaminated with excess organic matter or body fluids. If an AER is used, check the number of channels in each endoscope and ensure that they can all be connected to the washer disinfector using the correct connectors/connection sets according to the manufacturer's instructions to ensure exposure of all internal surfaces with the high-level disinfectant/chemical sterilant. All tank and fluid pathways in endoscope washer/disinfectors *must be regularly disinfected* to prevent microbial colonization of the fluid pathway which could be responsible for recontamination of processed endoscopes and subsequent misdiagnosis of infection. The final rinse water must be of a suitable quality with respect to hardness and freedom from microbiological contamination. A record must be kept of the number of machine cycles to ensure that the disinfectant is not unreasonably diluted or neutralized by organic matter. Single-use disinfectants are preferred.

Endoscopy accessories

Endoscopy accessories which are used for invasive procedures *must be sterile* after each use; alternatively single-use accessories may be used.

Process validation

Use only validated processes based on the local guidance. In the UK follow guidance in NHS Estates HTM 2030 Washer Disinfectors, MHRA Device Bulletin DB2002 (05) and MAC Manual on Decontamination. Report any equipment problems relating to endoscope, washer disinfector or disinfectant to the appropriate regulatory authority. In the UK, this should be reported to the UK Medicines and Healthcare products Regulatory Agency (http://www.mhra.gov.uk) and CCDC at your local health protection unit.

Chemical disinfectants

The problems associated with the use of the most commonly used disinfectant, glutaraldehyde, have prompted the development of non-aldehydes alternatives. However, it is important to note that before any new chemical disinfectant is introduced, a written approval must be obtained regarding the compatibility of the product with both the endoscopy and endoscope washer disinfector manufactures. For effective disinfection, the manufacturer's recommended time for immersion must be followed. Since the harmful effects of the new disinfectants are not fully evaluated it is essential that a risk assessment is carried out and they may have to be used under exhaust-ventilated conditions using appropriate PPE.

Serial processing of endoscopes in automated systems may reduce disinfectant potency due to carry over of fluid from the cleaning stage of the procedure. Therefore, the disinfectant should be changed frequently as per manufactures' recommendations taking into consideration the usage and its contamination with organic matter. Routine testing of the disinfectant solution should be performed to ensure minimal effective concentration of the active ingredient. Check the solution each day of use (or more frequently) and document the results. If the chemical indicator indicates that the concentration is less than the minimum effective concentration, the solution should be discarded.

For example, the concentration of glutaraldehyde in the solution should not be allowed to fall below 1.5% and solutions must not be used beyond the manufacturer's recommended post-activation life. Test kits are available which indicate glutaraldehyde concentration. The rinse water should also be changed regularly to avoid build-up of glutaraldehyde on the instrument and eyepiece assembly, as residues may cause skin and eye irritation.

Water quality

Quality of water is important as the hard water may result in the build-up of lime scale on the internal pipe work of the washer and/or disinfector. Poor microbiological quality of water may result in microbial contamination. Tap water contains microbes including *Pseudomonas* spp. and *Mycobacterium* spp. and its use has resulted in misdiagnosis of tuberculosis due to contamination of endoscopes with environmental mycobacteria (e.g. *M. chelonae*) present in the rinse water which subsequently contaminated bronchial washings sent for culture. Therefore, use of pre-sterilized bottled water for standalone machines and pre-treated water for machines connected to the main water supply is recommended. Sterile water is recommended for the final rinsing of all types of endoscope to be used for invasive procedures.

Water testing

Sampling of the final rinse water for the total viable count (TVC) is recommended to be carried out weekly to ensure the effectiveness of the water treatment system and the machine disinfection cycle. In Europe (EN 15883) the standard states that there should be less than 10cfu/100 mL of final rinse water. In the event that the water is contaminated a suggested action plan is shown in Table 6.4.

Environmental cleaning

Environmental contamination with microorganisms

It has been estimated that each individual sheds approximately 1 million (3–6 ounces) skin squames (dead skin cells) per day and approximately 10% of these squames carry between 1–5000 viable bacteria present as microcolonies. During human activity, they are constantly dispersed in the environment like 'flying saucers'. In addition, we also

Table 6.4 Sampling of the final rinse water for the total viable count (TVC) and suggested action plan

Aerobic colony count in 100 mL	Interpretation	Action
<1 cfu	Satisfactory	No action required
1–9 cfu on a regular basis	Acceptable: indicates that bacterial numbers are under a reasonable level of control	No action unless *Pseudomonas* spp. or *Mycobacteria* spp. Otherwise disinfect AER and repeat sampling
10–100 cfu	Unsatisfactory; investigate potential problems and super-chlorinate or repeat automatic endoscope reprocessor self-disinfect	Advise alcohol flush post rinsing for ERCP scopes, bronchoscopes and cystoscopes. Double strength disinfect machine and repeat sampling. If contamination continues—change bacterial filters, disinfect machine and resample. If problem remains contact manufacturer for advice
>100 cfu	Unacceptable: take automatic endoscope reprocessor out of service until water quality improved	Suspend ERCPs, cystoscopies, and bronchoscopies until situation resolved. Disinfect machine with double strength and repeat sampling. If contamination continues–change bacterial filters, disinfect machine and resample. If problem remains contact manufacturer for advice

cfu, colony forming unit.
Note: samples of rinse water are collected from all machines weekly (HTM 2030 Washer Disinfectors).
  Validation and verification states that there should be no organisms present in 100 mL of water.
Adapted with modification from Willis C. Bacteria-free endoscopy rinse water–a realistic aim? *Epidemiology and infection* 2005; **134**(2):279–84, and Department of Health. *Health Technical Memorandum 01–06: Decontamination of flexible endoscopes an automatic endoscope reprocessor*, London: Department of Health, 2010.

shed up to 210 particles while speaking, 3500 when coughing and 4500–1,000,000 particles when sneezing (Duguid, 1945). As a result, the health care environment is constantly contaminated by microorganisms from infected/colonized patients, staff, and visitors. The number and types of microorganisms present on environmental surfaces are determined by the number of people in the environment, and the amount of human activity and whether the surfaces are vertical or horizontal.

Current scientific evidence suggests that a contaminated environment plays an important role in the spread of microorganisms and if not cleaned/disinfected on a regular basis, may act as a reservoir for potential pathogens (Dancer, 2008; Weber et al., 2011). The transfer of microorganisms from patients to environmental surfaces and then back to patients can occur via contact with contaminated hands when hand hygiene is not performed and/or via contact of patients with environment, items, and equipment which has not be adequately clean and disinfected. Therefore, regular cleaning and disinfection of the environment is essential to reduce the bioburden of microorganisms to prevent cross-infection.

Survival of microorganisms

Survival of microorganisms in the environment depends on various factors, and survivals of various clinically relevant pathogens are outlined in Table 6.5. In general, dry and dusty conditions favour the persistence of Gram-positive cocci and bacterial spores (staphylococci, enterococci, *Clostridium difficile* spores, etc.) whereas moist, environments favour Gram-negative bacilli (Enterobacteriaceae, *Pseudomonas* spp., etc.). Fungi are also present on dust and proliferate in moist, fibrous material.

Table 6.5 Persistence of clinically relevant microorganisms on dry inanimate surfaces

Type of microorganisms	Duration of persistence	Type of microorganisms	Duration of persistence
Bacteria		**Viruses**	
Acinetobacter spp.	3 days to 5 months	Adenovirus	7 days–3 months
Bordetella pertussis	3–5 days	Astrovirus	7–90 days
Campylobacter jejuni	up to 6 days	Coronavirus	3 hours
Clostridium difficile (spores)	5 months	SARS-associated virus	72–96 hours
Chlamydia pneumoniae, C. trachomatis	≤30 hours	Coxsackie virus	>2 weeks
Chlamydia psittaci	15 days	Cytomegalovirus	8 hours
Corynebacterium diphtheriae	7 days–6 months	Echovirus	7 days
Corynebacterium pseudotuberculosis	1–8 days	Hepatitis A virus	2 hours–60 days
Escherichia coli	1.5 hours–16 months	Hepatitis B virus	>1 week
Enterococcus spp. including VRE and VSE	5 days–4 months	HIV	>7 days
Haemophilus influenzae	12 days	Herpes simplex virus, type 1 and 2	4.5 hours–8 weeks
Helicobacter pylori	≤90 minutes	Influenza virus	1–2 days
Klebsiella spp.	2 hours to >30 months	Norovirus and feline calici virus	8 hours–7 days
Listeria spp.	1 day–months	Papilloma virus 16	>7 days
Mycobacterium bovis	>2 months	Papovavirus	8 days

Table 6.5 (*continued*) Persistence of clinically relevant microorganisms on dry inanimate surfaces

Type of microorganisms	Duration of persistence	Type of microorganisms	Duration of persistence
Bacteria		**Viruses**	
Mycobacterium tuberculosis	1 day–4 months	Parvovirus	>1 year
Neisseria gonorrhoeae	1–3 days	Poliovirus type 1	4 hours–<8 days
Proteus vulgaris	1–2 days	Poliovirus type 2	1 day–8 weeks
Pseudomonas aeruginosa	6 hours–16 months	Pseudorabies virus	≥7 days
Salmonella typhi	6 hours–4 weeks	Respiratory syncytial virus	up to 6 hours
Salmonella typhimurium	10 days–4.2 years	Rhinovirus	2 hours–7 days
Salmonella spp.	1 day	Rotavirus	6–60 days
Serratia marcescens	3 days–2 months	Vaccinia virus	3 weeks–>20 weeks
Shigella spp.	2 days–5 months		
Staphylococcus aureus, including MRSA	7 days–7 months	**Yeasts**	
Streptococcus pneumoniae	1–20 days	*Candida albicans*	1–120 days
Streptococcus pyogenes	3 days–6.5 months	*Candida parapsilosis*	14 days
Vibrio cholerae	1–7 days	*Torulopsis glabrata*	102–150 days

With permission from Kramer A, Schwebke I, Kampf G. How long do nosocomial pathogens persist on the surfaces? A systematic review. *BMC Infectious Disease* 2006; **6**:130–8.

Frequency of cleaning

Housekeeping surfaces can be divided into two groups: 1) those surfaces which come into frequent contact with hands or '*hand touch surfaces*' (door handles, table tops, work surfaces, etc.), and 2) those surfaces that have minimal contact with hands (floors, walls, window sills, ceilings etc.). As a rule, '*hand touch surfaces*' must be cleaned and/or disinfected more frequently than surfaces that have minimal contact with hands. In addition to these factors, frequency of cleaning should take into account of the following factors:

- High risk units, ICU, NNU, Burns unit, etc.
- Potential of contamination of the surface with body and/or body fluids.
- Potential of contamination of environmental with dust, soil, and/or water.

The methods, frequency, and the products used are a matter for local policy. Guidance on the recommended frequency of cleaning is outlined in the *National Standards of Cleanliness for the NHS*, 2002 and *Revised Healthcare Cleaning Manual*, 2009. They are available from http://www.nrls.npsa.nhs.uk/resources.

Cleaning methods

Effective cleaning cannot be achieved by using water *alone*; it requires *detergents/surfactants*, and the physical action of scrubbing. Adding detergent aids cleaning because one end of the detergent molecule is hydrophilic and mixes well with water. The other end is hydrophobic and is attracted to non-polar organic molecules. If the detergents are electrically charged, they are called 'ionic detergents'. Anionic are negatively charged detergents and are only mildly bactericidal. They are used as laundry detergents to remove soil and debris but they also reduce the number of microorganisms associated with the item being washed. Cationics are positively charged detergents and are highly bactericidal.

Cleaning is *essential* as it removes organic matter, and visible soils, all of which interfere with microbial inactivation if chemical disinfectants are used. Warm water and detergent are sufficient for most purposes. In certain situation, after thorough cleaning of the environment use of disinfectants is also necessary as some pathogens (spores of *C. difficile*, MRSA, VRE, etc.) can survive in the environment for prolonged periods.

The following points should be taken into consideration when cleaning is undertaken:

♦ All personnel should be provided with and education and training so that they carry out their job effectively.

♦ They should wear appropriate PPE and follow local procedure and protocol.

♦ Cleaning must always be carried out from the cleanest and finish in the dirty area to prevent cross-contamination. The equipment used for the cleaning should be colour-coded accordingly.

♦ Special emphasis must be placed on cleaning and disinfecting contaminated surfaces which come into frequent contact with hands—'*hand touch surfaces*'—and these areas should be cleaned more frequently than surfaces with minimal hand contact.

♦ Damp dusting of horizontal surfaces should be done daily with cleaning cloths pre-moistened with water and detergent. Housekeeping surfaces require regular cleaning and removal of soil.

♦ Frequency of cleaning *must be increased* in an outbreak situation.

♦ Walls, blinds, and window curtains should be regularly cleaned to ensure that they are free from stains, splatters, dirt, or fungi.

♦ Dispersal of microorganisms in the air from the floor must be avoided. Dry sweeping with a broom should never be used as it disperses microorganisms from the floor into the air which will remain suspended for several minutes and contaminate the horizontal surfaces in the area.

♦ Room must be terminally cleaned when the patients are discharged (Box 6.4).

♦ Routine environmental swabbing to monitor the effectiveness of the cleaning process is *not* recommended.

Box 6.4 Procedure for terminal cleaning of a room

Terminal cleaning of a room should be done when a patient who has been under source isolation is discharged. Routine fumigation of the room is not necessary unless there is case of highly dangerous pathogens e.g. viral haemorrhagic fevers. Personnel should be trained to fulfil the standardized protocol. Cleaning should always be carried out from 'clean' to 'dirty' areas. Special emphasis must be placed on cleaning and disinfecting contaminated surfaces which come into frequent contact with hands. Environmental swabbing to monitor the effectiveness of the cleaning process is *not* recommended.

The following procedure should be followed:

◆ Domestic staff should wear appropriate PPE.

◆ Discard all disposable items or equipment into clinical waste bags which should be sealed *before* leaving the room.

◆ Remove any items or equipment to the dirty utility area for cleaning and disinfection.

◆ *Gently* place all linen into the appropriate laundry bags. Bags must be sealed *before* leaving the room or the area.

◆ Dust high ledges, window frames, and curtain tracks. If a vacuum cleaner is used then it must be fitted with HEPA air filters at the exhaust.

◆ Clean and disinfect all ledges, fixtures, and fittings, including taps and door handles.

◆ Wash sinks with warm water and detergent; hypochlorite/detergent cleanser may be used, if necessary. Rinse with water and dry thoroughly.

◆ Wash floors and spot clean walls with detergent solution. Rinse and dry thoroughly.

◆ The bed mattresses should be wiped with warm water and detergent, then disinfected with appropriate disinfectant (e.g. freshly prepared hypochlorite 1000 ppm av Cl_2) and then dried thoroughly.

◆ Open windows, if required, to facilitate thorough drying of all surfaces.

◆ The room may be re-used again by the next patient when all surfaces are dry.

Cleaning methods and equipment

It is essential that the chosen methods of cleaning produce minimal mists and aerosols or dispersion of dust in the patient-care areas. Bucket solutions become contaminated almost immediately during cleaning, and continued use of the solution transfers increasing numbers of microorganisms to each subsequent surface to be cleaned. Therefore it is essential that *fresh cleaning solution should be made daily* and any remaining solution discarded after use.

Another source of contamination in the cleaning process is the cleaning cloth or mop head, especially if left soaking in dirty cleaning solutions. Therefore it is essential that the detachable heads of used mops must be machine laundered, thermally disinfected, and dried daily. Mop buckets must be washed with detergent, rinsed, dried, and stored inverted when not in use. A simplified approach to cleaning involves replacing soiled cloths and mop heads with clean items each time a bucket of detergent is emptied and replaced with fresh, clean solution. If a scrubbing machine is used then the reservoir must be drained after use and stored dry. Colour-coded cleaning equipment should be used for each area, i.e. clinical, non-clinical, kitchen, and sanitary area according to the local policy.

Dry method

Dust-retaining materials, which are specially treated or manufactured to attract and retain dust particles, should be used as they remove more dust from dry surfaces. It represents a hygienic adaptation of the broom that it replaces and is ideal for avoiding the dispersion of contaminated dust in the environment.

A *microfibre cloth* (contains fibres smaller than 12 μm) can also be used for dry/dust mopping. When microfibre cloths are used for damp cleaning, *only clean water* should be used as addition of detergent is not necessary because grease and oil attach to the polymers of microfibre cloths. Therefore, these cloths are difficult to rinse out effectively and like conventional cleaning cloths, wet and dirty microfibre cloths provide an ideal growth medium for microorganisms. After use they must be washed.

Moist method

The *double bucket method* is the most commonly used method. One bucket is for clean water, to which a detergent and/or disinfectant solutions are added and the other bucket contains clean water for rinsing. This method helps minimize the recontamination of areas and is the preferred method of cleaning. When using the *single bucket method* the solution should be changed when it is dirty, even if cleaning of the area is not complete, and before moving to another area. Mop buckets should be emptied, and left upside down to drain and dry after each use. Mops should be disinfected in a thermal washing process once a day in high-risk areas and weekly in low-risk areas.

An alkaline detergent is recommended for daily cleaning of 'clean' and 'dirty' sanitary facilities. An acidic (descaling) agent is used to prevent and remove scale from washbasins, showers, bathtubs, and toilets.

Vacuum cleaner

There is the potential for vacuum cleaners to serve as dust dispersers if they are not operating properly. If a vacuum cleaner is used then it must be fitted with high-efficiency particulate (HEPA) air filters at the exhaust. Doors to patients' rooms should be closed when vacuuming areas where immunosuppressed patients are located. The collection bag of the vacuum cleaner may not be allowed to get too full. The vacuum cleaner (including the cord) must be cleaned every day if it is used daily. In addition, the dust filter in the exhaust opening must be checked. In the event of visible blocking (dusty layer on filters) it must be replaced and/or cleaned. Bacterial and fungal contamination of filters in cleaning equipment is inevitable, and these filters should be cleaned regularly or replaced according to the equipment manufacturer's recommendations.

Box 6.5 Methods to clean blood spills

Splashes and drips

- ◆ Wear non-sterile gloves for this procedure.
- ◆ Wipe the area immediately with a paper towel soaked in sodium hypochlorite (bleach) solution; alternatively a disposable alcohol wipe can be used.
- ◆ Clean the area with water and detergent.
- ◆ Dry the surface with disposable paper towels.
- ◆ Discard gloves and paper towels as clinical waste according to local policy.
- ◆ Wash hands with soap and water and dry hands immediately.

Larger spills

- ◆ Sprinkle the spill with NaDCC (a solid form of hypochlorite) granules until the fluid is absorbed (if the quantity is small i.e. ≤30 mL). Leave the spill for a contact period of about 3–5 min to allow for disinfection.
- ◆ Depending on the method used, either scoop up the absorbed granules or lift the soiled paper towels and discard into a yellow plastic waste bag as clinical waste.
- ◆ Wipe the surface area with fresh hypochlorite 1000 ppm av Cl_2 solution and rinse with clean water as the hypochlorite solution may be corrosive.
- ◆ Dry the surface with disposable paper towels.
- ◆ Remove gloves and plastic apron and discard as clinical waste according to local policy.
- ◆ Wash hands with soap and water and dry hands immediately.

Management of infectious spills

Spills of blood and high-risk body fluids should be removed as soon as possible and the area washed with detergent/disinfectant and dried as a part of good infection control practice (see Box 6.5).

Health care facilities should have written protocols in place for dealing with blood and body substance spills. It is not necessary to use hypochlorite solution (bleach) for managing 'low-risk' body fluids but it may be used if the circumstances indicate that it is necessary.

Key references and further reading

Bradley C. Physical and chemical disinfection. In: Fraise AP, Bradley C (eds). *Ayliffe's Control of Healthcare-associated Infection*, 3rd edn, pp.88–106. London: Hodder Arnold, 2009.

Canadian Guidelines. *Infection prevention and control guideline for Flexible Gastrointestinal Endoscopy and Flexible Bronchoscopy*. Public Health Agency of Canada, 2010. Available at: http://www.phac-aspc.gc.ca.

CDC and HICPAC Guidelines. Guidelines for Environmental Infection Control in Health Care Facilities. *Morbidity and Mortality Weekly Reports* 2003; **52** (RR10):1–42. 'Errata: Vol. 52 (No. RR10)' (Morbidity and Mortality Weekly Reports Vol. 52 [42]: 1025–6) on 24 October 2003 and as a 'Notice to Readers' scheduled to appear in December 2003).

CDC. *Guideline for Disinfection and Sterilization in Healthcare Facilities, 2008*. Atlanta, GA: CDC, 2008.

Dancer SJ. Importance of the environment in meticillin-resistant *Staphylococcus aureus* acquisition: the case for hospital cleaning. *Lancet Infectious Disease* 2008; **8**:101–13.

Department of Health. *Health Technical UK Memorandum 01–06: Decontamination of flexible endoscopes an automatic endoscope reprocessor*. London: Department of Health, 2010.

Duguid JP. The numbers and the sites of origin of the droplets expelled during expiratory activities. *Edinburgh Medical Journal*. 1945; **52**:385–401.

Fraise A, Bradley C. Decontamination of equipment, the environment and the skin. In: Fraise AP, Bradley C (eds). *Ayliffe's Control of Healthcare-associated Infection*, 3rd edn, pp.107–49. London: Hodder Arnold, 2009.

Hoffman P, Bradley C, Ayliffe GAJ. *Disinfection in Healthcare*. 3rd edn. Oxford: Blackwell Publishing, 2005.

Kramer A, Schwebke I, Kampf G. How long do nosocomial pathogens persist on the surfaces? A systematic review. *BMC Infectious Disease* 2006; **6**:130–8.

Medical Devices Agency. *Device bulletin: The purchase, operation and maintenance of benchtop steam sterilizers*. (MDA DB 9605). London: Medical Devices Agency, 1996.

Medical Devices Agency. *Device bulletin: The validation and periodic testing of benchtop vacuum steam sterilizers*. (MDA DB 9804). London: Medical Devices Agency, 1998.

Multisociety Guidelines on Reprocessing Flexible GI endoscopes. Infection Control and Hospital Epidemiology 2011; **32**(6):527–537.

National Patient Safety Agency. *UK National Standards of Cleanliness for the NHS, 2002 and Revised Healthcare Cleaning Manual*. London: NPSA, 2009. Available at: http://www.nrls.npsa.nhs.uk/resources.

Pan American Health Organization. *Sterilization manual for health centres*. Washington, DC: Pan American Health Organization, 2009.

Rutala WA, Weber DJ. How to assess risk of disease transmission to patients when there Is a failure to follow recommended disinfection and sterilization guidelines. *Infection Control Hospital Epidemiology* 2007; **28**(2):146–55.

Spaulding EH. Chemical disinfection of medical and surgical materials. In: Lawrence CA, Block SS (eds) *Disinfection, Sterilization and Preservation*, pp.517–31. Philadelphia, PA: Lea & Febiger, 1968.

Weber DJ, Rutala WA. The role of the environment in transmission of *Clostridium difficile* infection in healthcare facilities. *Infection Control and Hospital Epidemiology* 2011; **32**(3):207–9.

WHO. *Essential Environmental health Standards in Health Care*. Geneva: World Health Organization, 2009.

Willis C. Bacteria-free endoscopy rinse water–a realistic aim? *Epidemiology and infection* 2005; **134**(2):279–84.

Appendix 6.1 Disinfection procedures for individual items and equipment

Items/equipment	Method
Airways and laryngeal mask	Use single-use or heat disinfect in SSD.
Ampoules/vials	Wipe neck or rubber top with 70% isopropyl alcohol and allow to dry before opening or piercing. *Do not* immerse ampoules/vials in disinfectant solution.
Auroscope tip	Use single-use disposable tips. If reusable tips are used then send to SSD for sterilization. Chemical disinfectant should be used only when other methods are unavailable.
Babies' feeding bottles and teats	Teats and bottles must be cleaned and disinfected using heat treatment. Chemical disinfectant should be used only when other methods are unavailable in which case *wash thoroughly, rinse* and place in freshly prepared hypochlorite (125 ppm av Cl_2) solution for 30 min.
Baths/showers/shower chairs	Wash surfaces with detergent solutions and allow to dry. If disinfection is required, *non-abrasive* hypochlorite/detergent cream can be used. Seat pads are not recommended but if used they should be discarded after each patient use.
Bedpans and urinals	*Non-disposable*: reusable items must be heat disinfected in a washer/disinfector (80°C for 1 min). All bedpans and urinals must be stored dry on a rack, inverted and tilted forward to avoid trapping water. If this facility is not available, after thoroughly cleaning with detergent, disinfect with hypochlorite (1000 ppm av Cl_2) solution. Bedpan washer machine, bedpan holders, and storage racks/shelves must be cleaned with detergent on a daily basis. *Disposable*: use single-use disposable items and dispose of into a macerator unit. Carriers used with disposable bedpans should be washed in bedpan washer or cleaned after each use with detergent and water, rinsed, and stored inverted on a rack.
Beds and bed frames	For normal daily cleaning use detergent and hot water and allow to dry. Perform thorough cleaning *after discharge* of each patient. *Colonized/infected patients*. After cleaning with detergent, disinfect with hypochlorite 1000 ppm av Cl_2 solution.
Birthing pools	Use a single-use disposable pool liner. Discard pool liner and then thoroughly clean and disinfect (pay particular attention to the outlet) with hypochlorite (1000ppm av Cl_2).
Bowls (vomit)	Empty and rinse. Wash with detergent and hot water, rinse, and dry.
Bowls (washing)	Individual wash bowls should be available for each patient. After each use, wash with detergent and rinse. Keep dry by storing inverted and tilted forward to avoid trapping water. *Colonized/infected patients*. Heat disinfect in a washer/disinfector (80°C for 1 min). Keep dry by storing inverted and tilted forward to avoid trapping water.

Items/equipment	Method
Breast pumps	This must be for single patient use only. Wash with detergent and water and then rinse. Immerse in hypochlorite (125 ppm av Cl$_2$) solution for 30 min. Heat sterilize before use by other subsequent patients.
Cardiac and urinary catheters, intravascular devices, and all other invasive devices, i.e. needles, syringes	Use sterile single-use disposable item only.
Cardiac monitors, defibrillators, and ECG equipment	Use single-use disposable ECG pads. Clean and disinfect ECG leads and machine as per manufacturer's recommendations.
Carpets	Clean daily using vacuum cleaner with high efficiency filter on exhaust to minimize dispersal of microorganisms in the environment. They should also be cleaned using hot water extraction methods. For known contaminated spillage, clean with detergent and disinfect with chemical agent which does not damage carpet.
Cheatle forceps	Do not use. If used then autoclave daily and store in a clean container.
Cleaning equipment	*Mops:* the detachable heads of used mops must be thermally disinfected in a laundry machine or chemically disinfected and dried daily. *Mop bucket:* wash with detergent, rinse, dry, and store inverted when not in use. *Scrubbing machine:* drain reservoir after use and store dry. Colour coded cleaning equipment should be used for each area, i.e. clinical, non-clinical, kitchen and sanitary area according to the local policy.
Commodes	After each use, clean with detergent and disinfect using hypochlorite (1000ppm av Cl$_2$) solution; pay particular attention to the outlet. If faecal contamination has occurred, remove soil with tissue and wash with detergent and hot water and then disinfect using hypochlorite (1000ppm av Cl$_2$) solution. Pay particular attention to under the arms.
Cots	Routinely wash with detergent and dry with disposable wipe on a daily basis. *Colonized/infected patients*: After cleaning, disinfect with 70% isopropyl alcohol impregnated wipe or use hypochlorite (125 ppm av Cl$_2$) solution. *Do not* use phenolic disinfectants on infant cots, prams, or incubators as residual fumes may cause respiratory irritation.
Crockery and cutlery	Machine wash with rinse temperature above 80°C and dry or hand wash in detergent and hot water (approx. 60°C), rinse and allow to dry thoroughly. Patients who are infected with enteric pathogens and patients with open pulmonary tuberculosis, heat disinfect. If this is not possible consider use of single-use disposable items.

Items/equipment	Method
Curtains	Routinely launder curtains as per local proceudres; 2–3 times per year is considered sufficient. If soiled, send to the hospital laundry or use a washing machine which reaches thermal disinfection temperature.
	Colonized/infected patients: send to the hospital laundry or use a washing machine which reaches thermal disinfection temperature when the patient is discharged.
	Disposable curtains are available and should be considered for use only for infected patients or if you are unable to thermal disinfect.
Drains	Smelly drains require cleaning; contact your estates department.
Drip stands	Clean with detergent after each use.
Duvets	Cover duvets with water-impermeable cover and wash cover with detergent solution, and allow to dry. Launder to thermal disinfection temperatures after each patient use, weekly or if visibly soiled.
Endoscopes—invasive	Heat sterilize *only* if the endoscopes are heat tolerant. Heat sensitive endoscopes must be disinfected using a compatible high level chemical disinfectant (see 'Decontamination of endoscopes'). Endoscopy accessories which are used for invasive procedures *must be sterile* after each use; alternatively single-use accessories may be used.
Endoscopes—non-invasive	Heat-sensitive endoscopes must be disinfected using a compatible high-level disinfectant.
Endotracheal tubes	Use single-use or heat sterilize in SSD.
Fixtures, fittings and ledges	In clinical areas damp dust daily with detergent solution and dry. Pay particular attention to surfaces which are in frequent contact with hands to reduce bioload.
	Colonized/infected patients: after cleaning with detergent, disinfect with hypochlorite 1000 ppm av Cl_2 solution or other appropriate disinfectant and allow to dry.
Floors	*Dry cleaning*: use vacuum cleaner which is fitted only with high-efficiency filter on exhaust or use a dust-attracting dry mop. *Never* use brooms in clinical areas.
	Wet cleaning: wash with a detergent solution. Disinfection is *not* routinely required unless spillage of blood or body fluids occurs.
Furniture	*Non-fabric furniture:* routinely clean with detergent solution.
	Fabric furniture: use vacuum cleaner which is fitted only with high efficiency filter on exhaust.
Haemodialysis machines	Thoroughly clean between patients and disinfect at the end of the day per manufacturer's recommendations.
	Colonized/infected patients: after cleaning with detergent, disinfect with hypochlorite (1000 ppm av Cl_2) solution or other appropriate disinfectant as per manufacturer's recommendations.

Items/equipment	Method
Hoist/sling	Clean surfaces of the hoist with detergent solution. Wash sling with detergent, rinse and dry. Examine material for wear or damage before each use.
	Colonized/infected patients: use single-patient use sling and thermal disinfect using machine wash or use chemical disinfection which is compatible with the material as per manufacturer's recommendations.
Humidifiers	Clean and sterilize humidifiers between patients. Fill with sterile water, and change every 24 h or sooner, if necessary.
	Single-use humidifiers are available but they are expensive.
Hydrotherapy pools	Drain and clean regularly as part of routine maintenance. Maintain disinfectant levels in water as per recommended guidelines. Routine microbiological monitoring of water is recommended.
Infant incubators	Routinely wash with detergent and dry with disposable wipe on a daily basis.
	Colonized/infected patients: after cleaning, wipe with 70% isopropyl alcohol impregnated wipe or use hypochlorite (125 ppm av Cl_2) solution.
	When the baby is discharged, dismantle incubator and wash *all removable parts* and clean with detergent and then disinfect with hypochlorite (125 ppm av Cl_2) solution or other disinfectant as per manufacturer's recommendation and allow to dry. The cleaning and disinfection should be done in a separate area.
Laryngoscope blade	Clean the blade thoroughly with detergent and hot water. Dry thoroughly and wipe with a 70% alcohol impregnated wipe.
	Colonized/infected patients: in cases of suspected/confirmed infection or visible blood, the blade should be sent to SSD for sterilization before further use.
Locker tops	Damp dust daily with detergent solution and allow to dry.
	Colonized/infected patients: after cleaning with detergent, disinfect with hypochlorite (1000 ppm av Cl_2) solution or other appropriate disinfectant allow to dry.
Mattresses and pillows	Mattresses and pillows should be protected by a waterproof cover which should be routinely cleaned, disinfected, and dried. They must be inspected for damage and *replaced immediately*, if necessary.
	Contaminated mattresses and pillows can be disinfected with hypochlorite 1000 ppm av Cl_2 solution. Use of unnecessary and excessive disinfection damages the mattress and pillow covers and reduces life. Seek advice from manufacturer. Check the mattress regularly for signs of damage.
Mops	See *Cleaning equipment*.

Items/equipment	Method
Nail brushes (for surgical scrub only)	Do not use routinely; instead use a manicure stick to clean the nails before surgical scrub. To prevent skin damage, *never* use a nail brush to scrub skin. Use a sterile, pre-packed, single-use brush or send to SSD after each use for sterilization. *Do not* soak nail brush in a disinfectant solution as a method of 'sterilization'.
Nebulizers	Clean and sterilize nebulizers between patients or use high-level disinfection. Fill with sterile water only.
	Single-use disposable nebulizers are available but they are expensive.
Neurological test pins	Single-use only.
Oxygen tents	Wash with hot water detergent solution, rinse well and dry thoroughly. Store covered with clean plastic sheeting in a clean area.
Peak flow meters	Each patient should be supplied their own peak flow meter. They are not recommended for routine multi-patient use. Peak-flow meters with one-way valves can be used with bacterial/viral filter with 99.9% efficacy and can be used for 'one off' reading. Follow manufacture's recommendations regarding its use and decontamination methods.
Pillows	See *Mattresses and pillows*.
Razors	Avoid preoperative shaving if possible (see 'Preoperative patient care', Chapter 15). For clinical shaving use clipper.
	Safety razors: use disposable or autoclave razors with single-use disposable heads.
	Electric razors: detach head, clean thoroughly, and immerse in 70% isopropyl alcohol for 10 min, remove and allow to dry between each patient.
Rooms	Wash surfaces with detergent solution and allow to dry.
	Colonized/infected patients: After cleaning with detergent, disinfect with hypochlorite 1000 ppm av Cl_2 solution or other appropriate disinfectant and allow to dry.
Scissors	Surface disinfect with a 70% alcohol impregnated wipe before use. If visibly soiled clean first with a detergent solution.
Shaving brushes	*Do not* use for clinical shaving. Patients may use their own brush for face shaves; it should be rinsed under running water and stored dry.
Sphygmomanometer cuffs	Use dedicated item in high-risk areas (e.g. ICU) or on patients known to be *colonized/infected*. Wash sleeve and disinfect with 70% alcohol impregnated wipe to clean tubing and inflation bladder.
Splints and walking frames	Wash and clean with detergent and allow to dry.

Items/equipment	Method
Stethoscope	Surface disinfect with 70% alcohol impregnated wipe between patients. Use dedicated stethoscope in high-risk area e.g. ICU, NNU or patients with infection or colonized with MDROs.
Suction bottle/ equipment	Use single-use disposable, if possible. The suction catheters should be single use. *Non-disposable bottles:* wear a plastic apron and non-sterile disposable gloves for this procedure. Following use, the botttle should be emptied into the sluice hopper. Wash non-disposable bottles with detergent and allow to dry or heat disinfect in washing machine or send to SSD.
Surgical instruments	Transport safely in a closed rigid container to SSD for sterilization. Clean manually or use thermal washer-disinfector and then steam sterilize all instruments in SSD.
Surgical instruments	Steam sterilize if heat tolerant. Single use items may be used.
Thermometers	*Oral: single-patient use thermometers* must be dedicated for infected patients and patients in high-risk areas, e.g. ICU. They should be cleaned and wiped with a 70% isopropyl alcohol impregnated wipe after each use and stored dry. On discharge of patient, wash both thermometer and thermometer holder with detergent, immerse in 70% alcohol for 10 min. Wipe and store dry. *Communal thermometers:* wipe clean, wash in a cold neutral detergent, rinse, dry and immerse in 70% isopropyl alcohol for 10 min. Wipe and store dry. *Rectal:* clean and wash in detergent solution after each use, wipe dry and immerse in 70% alcohol for 10 min. Wipe and store dry. *Electronic:* where possible use a single-use sleeve. If not possible, use either single-use thermometer or clean and disinfect between use. Do not use without sleeve or on patients with an infectious disease. Single-use sleeve, single-patient use in high-risk areas or infected patient. Clean, then wipe with a 70% isopropyl alcohol impregnated wipe after each use. *Tympanic:* single-use sleeve.
Toilet seats and flush handle	Wash with detergent and disinfect with hypochlorite 1000 ppm av Cl_2 solution. Frequency of cleaning should be according to the local protocol. Increased frequency of cleaning is essential in an outbreak situation (especially of gastroenteritis) and in an area where soiling is more likely e.g. gynaecology, maternity, urology department.
Tonometer prisms	Use single-use or clean and disinfect with hypochlorite (500 ppm av Cl_2) solution for 10 min. Rinse thoroughly and dry.

Items/equipment	Method
Toys	*Soft toys:* avoid use of soft toys as they are difficult to disinfect. Individual toys for patients can be machine washed and dried using a tumble dryer. Heavily contaminated soft toys may have to be destroyed. Do not soak toys in a disinfectant solution.
	Hard toys: wash with detergent and disinfect with an alcohol impregnated wipe or use hypochlorite (1000 ppm av Cl$_2$) solution. For children with infectious diseases do not use communal toys or those which cannot easily be disinfected.
Trolleys	Clean and wipe trolley tops with a 70% isopropyl alcohol impregnated wipe before use. If contaminated, clean with detergent and then disinfect with a 70% isopropyl alcohol impregnated wipe and dry.
Ultrasound	Damp dust with detergent solution and allow surface to dry before use. Draw up local protocol for cleaning and disinfection based on the manufacturer's recommendations.
Urinals	See *Bedpans and urinals.*
Vaginal speculae	Send to SSD for sterilization or use single-use.
Ventilator breathing circuits	Use single-use or heat disinfect/sterilize in SSD.
	Infected patients: for patients with respiratory infection and other serious infection use disposable tubing. *Never* use glutaraldehyde to disinfect respiratory equipment.
Ventilators	After every patient, clean and disinfect ventilators. Dismantle and sterilize/disinfect (high-level) all re-usable components as per the manufacturer's recommendations.
Wash-hand basin	Routinely clean with detergent to remove stains, scum, etc. If disinfection is required *non-abrasive* hypochlorite/detergent cream can be used.
Wheel chairs	Clean with detergent, rinse and dry.
X-ray equipment	Damp dust with detergent solution and allow surface to dry before use. Draw up local protocol for cleaning and disinfection based on the manufacturer's recommendations.

Chapter 7

Isolation precautions

> ... by forseeing in a distance, which is only done by
> men of talents, the evils which arise from them are soon
> cured; but when, from want of foresight, they are suffered
> to increase to such a height that they are perceptible to
> everyone, there is no remedy.
>
> *Niccolò Machiavelli*

The separation of infected people in order to prevent the spread of infectious diseases is not new and is mentioned in the Bible (Leviticus chapter 13) in the Old Testament. However, the word 'quarantine' originated when bubonic plague struck Venice in 1403. In order to protect its population, it was decided that no one could enter the city until a waiting period ('quarantine') of 40 days had passed; 'quarantine' originates from the Italian word *quaranta*.

The advent of the HIV/AIDS epidemic by the mid 1980s created a panic both amongst the general public and HCWs. In response, the term 'universal precautions' for blood and body fluid was introduced by the US CDC for all patients. This term was ambiguous, leading to universal confusion in its interpretation. As a result, inappropriate use of gloves increased substantially and has contributed to a rise in the incidence of latex allergy amongst HCWs. In addition, once the HCWs wore gloves, they thought they were 'protected' and could provide a substitute for hand hygiene. Failure to decontaminate hands after removing gloves is not uncommon and has probably contributed to an increase in the transmission of multiresistant microorganisms in health care facilities.

The term 'universal precautions' has now been abandoned by the CDC and has been replaced by 'standard precautions' in the isolation guidelines and these precautions should be part of the routine care of all patients irrespective of their infectious status (CDC/HICPAC guidelines 2007). Instead of 'standard precautions', some countries have adopted the term 'routine precautions', or 'basic precautions' but for the purpose of this chapter the term 'standard precautions' will be used. The rationale for implementing standard precautions for the care of *all patients* at *all times* is as follows:

1. Patients may be infectious but show no signs or symptoms of infection at the time of admission as s/he may be incubating the infectious disease.

2. S/he may not show signs or symptoms of infection as the patient may be an *asymptomatic carrier* (e.g. hepatitis B and C, *Salmonella typhi*) or *colonized* with multiresistant microorganisms (e.g. MRSA, ESBL, or VRE).

3. Infectious status is often determined by laboratory tests that cannot be completed in time to provide emergency care due to lack of laboratory facilities, and/or appropriate tests are not requested due to lack of proper history taking which fails to raise the suspicion of possible infective causes.

In addition to the application of standard precautions, HCWs should be immunized against vaccine-preventable diseases both for their own protection and the protection of others. It is the responsibility of employers to ensure that there is adequate provision of hand-hygiene facilities and availability of PPE. All HCWs must be given adequate education and *practical training* in IPC. The education programme should be part of an induction programme and cover all staff and should be regularly updated in view of changing knowledge and work practices.

Risk assessment

Whenever isolation of a patient is considered, assessment of risk should be carried out and the disadvantages must be weighed against the benefits. The placement of a patient into isolation should never be undertaken as a matter of convenience. The patient's underlying condition is the driver for determining the provision of care and where it should be delivered. Isolation of patients may not only have a psychological impact on the patient, but putting a patient in an isolation ward may also have an adverse influence on the quality of care by distancing the patient from specialist care. In addition, in certain cultures and religions, the concepts of pestilence and contagion are still inextricably intertwined with beliefs that such diseases are divine punishments for sinners and for those who live dissolute lives. Therefore, it is essential that the need to continue isolation should be reviewed on a daily basis.

Types of isolation

Isolation procedures can be divided into two main categories, i.e. source isolation and protective isolation. Please refer to Chapter 19 for discussion of requirements for building source and protective isolation rooms.

Source isolation

The aim of source isolation is to prevent exogenous infections, i.e. the transfer of microorganisms from an infected/colonized patient to other staff, patients, and visitors (see 'Chain of infection', Chapter 1). The two-tier approach is recommended— the first tier is application of *standard precautions* for all patients regardless of their infectious status and the second tier or *additional precautions* are transmission-based measures that are applied for patients who are known/suspected to have communicable disease or infected and/or colonized with multi-resistant microorganisms. Table 7.1 summarizes the infection control precautions for various categories based on transmission modes. It is important to remember that some microorganisms may have more than one mode of transmission. The duration of isolation precautions along with additional measures for various infectious conditions and incubation periods of various infectious diseases are summarized in Appendix 7.1 and Appendix 7.2 respectively.

Table 7.1 Summary of infection control precautions for various categories

Activity	Standard precautions	Contact transmission	Droplet transmission	Airborne transmission
Isolation room	Single room not required	Single room and minimize time outside	Single room, minimize time outside when patient may wear mask	Single room with negative pressure ventilation,* minimize time outside when patient may wear mask. Exclude non- essential susceptible people
Hand hygiene	Yes	Yes	Yes	Yes
Gloves	When likely to touch blood, body fluids and contaminated items	Wear gloves on entering room to provide patient care and when likely to touch blood, body fluids and contaminated items	As per *Standard precautions*	As per *Standard precautions*
Apron/gown	If soiling likely, i.e. during procedures likely to generate contamination from blood and body fluids	Wear it on entering room if clothing will have substantial contact with the patient, environmental surfaces or items in the patient's room	As per *Standard precautions*	As per *Standard precautions*
Mask	Wear regular mask during procedures likely to generate contamination with aerosols**	As per *Standard precautions*	As per *Standard precautions*	Wear high efficiency filtration mask (FFP3 or N95) on entering the room (see 'Respirators', Chapter 9)
Eye protection/ face-shields	During procedures likely to generate contamination with blood and body fluids	As per *Standard precautions*	As per *Standard precautions*	As per *Standard precautions* Non-essential susceptible people should be excluded

Equipment decontamination	Yes	Yes	Yes	Yes
Environment cleaning	Yes	Yes	Yes	Yes
Miscellaneous	Avoid contaminating environmental surfaces with gloves	Remove gloves and gown, wash hands before leaving patient's room	Provide at least 1 metre of separation between patients in cohort	Advise patient to cover nose and mouth when coughing or sneezing

*Keep room vacant for 1 h post-discharge of patient and 2–3 h for measles.

**Only for situations that may provoke contamination of mucous membrane. Procedures that are likely to create significant aerosols; suctioning, dentistry, intubation, chest physiotherapy, etc.

Protective isolation

The aim of *protective isolation* is the reverse of source isolation, i.e. to prevent transfer of infection from personnel and the inanimate environment (exogenous source) to immunosuppressed patients. It is important to note that immunosuppressed patients are also at increased risk of *endogenous infections* (see 'Chain of infection', Chapter 1) where the most common source of infection is their *own gut flora* which is damaged by chemotherapy. Isolation in a single room is not required unless these patients are profoundly immunosuppressed, e.g. patients receiving chemotherapy and/or radiotherapy as part of cancer treatment or on immunosuppressive agents for transplant patients to prevent rejection of donor organs. The patients who are at *greatest risk* are the individuals who are severely neutropenic (i.e. <1000 polymorphonuclear cells/mL for 2 weeks or <100 polymorphonuclear cells/mL for 1 week), patients undergoing any transplantation, and those who have received intensive chemotherapy. These patients are also susceptible to environmental contaminants, such as aspergillosis or Legionnaires' disease (see Chapter 11). A specialized room with positive pressure ventilation and high efficiency particulate air filtration is required (see 'Protective isolation room', Chapter 19).

In addition to the above precautions, the following precautions should be implemented when dealing with immunocompromised patients:

- In an outpatient waiting room, additional precautions for the control of airborne transmission of disease may be required. These patients should be seen ahead of others in the waiting room to minimize the time they are exposed to other patients in the waiting area.

- Where invasive medical or dental procedures are involved, it would be reasonable to place immunocompromised patients at the start of the operating schedule, if possible.

Practical issues and considerations

Isolation and management of infected patients

Accident and emergency

The initial point of contact between a hospital and the infectious patient may be the A&E department. There is a greater risk of transfer of microorganisms in A&E as they are often crowded and patients may have to wait for prolonged periods in a communal waiting area with other patients, thus increasing the risk of transmission of infections. This risk *must* be minimized by establishing a fast track or triage system for potentially infectious patients with early isolation in a single room with en suite toilet and implementation of appropriate infection control precautions until they are transferred to other wards or departments.

Admissions policy

An admissions policy and procedure to deal with potentially infectious patients, interhospital transfers, and patients from overseas should be drawn up to reduce the risk of not only infectious diseases but to reduce the risk of transmission of multiresistant pathogens.

The admissions policy should include direct admission of patients to a single room with suspected/proven infection or patients with multi-resistant microorganisms.

Patient placement and cohorting

All patients with suspected/proven infection must be isolated in a single room, preferably with en suite toilet facilities, and this must be done at the time of admission. However, if the facilities are available, then certain types of patients (e.g. open case of pulmonary tuberculosis) should be nursed in a negative pressure ventilation room to protect other patient, staff, and visitors. The aim of positive pressure ventilation is to *protect the patient* and only severely immunosuppressed patients should be nursed in these rooms (see 'Protective isolation room', Chapter 19) (see Figure 7.1).

It is essential that, for patients who are nursed in a single room/cohorted, staff should ensure that visitors and other staff are made aware of the infection risk and precautions to take to prevent cross-infection. Doors should be kept closed at all times. The number of personnel who have contact with the patient (which includes both visitors and HCWs) *must* be kept to absolute minimum. If possible, consideration should be given that only HCWs who are immune to the infectious disease either through vaccination or exposure to the disease should provide care to the patient.

A suitable door sign must be placed on the entrance door to alert both staff and visitors. The sign should be prominently displayed, providing sufficient information whilst ensuring that there is *no breach of confidentiality*. Some health care facilities prefer to use door signs which specify the type of isolation precautions and this can be used according to local policy but care must be taken not to stigmatize the patient in isolation.

If the hospital lacks single rooms for isolation of patients, it is essential that they have a written guideline which outlines the priorities for isolation of patients based on local epidemiology and the risk assessment.

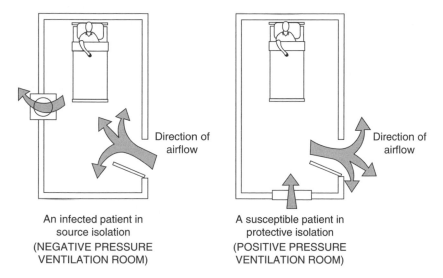

Direction of airflow	Direction of airflow
An infected patient in source isolation (NEGATIVE PRESSURE VENTILATION ROOM)	A susceptible patient in protective isolation (POSITIVE PRESSURE VENTILATION ROOM)

Fig. 7.1 Rooms showing isolation of patients in negative (source isolation) and positive (protective isolation) pressure ventilation rooms.

In an outbreak situation, when single rooms for isolation are not available, patients who have active infection and/or colonization with the same microorganism can be *cohorted* in a designated ward. If there is no dedicated ward, consider cohorting patients into bays within a ward. The dedicated rooms, bays, and areas used for isolated patients must have dedicated hand hygiene and toilet facilities. For effective isolation, bays should have doors that can be closed to provide physical separation from other patients. When a side room or cohorting is not possible, maintain a spatial separation of at least 1 metre (3 feet) between the infected patient and other patients and visitors. Fans should not be used to control the patient's temperature and the patient's notes and charts should be kept outside the room/bay/area. It is important that cohort patients should be cared for *only* by designated staff and 'top-up' training can be provided to ensure that staff adhere to the infection control precautions.

Patients with highly transmissible and dangerous infections, (e.g. viral haemorrhagic fevers) must be admitted or transferred to a local Infectious Diseases Unit under strict isolation precautions. Certain categories of patients require negative pressure ventilation (e.g. patients with M/XDR tuberculosis) should be nursed in negative pressure ventilation in relation to the surrounding areas. Mechanically ventilated rooms should achieve 6–12 exchanges of air per hour and there should be adequate temperature and humidity regulation, such that windows need not be opened and doors can be kept closed when the rooms are in use. No recirculation of air should be permitted for respiratory isolation rooms. The exhaust air from isolation rooms should be vented to the exterior (see 'Isolation rooms', Chapter 19).

Notification

It is the responsibility of the clinical team to notify the IPC team and other appropriate local officers (e.g. CCDC in the UK). Notification should be made on clinical suspicion of the disease, it is not necessary to wait for laboratory confirmation of the infection. Depending on the type of infection, initial notification should be made by telephone to initiate the proper follow-up process as soon as possible. Please refer to local policy for a list of notifiable diseases.

The patient's medical notes should be suitably tagged with appropriate stickers and flagged on the hospital's computer so that they can be easily identified on their next admission. The top 'Alert' sticker should be put on the front and the second sticker indicating the microorganism should be put on the inside of the patient's notes to protect the patient's confidentiality.

Collection and transport of pathology specimens

Collection, labelling, and transportation of laboratory specimens from patients in isolation rooms should follow written policies that reflect national guidelines. The specimens should be taken before starting antimicrobial therapy. Laboratory specimens must be correctly labelled and packaged, i.e. the request form must be kept separate from the specimen in a self-sealing plastic bag. Specimens must be handled carefully, ensuring that the outside of the container is not contaminated. Specimens from a patient with known or suspected infectious disease should have a 'Danger of Infection – Take special care' label both on the request form and on the specimen.

Specimens from highly dangerous and fatal infectious diseases must *not* be sent to the laboratory without prior arrangement with laboratory staff.

When a specimen pneumatic tube system exists, this should only be used after appropriate consideration of the risks. Porters and others who transport specimens must be aware of the procedures for transportation and follow appropriate procedures in the event of spillage or breakage of specimen containers. Up-to-date standard operating procedures should be available for all these processes.

Commercial containers are available for safe transportation of specimens. Transportation of infectious material from one laboratory to another should follow local guidelines. International and national transport of infectious material by post, road, rail, and air is subject to strict controls and must follow the most up-to-date guidelines.

Movement of patient

Once admitted, every effort should be made to limit the movement of infectious patients unless it is necessary for clinical reasons only. If transport or movement is necessary, minimize patient dispersal of droplet nuclei by placing a surgical mask on the patient if possible. The receiving area/ward must be informed so that appropriate infection control measures can be put into place on arrival. If the patient is transported out of the room, ensure that precautions are maintained to minimize the risk of transmission of microorganisms to other patients or environments.

Ward rounds

It is essential that senior medical staff act as role models for good infection control practice. During the ward round they must observe all the necessary infection control precautions, wear appropriate PPE, and *must* disinfect before and after touching patients, after touching the environment, and after contact with blood/body fluids.

During ward rounds, the number of staff visiting the patient in source isolation must be kept to an absolute minimum and, if possible, the infected patients should be visited *last*, after dealing with all non-infected patients. The patient in isolation must have dedicated items (stethoscope, etc.) and medical notes and x-rays must not be brought into the isolation room; other charts must be kept outside the isolation room.

Infection control precautions

Hand hygiene

Hand hygiene is absolutely essential to reduce the risk of cross-infection (refer to Chapter 8 for details). For visibly clean hands, alcoholic hand rub should be used to disinfect hands. Wash hands with soap and water if the hands are soiled or for patients with diarrhoeal diseases. Hands *must* be disinfected after removing gloves.

Personal protective equipment

Based on the risk assessment appropriate PPE must be worn. Refer to Chapter 9 for details.

Gloves: wear clean, non-sterile disposable gloves for procedures that may involve contact with blood or body fluids, secretions, excretions, or non-intact skin or mucous membranes. They should be *changed between tasks* and procedures undertaken on the *same patient* to prevent transfer of microorganisms between body sites. A separate pair of gloves should be used for the next patient. Remove gloves promptly after use and wash hands with soap and water or disinfect visibly clean hands with an alcoholic hand rub *immediately* after removing gloves.

Masks and eye protection: masks and eye protection help to guard the mucous membranes of the eyes, nose, and mouth from exposure to blood or body fluids that may be splashed, sprayed, or splattered into the face. Wear such protective gear if splashing of blood or high-risk body fluid is anticipated. Eye protection may be in the form of a mask with attached visor or protective spectacles. In the case of cross-contamination, it may be appropriate to wear a full-face visor. Masks are single-use items and should be disposed of as clinical waste.

Plastic aprons and gowns: the decision of whether an apron or gown is more appropriate will depend on the procedure or activity and the amount of fluid contamination which is anticipated.

Aprons: the apron should be of a size which provides coverage to the front of the body and clothing. Single-use disposable plastic aprons should be worn by all staff and visitors assisting in the care of the patient or having contact with their immediate environment or when handling blood, body fluids, secretions, and excretions. Plastic aprons should be worn as single-use items for one procedure or episode of patient care only. They should be removed immediately after use by tearing the neck strap and the waist tie and discarded into clinical waste bag before leaving the room. Hands must be washed immediately after removing and bagging the soiled plastic apron.

Gowns: clean, non-sterile gowns should be worn during procedures which are likely to expose HCWs with spraying or splashing of blood, body fluids, secretions, or excretions. Gowns should be impermeable and made of a water-repellent type of fabric. Both aprons and gowns should be removed after use and discarded and the hands washed to prevent the transfer of microorganisms to other patients or environments.

If the gown is expected to become wet during the procedure and if a water-repellent gown is not available, a plastic apron should be worn over the gown. Grossly soiled non-disposable gowns should be promptly removed and placed in the designated leak-proof laundry bag. Hands should be washed immediately after removing and bagging of the soiled gown.

Decontamination of equipment and environmental issues

Decontamination of items and equipment

Where possible, equipment should be single-patient use and should be discarded after use as per local policy. If the use of communal equipment is unavoidable, then it *must* be decontaminated before use on each patient. If the equipment is soiled with blood, body fluids, secretions, or excretions, wear appropriate PPE when cleaning or handling it. Excreta from infected patients should be disposed of as soon as practicable; prior soaking of bedpans in disinfectant is not required. Commodes, bed pan carriers, urine measuring jugs, and toilets are a risk particularly for pathogens and must be regularly and adequately cleaned according to local policy. Single-use bedpans and urinals can be employed and should be disposed of in a macerator. Reusable bedpans/urinals should be cleaned and heat disinfected in a bedpan washer. The bedpan washer must be included in a planned preventative maintenance programme.

Linen

Wear appropriate PPE when handling linen contaminated with blood, body fluids, secretions, or excretions. Handle soiled linen as little as possible and place *gently* in appropriate laundry bag as per local policy. To avoid contaminating a uniform, soiled linen should be held away from body.

Environmental cleaning

The room and its items/equipment should be cleaned according to local cleaning procedures. Hot water and detergent is sufficient for most purposes, however 'hand-touch' surfaces and patient care items/equipment must be cleaned and disinfected using appropriate disinfection on a daily basis to reduce the bioburden of microorganisms. All baths and shower facilities and associated equipment must be decontaminated after each patient use. The methods and frequency for these processes, and the products used should be according to local policy.

Staff employed for these purposes should receive specific training in the relevant aspects of infection control, which includes issues for specific areas such as isolation rooms. Spillage of blood and body fluids should be disinfected and cleaned promptly using a safe method (see Chapter 6). Appropriate personal protective clothing should be worn and waste should be discarded as clinical waste.

When the patient is discharged from an isolation room, the room must be thoroughly cleaned. Single-use items must be discarded and other items/equipment must be decontaminated as per local policy. Items which require high-level disinfection/sterilization must be sent to the sterile supply department for sterilization. After cleaning, once the room is dry, it can be occupied by the next patient.

Clinical waste

All clinical waste should be put into yellow plastic bags according to local policy. All used sharps must be discarded into an approved container which should be readily accessible and must be securely fastened. Clinical waste should be segregated, stored, and transported according to local policy.

Key references and further reading

CDC/HICPAC. Guideline for isolation precautions: Preventing transmission of infectious agents in healthcare settings 2007. *American Journal of Infection Control*, 2007; **35**(10):S65–S164.

Department of Health. *Isolating patients with healthcare-associated infection: A summary of best practice*. London: Department of Health, 2007.

Heymann DL. *Control of communicable disease manual*, 19th edn. Washington, DC: American Public Health Association, 2008.

Pratt RJ, Pellowe CM, Wilson JA, *et al. epic2*: National evidence- based guidelines for preventing healthcare-associated infections in NHS hospitals in England. *Journal of Hospital Infection*, 2007; **65**:S1–S64.

Appendix 7.1 Type and duration of isolation precautions

Infectious diseases	Infectious agents and incubation period (IP)	Infection control precautions	Transmission route	Source of infection and period of infectivity (PI)	Additional information
Acquired immune deficiency syndrome(AIDS)/ human immune deficiency virus (HIV) infection	HIV. IP: variable: 1–3 months from exposure to appearance of transfusion of	Standard	Person-to-person by sexual contact, percutaneous inoculation (see 'HIV infection', Chapter 11), infected blood or blood products, and vertical transmission	Human blood and 'high- risk' body fluids PI: lifelong	Patients with HIV infection must not donate blood, plasma, or organs for transplant, tissues, cells, semen for artificial insemination (see 'HIV infection', Chapter 11)
Actinomycosis	*Actinomyces israelii* is the usual human pathogen although other types have been reported	Standard	The source of clinical disease is endogenous	The natural reservoir is the human mouth and gut	Common commensal of the human mouth and gut
Amoebiasis (dysentery)	*Entamoeba hystolitica* IP: 2–4 weeks (variable from a few days to several months)	Standard	Faecal–oral route, usually due to the ingestion of faecal contaminated food or water containing amoebic cysts	A protozoan parasite, which exists in two forms: the infective cyst and the potentially pathogenic trophozoites. PI: as long as cysts appear in faeces which may be for years	Patients with amoebic dysentery pose only a limited risk of transmission to others under normal sanitation conditions due to the absence of cysts in dysenteric stools and the fragility of trophozoites

Disease	Organism/IP	Precautions	Transmission	Period of infectivity	Comments
Anthrax	*Bacillus anthracis* IP: 1–7 days although periods of up to 60 days are possible	Standard for both cutaneous and pulmonary anthrax	*Cutaneous*: inoculation from contaminated animal tissue and hides *Pulmonary*: from inhalation of *B. anthracis* spores	Articles and soil contaminated with spores, which may remain infective for decades Patients with pulmonary disease may be more infectious but person-to-person spread is very rare PI: duration of hospitalization; until off antibiotics and cultures are negative	On exposure to air this organism forms spores which may remain viable in the environment for years. Contact the laboratory *before* sending samples Antibiotic therapy renders a skin lesion non-infectious within 24 h
Ascariasis (roundworm which have infestation)	*Ascaris lumbrocoides* IP: the life cycle takes 4–8 weeks to be mature fertilized	Standard	By ingestion of mature eggs in water or uncooked food-stuff which have been contaminated with soil containing infected faeces	Humans: ascarid eggs in soil PI: as long as mature fertilized worms are present in the intestine	The usual lifespan of adult is 12 months. Under favourable conditions embryonated eggs can remain viable in soil for years
Aspergillosis (pulmonary)	*Aspergillus fumigatus* or *Aspergillus flavus* IP: unknown, probably a few days to few weeks	Standard	Caused by inhalation of *Aspergillus* spp. spores usually associated with building work	Ubiquitous within the environment No person-to-person spread	May present in several clinical conditions, e.g. allergic bronchopulmonary aspergillosis, aspergilloma, and as a concomitant organism in a lung abscess or empyema. May also cause invasive disease in immunocompromised patients

Infectious diseases	Infectious agents and incubation period (IP)	Infection control precautions	Transmission route	Source of infection and period of infectivity (PI)	Additional information
Bornholm disease (Pleurodynia Epidemic myalgia)	Coxsackie A and B viruses, types 1, 2, 3, 5 and 6 Echo virus 1 and 6. IP: usually 3–5 days	Standard, droplet, and contact	Person-to-person spread by direct or indirect contact with respiratory droplets or faeces from an infected person	PI: during the acute stage of the illness organism may be isolated from the faeces for as long as 3 weeks after recovery	
Botulism	Caused by toxins of *Clostridium botulinum* IP: neurological signs become apparent 12–36 h after ingesting contaminated food	Standard	Three forms of botulism *Food borne:* ingestion of toxin *Wound botulism:* contamination of a wound with soil or earth *Intestinal botulism:* ingestion of botulinium spores which germinate in the gut producing toxin	Ubiquitous spores of *C. botulinum* are in soil No person-to-person transmission	Outbreaks associated with a contaminated food source, usually contaminated canned food
Brucellosis	*Brucella* spp. IP: uncertain. 1–2 months common; occasionally several months	Standard and contact precautions if there are draining lesions	By direct or indirect *contact* with tissues, blood, urine, vaginal discharges, aborted foetuses and placentae of infected animals through breaks in the skin or, by *ingestion* of unpasteurized milk and dairy products of infected animals and airborne by *inhalation* of the organism in laboratories or in slaughter houses	No person-to-person transmission Reservoir cattle, sheep, swine, or goats	Preventative measures include: Promoting good practice in the handling and disposal of placentae, discharges and fetus from aborted animals Do not consume unpasteurized dairy products

Campylobacter gastroenteritis	*Campylobacter jejuni* or *coli* IP: usually 2–5 days (1–10 days depending on the dose ingested)	Standard	Ingestion of contaminated food usually unpasteurized milk, undercooked poultry, and non-chlorinated water Also by contact with infected puppies, kittens, and farm animals	Person-to-person transmission is rare but can occur. Source of infection is usually poultry, cattle, puppies and kittens	Most raw poultry meat is contaminated with *Campylobacter jejuni*. Thorough cooking renders it safe to eat
Candidiasis (thrush)	*Candida* spp. IP: variable 2–5 days for thrush, in infants.	Standard	Usually endogenous The organism is part of the normal human flora Nosocomial spread can occur in high-dependency units such as SCBU and ICU by contact with secretions or excretions of mouth, skin, vagina and faeces from carriers	Humans	Clinical disease occurs when host defences are low. Predisposing factors for superficial candidiasis include: diabetes, broad-spectrum antibiotic therapy, steroid therapy and HIV infection. Predisposing factors for deep candidiasis include immunosuppression, neutropenia, haematological malignancy and very low birth weight in neonates

Infectious diseases	Infectious agents and incubation period (IP)	Infection control precautions	Transmission route	Source of infection and period of infectivity (PI)	Additional information
Chickenpox (varicella)	Varicella zoster virus (VZV) IP: 10–21 days	Standard, airborne, and contact	From person to person by *direct contact, droplet* or *airborne* spread of vesicle fluid or secretions of the respiratory tract of chickenpox cases or of vesicle fluid of patients with herpes zoster (shingles). May also be spread by *indirect contact* have been freshly contaminated with discharges from vesicles and mucous membranes of infected people	Humans: susceptible persons should be considered to be infectious 10–21 days following exposure. The patient is infectious from as long as 5 but usually within 1–2 days before the onset of the rash and continues until all lesions are crusted or scabbed usually 5 days after the rash appears	Discharge patient home if clinical condition permits. Only those HCWs who have immunity (established either by a clear history of having had chickenpox or shingles or by serological testing for immunity) should care for patients who have chickenpox Visitors who do not have immunity to chickenpox should be made aware of the risk of acquiring infection by contact with an infectious individual. (see 'Varicella zoster virus', Chapter 11)
Chlamydia infection	*C. trachomatis* IP: poorly defined, 7–14 days or longer	Standard and contact	Sexual contact with infected secretions. Untreated infection during pregnancy can cause eye infection and respiratory infection in the neonate during the birthing process	Humans	Treat sexual contacts

Cholera	*Vibrio cholerae* IP: few hours to 5 days	Standard and contact	By ingestion of food or water which has been either directly or indirectly contaminated with faeces or vomit of infected persons spread Person-to-person is unusual	Humans PI: the infectivity is thought to last until faecal samples are negative, which is usually a few days after clinical recovery or after antibiotic treatment Carrier states may persist for several months in some cases	
Clostridium difficile-associated diarrhoea	*C. difficile* IP: 5–10 days	Standard and contact	*Endogenous* infection, precipitated by antibiotic therapy due to overgrowth of *C. difficile* in the gut and toxin production *Exogenous* infection by ingestion of spores from a contaminated environment Person-to-person spread is possible in the case of active diarrhoea	Humans: endogenous, gut commensal PI: duration of diarrhoea	*C. difficile* is a part of normal gut commensal. Do not send stool specimens for clearance as the *C. difficile* toxin may be present in the stool after the diarrhoea has settled. See '*Clostridium difficile* infection', Chapter 11, for treatment of symptomatic patients
Clostridium food poisoning	*Clostridium perfringens* IP: 6–12 h	Standard	By ingestion of food that has been contaminated with soil or faeces and held under conditions which permit multiplication of the organism. Usually associated with inadequately heated or reheated dishes	Heavy contamination ($>10^5$) is required to produce clinical disease No person-to-person spread	*C. perfringens* is found in the soil and GI tract of healthy people. Spores survive normal cooking temperatures, germinate and multiply during slow cooling, storage at ambient temperatures and/or inadequate re-warming

Infectious diseases	Infectious agents and incubation period (IP)	Infection control precautions	Transmission route	Source of infection and period of infectivity (PI)	Additional information
Conjunctivitis	Bacterial infection IP: 24–72 h *Haemophilus*, *Streptococcus*, *Moraxella* and *Branhamella* spp.	Standard and contact	Contact with the discharge from the conjunctivae or respiratory tracts of infected persons from contaminated fingers, clothing or other articles	Humans PI: during the period of active infection	Children under 5 years are more likely to have infection The very young, the elderly, and debilitated appear to be particularly susceptible to staphylococcal infections Eradication should be confirmed by culture after treatment
	Ophthalmia neonatorum *N. gonorrhoeae* IP: 1–5 days	Standard and contact	By direct contact with the infected cervix and secretions during the birthing process	Humans: infected maternal cervix and secretions PI: whilst the discharge is present if untreated until 24 h after starting antibiotic therapy	Advise patient to avoid hand-to-eye contact. In the home care setting avoid the use of communal towels and toilet articles. Clinical staff who have acute infection should not have patient contact until the condition resolved
	Viral epidemic kerato-conjunctivitis, or shipyard eye. Usually caused by various adenovirus types IP: 5–12 days; may be longer	Standard and contact	Direct contact with eye secretions of an infected person and indirectly, through contaminated surfaces instruments or eye preparations	Humans PI: the condition is considered infective from late in the incubation period until 14 days after onset. Prolonged viral shedding has been reported	

Cryptococcosis (usually presents as a subacute or chronic meningitis)	Cryptococcus neoformans IP: 1–12 days (average of 7 days)	Standard	Transmitted probably by inhalation from an external environmental source	No person-to-person spread. Saprophytic growth in the external environment. Associated with old pigeon nests and droppings	Susceptibility is increased during steroid therapy, immune deficiency disorders especially AIDS and disorders of the reticuloendothelial system
Cryptosporidiosis	Cryptosporidium parvum IP: 1–12 days (average of 7 days)	Standard	Transmitted by the faecal–oral route by ingestion of oocysts. This includes person-to-person, animal-to-person, waterborne and foodborne routes. One or more autoinfectious cycles may occur in humans	Humans: cattle and other domestic animals. PI: oocysts, the infectious stage, appear in the stool at the onset of symptoms and continue to be secreted in the stool for several weeks after the symptoms resolve	Cryptosporidium oocysts are highly resistant to chemical disinfectants used to purify drinking water. Only filters which can remove particles 0.1–1.0 mm in diameter should be used. Boiling drinking water for 1 min will destroy oocysts. Oocytes may remain infectious for 2–6 months in a moist environment
Creutzfeldt–Jakob disease	Prions IP: 2–50 years	Standard and contact	No person-to-person transmission. Iatrogenic cases have been recognized	Humans PI: infectivity during the incubation period is not known	Transmission of variant vCJD is believed to be caused by the consumption of beef from cattle infected with bovine spongiform encephalopathies (see 'Prion disease', Chapter 11)

Infectious diseases	Infectious agents and incubation period (IP)	Infection control precautions	Transmission route	Source of infection and period of infectivity (PI)	Additional information
Cytomegalovirus infection	Cytomegalovirus virus (CMV) IP: 3–8 weeks for transplant and infusion 2–12 weeks for infection acquired during birth	Standard and contact	Intimate exposure by mucosal contact with infectious tissues, secretions and excretions The fetus may be infected *in utero* or virus may be transmitted to the infant during the birthing process	Humans: CMV is excreted in urine, saliva, breast milk, cervical secretions and semen during primary and reactivated infections PI: virus is excreted for many months after primary infection and may persist or be episodic for years After neonatal infection, excretion of virus may be present for 6 years Excretion recurs with immunodeficiency and immunosuppression	Women of childbearing age who work in hospitals (esp. delivery and paediatric wards), day care centres, nurseries and similar health care settings must at all times employ standard infection control precautions This includes hand washing after nappy changes and toileting
Dengue fever	Flaviviruses (serotypes 1,2,3 & 4) IP: 3–14 days; commonly 4–7 days	Standard	Transmitted by bite of infective mosquitoes esp. *Aedes aegyptis* No direct person-to-person transmission	Can present as dengue haemorrhagic fever	This is a day-biting species, with increased biting activity for 2 h *after* sunrise and several hours *before* sunset Dengue haemorrhagic fever can be misdiagnosed as viral haemorrhagic fevers

Disease	Organism / IP	Precautions	Reservoir / Transmission	Period of infectivity	Comments
Diphtheria	Cutaneous: *Corynebacterium diphtheriae* IP: 2–5 days or longer	Standard and contact	Humans Direct contact with a patient or carrier, or contact with articles, which have been contaminated with discharge from lesions of infected people	PI: until off antibiotics and three swabs are culture negative from skin lesions taken at least 24 h apart after antibiotic therapy	Throat and nasal swabs should be taken from all close contacts Notify laboratory *before* sending samples Culture positive carriers of toxigenic *C. diphtheria* should receive chemoprophylaxis with erythromycin and swabs repeated after treatment
	Pharyngeal	Standard and droplet		PI: until off antibiotics and three consecutive swabs from nose and throat are culture negative Where culture facilities are not available, isolation may be discontinued after 14 days of appropriate antibiotic treatment	
Dysentery: (bacillary or shigellosis)	*Shigela* spp. IP: 1–3 days (from 12 h–1week)	Standard and contact	Faecal–oral by direct or indirect contact with a symptomatic person or a short-term asymptomatic carrier Flies can transfer organisms from a contaminated source on to uncovered food items The infectious dose varies, 10–100 organisms	Humans PI: duration of diarrhoea	Advise the patient of the importance of good hand hygiene, using soap and running water, especially after going to toilet or handling contaminated items Persons with shigellosis who are food handlers, provide care to infants and HCWs should refrain from work until recovery and faecal samples are clear

Infectious diseases	Infectious agents and incubation period (IP)	Infection control precautions	Transmission route	Source of infection and period of infectivity (PI)	Additional information
Echinococcosis (tapeworm infestation)	*Echinococcus granulosus* IP: 12 months to many years depending on the number of cysts and how quickly they grow	Standard	Direct transmission by hand to mouth, transfer of eggs after contact with infected dogs or indirectly through contact with contaminated food, water, or soil	The adult worm which is in the small intestine of an infested dog produces eggs containing infective embryos (oncospheres), which are excreted in the animal's faeces Eggs may survive for several months in garden soil and when ingested by the intermediate host (people) the eggs hatch releasing the oncospheres	Educate the public to avoid exposure to dog faeces Hand washing with soap and water is an important protective measure
Haemophilis meningitis (also cause epiglottitis and other infections)	*H. influenzae* type b IP: 2–4 days	Standard and droplet	Transmitted by droplets and discharges from the nose and throat during the illness and carriage	It is transmissible so long as organisms are present in the nasopharynx Not transmissible after 48h effective antibiotic therapy	Close contacts should be given chemoprophylaxis (see 'Meningitis') Hib vaccination has substantially reduced the number of cases of invasive infection
Gas gangrene	*Clostridium perfringens* and other anaerobic organisms IP: variable	Standard	By contamination of a wound by soil or faecal material Acquired from endogenous route; no person-to-person spread	The organisms are found in soil and in the GI track of healthy individuals	

Disease	Organism / IP	Precautions	Spread	PI	Comments
Gastroenteritis	Various agents including viral, bacterial and protozoal infections. See 'Gastrointestinal infections', Chapter 11.	Standard and contact	Often from contaminated food or water. Person-to-person spread is possible for most infectious causes	PI: duration of diarrhoea	If the patient has diarrhoea, they should be nursed in a side ward. Educate the patient in hand washing with soap and water. In hospital, inform IPCT if outbreak is suspected. In the community inform the appropriate authority (CCDC in UK). Refer to 'Outbreak control measures', Chapter 4
Glandular fever (infectious mononucleosis)	Epstein–Barr virus IP: 4–6 weeks	Standard	Person-to-person spread by direct contact with the saliva of an infected person	Humans: saliva. PI: Until acute phase is over	Sometimes referred to as kissing disease
German measles (rubella) Acute rubella, and congenital rubella syndrome	Rubella virus IP: 14–21 days	Standard, droplet and contact	Direct contact with the nasopharyngeal secretions of infected persons, or by droplet spread	PI: from 7 days before up to 10 days after onset of rash. Infants who have congenital rubella syndrome may shed virus in the nasopharyngeal secretions and the urine for several months	In the case of congenital rubella contact precautions must be used in the health care setting until the baby is 1 year old or pharyngeal and urine cultures are negative
Gonorrhoea	N. gonorrhoea IP: 2–7 days	Standard and contact	During sexual activity with an infected person	Humans. PI: for 24 h after the start of effective antibiotic therapy	Refer to genito-urinary clinic for follow-up and treatment of sexual contacts

Infectious diseases	Infectious agents and incubation period (IP)	Infection control precautions	Transmission route	Source of infection and period of infectivity (PI)	Additional information
Hepatitis (viral)	Type A Hepatitis A virus IP: 25–30 days	Standard and contact	Faecal–oral	Humans PI: 7 days before to 7 days after onset of jaundice	Hepatitis A is most contagious *before* jaundice and is infectious in the early febrile phase of illness Close contacts may be given gamma globulin within 14 days to abort or attenuate clinical illness
	Type B and C IP: HBV: 75 days HCV: 20 days–13 weeks	Standard and contact	Sexually transmitted or by blood inoculation, e.g. needle stick accident or shared needles in IV drug misuse	Humans PI: blood and high-risk body fluids so long as viraemia persists	
	Type E Hepatitis E virus IP: 15–64 days (3–6 weeks)	Standard and contact	Faecal–oral Food-borne via drinking water contaminated with faeces from infected individuals or animals Parenteral spread, via blood products and solid organ transplantation has also been documented.		Severe, life-threatening hepatitis may occur in ~1% of cases. However, severe morbidity and mortality rates are highest in pregnant women. Diagnosis is made by detecting anti-HEV antibody (IgG and IgM).

Herpes	Herpes simplex virus IP: 2–14 days	Standard and contact	Direct transmission by contact with the active lesions of infected individuals	Humans: infected vesicle fluid PI: until vesicles healed	Protect immunologically compromised patients. Wear gloves when hands are in contact with oral or genital secretions Staff with cold sores should not work with compromised patients, neonates, or burns patients
Herpes zoster (shingles)	Varicella virus IP: not applicable	Standard and contact	Endogenous type infection—reaction of latent varicella infection	Human: caused by reactivation of varicella (herpes) virus PI: until vesicles are dry and healing	As herpes zoster may cause chickenpox in susceptible individuals only those HCWs who have immunity (established either by a clear history of having had chicken-pox or shingles or by serological testing for immunity) should care for patients with shingles. Visitors who do not have immunity should also be warned of the risks of infection
Impetigo	Staphylococci and streptococci IP: 7–10 days for streptococcal; 1–10 days for staphylococcal	Standard and contact	By direct contact with infected people or indirectly by contaminated articles	Humans PI: for 24 h after start of effective antibiotic therapy	

Infectious diseases	Infectious agents and incubation period (IP)	Infection control precautions	Transmission route	Source of infection and period of infectivity (PI)	Additional information
Infectious mononucleosis (glandular fever)	Epstein–Barr virus IP: 4–6 weeks	Standard	Person-to-person spread by direct contact with the saliva of an infected person	Humans: saliva Until acute phase is over	Sometimes referred to as kissing disease
Influenza	Influenza virus IP: 1–3 days	Standard, airborne and droplet	Airborne spread by inhalation or by direct inoculation to the mucous membranes through indirect contact with infectious respiratory secretions	Humans	Immunization can be offered to a selected group (see 'Respiratory viral infections', Chapter 11)
Lassa fever (viral haemorrhagic fever)	Lassa virus IP: 6–21 days	Standard, airborne, droplet and contact	By aerosol or direct contact with infected materials	Humans and rodents	(see 'Viral haemorrhagic fevers', Chapter 11)
Legionnaire's disease	Legionella pneumophilia IP: 5–6 days	Standard	Inhaled infected aerosol	Organism ubiquitous in the aquatic environment No person-to-person spread	(see 'Legionnaire's disease, Chapter 11)

Disease	Organism	Precaution	Transmission	Notes
Leptospirosis (Weil's disease)	*Leptospira interrogans* (various servars) IP: 10 days (range of 4–19 days)	Standard	By contact of the skin and mucous membranes with water, moist soil or vegetation which is contaminated with the urine of infected animals. By inhalation of droplet aerosols and or ingestion of food which has been contaminated with the urine of infected rats	Infected animals, usually rats. Not transmitted from person to person
Listeriosis	*Listeria monocytogenes* IP: 3 days–10 weeks (average 3 weeks)	Contact	By ingestion of unpasteurized or failed pasteurization, infected dairy products, contaminated food. Neonatal infections can be transmitted to the fetus *in utero* or at the time of delivery	The prime reservoir is infected soil, mud, and water. Other reservoirs are infected animals and humans. Also acquired from eating contaminated food (esp. soft cheese). Person-to-person spread rare
Lyme disease	*Borrelia burgdorferi* IP: 7–10 days	Standard	Tick bite	Tick-borne. No person-to-person spread

Infectious diseases	Infectious agents and incubation period (IP)	Infection control precautions	Transmission route	Source of infection and period of infectivity (PI)	Additional information
Malaria	IP: *P. falciparum* 7–14 days *P. vivax* 8–14 days *P. ovale* 8–14 days *P. malariae* 7–30 days	Standard	Mosquito bite. Blood transfusion	Human reservoir Mosquito-borne vector No person-to-person spread	
Measles	Measles virus IP: 8–12 days	Standard and droplet	Close contact and direct inoculation of mucous membranes with secretions of an infected person's respiratory tract	Humans PI: for 5 days from the appearance of the rash, except in immunocompromised patients with whom precautions should be maintained for duration of illness	Discharge patient home if clinical condition permits Immunoglobulin for exposed immunocompromised patient If an outbreak in a paediatric ward, do not admit children who are immunosuppressed until 14 days after the last contact has gone home
Meningitis	'Coliforms' *Listeria monocytogenes* IP: 3 days–10 weeks	Standard	Respiratory tract Close contact, direct inoculation of mucous membranes		See 'Listeriosis'
	Neisseria meningitidis (meningococcal) IP: 2–10 days (average 3–4 days)	Standard and droplet		For 48 h after start of effective antibiotic therapy and patient has received chemoprophylaxis	Visiting by all children should be discontinued. In the case of a HCW being exposed to the patient's oropharyngeal secretions—refer for post-exposure chemoprophylaxis

Organism	Precautions	Source/transmission	Reservoir	Period of infectivity	Comments
Haemophilus influenzae (type b) IP: 2–4 days	Standard and droplet	Respiratory	Humans	Duration of illness	Close contacts should be given rifampicin as prophylaxis *Adult*: rifampicin 600 mg once daily for 4 days *Child*: 1–3 months 10 mg/kg once daily for 4 days; over 3 months 20 mg/kg once daily for 4 days (max. 600 mg daily)
S. pneumoniae (pneumococcal)	Standard	Respiratory tract			
Tuberculosis IP: 4–12 weeks	Standard and airborne (as pulmonary TB)	Respiratory tract	Humans		Isolate if patient has open pulmonary TB (see 'Tuberculosis', Chapter 11)
Viral IP: variable	Standard and droplet	Person-to-person by inhalation		Until virus no longer present in stool	Seek advice from a member of IPC team
Meningococcal septicaemia IP: 2–10 days (average 3–4 days)	Standard and droplet	By contact with the respiratory secretions of the infected patient		PI: for 48 h after start of effective antibiotic therapy and patient has received chemoprophylaxis	(see 'Meningococcal infections', Chapter 11)
MRSA (meticillin resistant *S. aureus*)	Standard and contact	*S. aureus* By direct contact with the infected site and indirectly by contact with fomites and the hands of health care workers	Humans		(see 'Meticillin resistant *Staph. aureus*', Chapter 10)
Multi-resistant Gram-negative organisms	Standard and contact	'Coliforms', pseudomonas and other Gram negatives			(see 'Multi-resistant Gram negative', Chapter 10)

Infectious diseases	Infectious agents and incubation period (IP)	Infection control precautions	Transmission route	Source of infection and period of infectivity (PI)	Additional information
Mumps (infectious parotitis)	Mumps virus IP: 16–18 days (range 14–25)	Standard, airborne, droplet, and contact	Airborne transmission or by droplet spread and direct contact with the saliva of an infected person	Humans 7 days before to 9 days after onset of parotid swelling Maximum infectiousness 2 days before to 4 days after the onset of illness	Exclude non-immune staff Inform visitors who are not immune Persons with subclinical infections may be infectious
Mycoplasma (primary atypical pneumonia)	Mycoplasma pneumoniae IP: 6–23 days	Standard	Respiratory secretions. Direct contact with an infected person and indirectly by inoculation of mucous membranes	Humans	
Orf	Orf virus IP: 3–6 days	Standard and contact	By direct contact with an infected animal lesion	PI: while the vesicles are active Isolation of patient is not necessary	Contact precautions for exudates
Parvovirus	Parvovirus B19 (IP: 13-18 days)	Respiratory route	Respiratory secretions. Attack rate is about 50% amongst susceptible household members.	PI: 6 before to 3 days after symptoms	Common childhood illness. Presents with erythema infectiosum which is characterized by fever and a rash with erythematous cheeks (slapped cheek disease) Diagnosis is by serology and/or viral DNA detection. Refer to p. 317 for more details.

Pertussis (see Whooping cough)				
Plague (Bubonic)	*Yersinia pestis* IP: 2–6 days	Standard and contact	Bites of infected fleas are the most common mode of transmission or contact with material from infected buboes	Infected rodents and mammals
Poliomyelitis	Polio virus IP: 7–14 days	Standard and contact	Infected respiratory secretions, faeces. Direct, respiratory, faecal–oral	Humans PI: until stools negative for polio virus or 7 days from onset	Droplet spread is possible during the first week; masks should be worn. Subsequently, faecal excretion is more important. Visitors and staff should be immunized Gamma globulin for non-immune contacts; booster for immunized Contacts. No elective surgery on non-immunized contacts Virus shedding may follow vaccination with a live oral polio vaccine for several weeks. Wash hands after changing babies' nappies

Infectious diseases	Infectious agents and incubation period (IP)	Infection control precautions	Transmission route	Source of infection and period of infectivity (PI)	Additional information
Psittacosis	*Chlamydia psittaci* IP: 1–4 weeks	Standard; airborne if active coughing	By inhalation of the infectious agent from desiccated bird droppings, secretions, and dust from feathers of infected birds	For 7 days after onset of symptoms	
Rabies	Rabies virus IP: 2–8 weeks	Standard and contact	The virus laden saliva of an infected animal is introduced usually by a bite or in some cases a scratch or rarely through a break in the skin or intact mucous membranes	In dogs and cats the period for communication is for the duration of the illness	Immunize staff in close contact Theoretical transmission from the saliva of an infected person is possible.
Ringworm	*Tinea* spp. IP: 10–14 days scalp ringworm; 4–10 days body ringworm; unknown athlete's foot	Standard and contact	Animal and human contacts	During the presence of the lesion	
Rubella (German measles)	Rubella virus IP: 14–17 days with a range of 14–21 days	Standard and droplet	Transmitted by droplet or by contact with the nasopharyngeal secretions of infected people	Humans: PI: from 7 days before up to 10 days after onset of rash	Discharge patient home if clinical condition permits Exclude non-immune women (staff or visitor) of child bearing age

Salmonellosis	*Salmonella* spp. IP: 12–36 h (Range 6–72 h)	Standard and contact	Faecal–oral by ingestion of contaminated food. Person-to-person spread is common	Contaminated food especially poultry PI: duration of diarrhoea	(see 'Gastrointestinal infections', Chapter 11)
SARS (severe acute respiratory syndrome)	IP: 2–10 days	Standard and contact	Close person-to-person spread is common	PI: duration of illness	
Scabies	*Sarcoptes scabiei* IP: 2–6 weeks before itching in people who have not had previous exposure and 1–4 days in people who have had previous infestation	Standard and contact	By direct contact with infested skin and indirectly by contact with undergarments and bedclothes if these have been contaminated by infested people immediately beforehand	Humans PI: until completion of appropriate treatment	Persons with Norwegian or crusted scabies are highly contagious (see 'Scabies and Pediculosis', Chapter 11)
Smallpox	Small pox virus IP: 12–14 days (range 7–17 days)				Smallpox has been eradicated from the world since 1977. If you suspect a case please contact local health authority (CCDC in the UK) and a member of the IPC team as a matter of urgency
Streptococcal infection	Group A (*S. pyogenes*)	Standard and contact	Throat carriage, respiratory and direct contact from infected lesions	Until off antibiotics and cultures are negative	Can cause outbreaks in maternity units
	Group B (*S. agalactiae*)	Standard and contact			Cross-infection can occur in SCBU

Infectious diseases	Infectious agents and incubation period (IP)	Infection control precautions	Transmission route	Source of infection and period of infectivity (PI)	Additional information
	Group C and G	Standard and contact	Direct contact from infected lesions	Until off antibiotics and cultures are negative	
Syphilis	*Treponema pallidum* IP: 10 days–3 months (average 3 weeks)	Standard and contact	Acquired by *direct contact* with the infectious exudates of obvious or concealed, moist, early lesions of skin and mucous membranes of infected people during sexual contact. Also transplacental	Human PI: whilst moist mucotaneous lesions of primary and secondary syphilis are present Transmission of infection is rare after 1 year in untreated cases.	Patients should be advised to avoid sexual contact until treated Follow-up and treatment of sexual contacts is necessary to prevent onward transmission.
	Congenital, primary and secondary	Standard and contact		For 48 h after start of effective therapy	
	Latent and tertiary	Standard			
Tetanus	*Clostridium tetani* IP: 1 day to several months (average 10–14 days)	Standard	Direct inoculation from contaminated soil, usually associated with a puncture wound or by injecting contaminated street drugs	Intestines of horses and other animals including humans. Tetanus spores are ubiquitous within the environment. No person-to-person transmission	

Toxocariasis	Standard	*T. canis* and *T. cati* IP: weeks to several months	By ingestion of *Toxocara* eggs from contaminated soil or by ingestion of larvae in raw liver from infected chickens, cattle and sheep	Dogs and cats are the reservoir of infection No person-to-person transmission	De-worm dogs and cats. Dispose of pet faeces in a sanitary manner. Wash hands after handling soil and before eating. Teach children not to put dirty objects in their mouth
Toxoplasmosis	Standard	*Toxoplasma gondii* IP: 7 days	Ingesting viable ova in (old) cat faeces or cysts in undercooked meat.	Cats and other felines are the reservoir. No person-to-person transmission	
Tuberculosis	Standard and airborne	Pulmonary (open) *Mycobacterium tuberculosis* IP: 4–12 weeks	Inhalation vis air-borne route	Fully sensitive strain: 2 weeks after start of effective anti-TB treatment. 4 weeks in neonatal and paediatric wards or if immunosuppressed patients are present. MDR/XDR till three sputums are negative for AAFB. Isolate patient in a negative pressure ventilation room.	Staff and visitors who are not immune should be warned of the risk of infection. Facemasks should be worn. Refer to 'Tuberculosis', Chapter 11 for details.
	Closed				Isolation of patient not necessary
Typhoid and paratyphoid (See salmonellosis)	Standard and contact	*Salmonella typhi* and *paratyphii* IP: 3 days–1 month usually 8–14 days paratyphoid 1–10 days	Faecal-oral and by ingestion of contaminated food and water contaminated by faeces and urine of patients and carriers.	Humans: patients and convalescent carriers. PI: duration of diarrhoea.	

Infectious diseases	Infectious agents and incubation period (IP)	Infection control precautions	Transmission route	Source of infection and period of infectivity (PI)	Additional information
VRE (vancomycin resistant enterococci)	*Enterococci faecium* and *E. faecalis*	Standard and contact	By direct and indirect contact with an infected or colonized person.		Refer to 'Vancomycin-resistant enterococci', Chapter 11 for details.
Whooping cough (pertussis)	*Bordetella pertussis* IP: 7–10 days	Standard and droplet	By contact with the discharges from respiratory mucous membranes of an infected person	Humans PI: until 3 weeks after onset of paroxysmal cough or 7 days after start of effective antibiotic therapy	Discharge patient home if clinical condition permits. Visiting by children should be restricted to those who are immune. Prophylactic erythromycin to close contacts
Viral haemorrhagic fever (also see Lassa fever)	Marburg and Ebola virus IP: 3–9 days for Marburg; 2–21 days for Ebola virus	Standard, contact and droplet	Person-to-person transmission occurs by direct contact with infected blood, secretions, tissue, organs, or semen	Blood and secretions are highly infectious Risk of transmission during the incubation period is low but increases during the later stages of the illness when the patient is vomiting, having diarrhoea or haemorrhage	Patients require transfer to a regional infectious disease unit Staff who have had contact with a patient must remain under health surveillance A major public health issue, notify health authority (CCDC in UK) on suspicion of this condition (see 'Viral haemorrhagic fever', Chapter 11)

Appendix 7.2 Incubation periods of infectious diseases

Diseases	Average period (range)
AIDS/HIV	Variable; usually 1–3 months from exposure to appearance of HIV antibodies
Amoebic dysentery	2–4 weeks. Range: few days to several months
Anthrax	A few hours to 7 days; most cases occur within 48 h after exposure
Ascariasis	4–8 weeks
Aspergillosis	Unknown
Botulism	12–36 h; can be up to several days
	Infant botulism 3 days to 2 weeks
Brucellosis	5–60 days; can be up to several months
Campylobacter enteritis	3–5 days. Range: 1–10 days
Candidiasis	2–5 days
Cat-scratch disease	3–10 days to appearance of primary lesion, further 2–6 weeks to appearance of lymphadenopathy
Chancroid (*H. ducreyi*)	3–5 days; can be up to 14 days
Chickenpox (varicella)	10–21 days; may be prolonged after passive immunization against varicella and in the immunodeficient
Chlamydial conjunctivitis *Chlamydia trachomatis*	5–12 days. Range: 3 days to 6 weeks in newborns; 6–19 days in adult
Cytomegalovirus (CMV)	Within 3–8 weeks after transplant or transfusion with infected blood; infection acquired during first birth is demonstrable within 3–12 weeks in newborn after delivery
Dengue fever	7–10 days. Range: 3–14 days
Dermatophytoses	*See* Tinea
Diphtheria	2–5 days. Range: 2–7 days
Erytherma infectiosum	4–10 days (variable)
Fifth disease or parvovirus	
Gastroenteritis (viral)	
Astrovirus	1–2 days
Calcivirus	1–3 days
Norwalk	12–48 h
Rotavirus	1–3 days

Diseases	Average period (range)
Gastroenteritis (bacterial food poisoning)	
Salmonellosis	12–36 h. Range: 6–72 h
Shigellosis (Bacillary dysentry)	1–3 days. Range: 12–96 h
Campylobacter jejuni/coli	3–5 days. Range: 1–10 days
Staph. aureus	2–4 h. Range: 30 min to 7 h
Clostridium difficile	5–10 days. Range: few days to 8 weeks after stopping antibiotic therapy
Clostridium perfringens	10–12 h. Range: 6–24 h
Clostridium botulinum	12–36 h. Range: 12–96 h
Cryptosporidiosis	7 days. Range: 2–14 days
Giardiasis (*Giardia lamblia*)	7–10 days. Range: 5–25 days
Bacillus cereus	1–6 h where vomiting is predominant symptom; 6–24 h where diarrhoea is predominant
Cholera	1–3 days. Range: few hours to 5 days
Escherichia coli:	
E. coli Entero-invasive [EIEC]	10–18 h
E. coli Enterotoxigenic [ETEC]	1–5 days
E. coli Enteropathogenic [EPEC]	9–12 h (probably)
E. coli 0157:H7(Verocyotoxin [VTEC])	1–3 days Range: 12–60 h
Vibrio parahaemolyticus	12–24 h. Range: 2–96 h
Yersinia enterocolitica	24–36 h Range: 3–7 days
Aeromonas hydrophila	12–48 h
Listeria monocytogenes	48 h to 7 weeks
Gonorrhoea	2–7 days genito-urinary; 1–5 days ophthalmia neonatorum
Haemophilus influnenzae type b infection	2–4 days (probably)
Hand, foot and mouth disease	3–5 days
Hepatitis	
Hepatitis A	25–30 days. Range: 15–50 days
Hepatitis B	75 days. Range: 45–180 days
Hepatitis C	20 days to 13 weeks. Range: 2 weeks to 6 months
Hepatitis D	35 days. Range: 2–8 weeks
Hepatitis E	15–64 days. Range: 26–42 days
Herpes simplex infection (perinatal)	2–14 days. Range: 2–28 days
Impetigo	
Streptococcal	7–10 days
Staphylococcal	1–10 days

Diseases	Average period (range)
Infectious mononucleosis Glandular fever	4–6 weeks
Influenza	1–5 days
Legionnaires' disease	5–6 days (2–10 days for pneumonia)
	1–2 days for Pontiac fever
Leishmaniasis	
Visceral	Few weeks to 6 months
Cutaneous	Few weeks
Leptospirosis	10 days. Range: 4–19 days
Listeriosis	3 days to 10 weeks
Lyme disease	7–10 days. Range: 3–32 days after tick exposure
Lymphocytic choriomeningitis	8–13 days. Range:15–21 days
Lymphogranuloma venereum	3–30 days
Malaria	
P. falciparum	7–14 days
P. vivax	8–14 days
P. ovale	8–14 days
P. malariae	7–30 days
Measles	8–12 days. Range: 7–18 days
Meningococcal disease	3–4 days. Range: 2–10 days
Molluscum contagiosum	2–7 weeks. Range: 7 days to 6 months
Mumps	16–18 days. Range: 12–25 days
Mycoplasma pneumoniae	6–23 days
Pertussis (whooping cough)	7–10 days. Range: 6–20 days
Plague	
Bubonic	2–6 days
Pneumonic	2–4 days
Pneumocystis carinii	Unknown
Poliomyelitis	7–14 days. Range: 3–35 days
Psittacosis (*Chlamydia psittaci*)	1–4 weeks
Prion disease	Up to 50 years
Q fever (*Coxiella burnetii*)	2–3 weeks (depends on size of infecting dose)

Diseases	Average period (range)
Rabies	2–8 weeks. Range: 5 days to a year or more, depends on the site and severity of the wound; injury closer to brain has shorter incubation period
Relapsing fever (*B. recurrentis*)	8 days. Range: 5–15 days
Respiratory syncytial virus	4–6 days. Range: 2–8 days
Ringworm	
Tinea capitis (scalp ringworm)	10–14 days
Tinea corporis (body ringworm)	4–10 days
Tinea pedis (athlete's foot)	Unknown
Tinea unguim	Unknown
Roseola infantum	8–10 days
Rubella (German measles)	16–18 days. Range: 14–32 days
Salmonellosis	12–36 h. Range: 6 h to 3 days
SARS	2–10 days
Scabies	2–6 weeks without previous exposure; 1–4 days re-infection
Shigellosis	1–3 days. Range: 12 –96 h
Syphilis	3 weeks. Range: 10 days to 3 months
Tetanus	3–21 days. Range: 1 day to several months depending upon the character, extent and the location of wound
Threadworms	Unknown
Toxic shock syndrome	2 days
Toxocariasis	Weeks to several months depending on the intensity of infection. Up to 10 years for ocular symptoms
Toxoplasmosis	7 days. Range: 4–21 days
Tuberculosis	4–12 weeks (variable)
Typhoid & paratyphoid fevers	1–3 weeks. Range: 3–60 days
Typhus fever	12 days. Range: 1–2 weeks
Viral haemorrhagic fevers	
Marburg	3–9 days
Ebola	2–21 days
Lassa	6–21 days
Yellow fever	3–6 days

Chapter 8

Hand hygiene

> What, will these hands ne'er be clean?
>
> Macbeth, *William Shakespeare*

More than 150 years ago, Ignaz Semmelweis (1818–1865) demonstrated that puerperal fever was a contagious disease and was spread by 'cadaverous particles' from patient to patient by the hands of HCWs. This led to the introduction of hand dips with chlorinated lime at Vienna General Hospital. Since then, many studies have demonstrated that contaminated hands are responsible for transmitting infections. Therefore, the importance of regular hand hygiene must be emphasized as one of the most crucial interventions to prevent cross-infection in health care facilities. It is the responsibility of health care establishments to ensure that adequate numbers of hand washing facilities and alcohol hand rub products are readily available in *all* clinical areas. They should be located in areas where there is significant patient contact.

Beside preventing cross-infection, it is interesting to note that cleaning with water to 'wash away our sins' is deep rooted in many cultures and religions, including Islam, Hinduism, and Christianity. Water is a cornerstone of baptism ceremonies and, in the Bible, Pontius Pilate—the man who authorized the crucifixion of Jesus—washed his hands after condemning Jesus to death. Shakespeare also subscribed to the idea, making Lady Macbeth attempt to wash away her guilt of plotting King Duncan's murder. Recent study found that washing our hands frees us from taking the blame for any unhappy outcome of a difficult decision and it 'wipes the slate clean', removing doubts about recent choices. They found that people who washed their hands immediately after making an agonizing decision were happier with their choice compared with those who didn't (Lee et al., 2010).

Microorganisms on the hands

Price (1938) has classified bacteria recovered from the hands into two categories:

Resident organisms: the resident flora consists of microorganisms living under the superficial cells of the stratum corneum and can also be found on the skin's surface. These microorganisms are normal flora of the skin and include coagulase-negative staphylococci (mainly *Staphylococcus epidermidis*), members of the genus *Corynebacterium* (commonly called 'diphtheroids'), and *Propionibacterium* spp. Since resident flora is usually deep-seated in the epidermis, they are not easily removed by a single hand washing procedure. The reduction of resident flora is required before aseptic/surgical procedures and this is achieved by performing surgical scrub (see Box 15.2, Chapter 15).

Transient organisms: transient flora is not part of the normal flora and colonizes the superficial layers of the skin. It is often acquired by HCWs during direct contact with patients or by contaminated environmental surfaces. These microorganisms usually survive only for a limited period of time and are easily removed by hand washing or use of alcoholic hand rub on physically clean hands. The transient flora includes most of the organisms responsible for cross-infection, e.g. Gram-negative bacilli (*Escherichia coli, Klebsiella* spp., *Acinetobacter baumannii, Pseudomonas* spp., *Salmonella* spp., etc), *Staph. aureus*, vancomycin resistant enterococci, *Clostridium difficile*, and viruses (norovirus, influenza, etc.).

Hand washing using soap and water

Hand washing refers to the application of soap (plain or antimicrobial) and water on the hands. Despite the fact that plain soap has minimal antimicrobial activity, it can be used for routine hand washing (WHO, 2009). Soap acts through its detergent properties and by mechanical action which removes dirt, organic material, loosely adherent transit and a small portion of the resident flora from the hands.

Water: although water is considered the 'universal solvent', water alone is not suitable for cleaning dirty hands as soap or detergent is needed with water to remove hydrophobic substances such as fats and oils which are often present on soiled hands. Despite common belief, water temperature does not appear to be a critical factor for removal of microorganisms from hands being washed. However, use of very hot water for hand washing should be avoided as it increases skin irritation and may cause damage. After hand washing, thorough rinsing and drying is necessary.

Soap: plain, neutral pH soap can be used for routine hand washing. Added substances, (including antimicrobial agents) should be avoided as they have *no added benefit* and may cause allergies, irritation, or dryness of the skin; humectants should be added to the soaps to reduce skin irritation and dryness.

If a bar of soap is used then the bar should be small in size to allow frequent changing. In order to avoid contamination with microorganisms, it should be kept dry (in a soap rack or on a magnet or ring) to promote drainage of water. However, the actual hazard of transmitting microorganisms with previously used soap bars is negligible as they are frequently washed away during hand washing.

Liquid soap should be stored in closed containers and the dispensers should be *regularly cleaned*. If liquid soap is dispensed from reusable containers, these *must be cleaned* when empty and *dried before refilling* with fresh soap to avoid microbial contamination. Special attention should be taken to clean pump mechanisms as these have been implicated as sources of cross-infection.

Antiseptic preparations: preparations containing antiseptics (chlorhexidine gluconate-detergent, povidone iodine solution, triclosan, etc.) are more effective in removing resident microorganisms and are used for surgical scrub but their use is *not* normally necessary for everyday clinical practice.

Hand drying: ideally, hands should be dried using individual *good quality* paper towels. Reusing or sharing of cloth/fabric towels *must be avoided* in health care facilities as they are recognized as a source of cross-infection. If cloth/fabric towels are used, then they *must be single-use* and sent to the laundry. When towels (paper or fabric) are used to dry hands, it is important to pat the skin rather than rub it, to avoid cracking of skin. Air dryers are slow, noisy, and can be used by only one individual at a time therefore their use in health care facilities is not recommended.

Nailbrushes: routine use of nailbrushes is *not* recommended because they damage the skin, encouraging the proliferation and persistence of microorganisms on the skin.

Hand hygiene using alcohol hand rub

In 1888, P. Furbringer was the first to recommend alcohol for hand disinfection of surgeons and medical staff. Numerous reports confirm that alcohol-based formulations have better efficacy, shorter application time, are well tolerated, and therefore have better acceptability than hand washing. In addition, they can be easily available *at the point of care* and this has resulted in improved compliance with hand hygiene. According to WHO guidelines, alcohol-based hand rub is the *preferred* means for routine hand antisepsis (WHO, 2009). However, there are a few situations where hand washing should be preferred, e.g. when hands are visibly dirty or soiled with blood or other body fluids, or where exposure to potential spore-forming pathogens is strongly suspected or proven, and after using the toilet.

The hygienic hand rub method is convenient and useful especially in areas where a hand-wash basin is not readily available, e.g.:

* Emergency situations where there may be insufficient time and/or hand washing facilities.
* When hand washing facilities are inadequate.
* In the community or when return to a hand-wash basin is impractical.
* During a ward round where there is a need for rapid hand disinfection.

Hand rub products

Hand rubs are available as gels, rinses, or foams. In general, gels are more expensive and may produce a feeling of humectant 'build-up'. Some gel formulations may have reduced antimicrobial efficacy compared with rinses. Hand rub rinses are less viscous and often dry more quickly than gels or foams, therefore they are less likely to produce a feeling of humectant 'build-up' but they often have a stronger smell of alcohol than gels. Like gels, foams are more expensive, may produce a stronger feeling of 'build-up' with repeated use, and may take longer to dry.

The promotion of hand hygiene is highly cost-effective, and the introduction of alcohol-based hand rub is a cost-effective measure. In resource limited countries, the cost of hand rub can be prohibitive if the product is purchased from a commercial supplier. In such cases, consideration should be given to producing hand rub locally based on WHO formulations (WHO, 2009).

Efficacy of alcohol-based hand rub products

Alcohol-based hand rubs are *more effective* in decontaminating hands than soap and water (Figure 8.1). However, the efficacy of alcohol-based, hand hygiene products is affected by the type of alcohol used, concentration of alcohol, contact time, volume of alcohol used, and whether the hands are wet when the alcohol is applied. Alcohol solutions containing 60–80% ethanol are most effective. Higher concentrations are less effective as proteins are more difficult to denature in the absence of water.

One mL of alcohol is significantly *less effective* than 3 mL. Although ideal volume applied to the hands is not known (as it may vary for different formulations), in general, if the hands feel dry after being rubbed together for less than 10–15 seconds, it is likely that an insufficient volume of alcohol rub was applied. The recommended duration of the entire procedure for hand hygiene using alcohol hand rub is 20–30 seconds.

Alcohol has no activity against bacterial spores or protozoan oocysts and has poor activity on some non-enveloped viruses (such as norovirus, rotaviruses, or enteroviruses) and may require higher ethanol concentrations (90%). As a result, some health care facilities have adopted guidelines to wash hands when dealing with suspected/confirmed cases of patients with diarrhoeal illness. In recent years, widespread use of alcohol-based hand rubs has been thought to be associated with the increase of

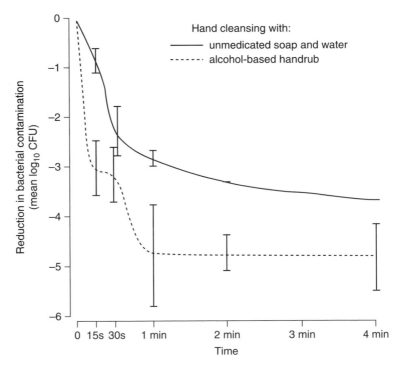

Fig. 8.1 Time-course of efficacy of unmedicated soap and water and alcohol-based hand rub in reducing the release of test bacteria from artificially contaminated hands. With permission from Pittet D, Allegranzi B, Sax H, *et al*. Evidence-based model for hand transmission during patient care and the role or improved practices. *Lancet Infectious Diseases* 2006; **6**:641–52.

C. difficile-associated infection. However, it is important to note that *C. difficile* infections began to rise in the USA long before the widespread use of alcohol hand rub. It is important to note that alcohol hand rub is effective against vegetative form but not against spores of *C. difficile*.

Indications and technique of hand hygiene

The WHO guidelines have simplified the recommended indications to perform hand hygiene into the concept of 'My Five Moments' which is summarized in Table 8.1

Table 8.1 Five moments for hand hygiene and examples of clinical situations

The five moments	Examples
1. Before touching a patient	◆ Shaking hands, helping a patient to move around, get washed ◆ Applying oxygen mask, giving physiotherapy, taking pulse, blood pressure, chest auscultation, abdominal palpation, recording ECG, etc.
2. Before clean/aseptic procedure	◆ Skin lesion care, wound dressing, subcutaneous injection, catheter insertion, opening a vascular access system or a draining system, secretion aspiration, preparation of food, giving medication, instilling eye drops, pharmaceutical products, sterile material etc ◆ Before handling an invasive device for patient care, regardless of whether or not gloves are used ◆ Before moving from a contaminated body site to another body site during care of the same patient
3. After body fluid exposure risk	◆ Skin lesion care, wound dressing, subcutaneous injection, drawing and manipulating any fluid sample, opening a draining system, endotracheal tube insertion, removal and secretion aspiration, clearing up urines, faeces, vomit, handling waste (bandages, napkins, incontinence pads), cleaning of contaminated and visibly soiled material or areas (soiled bed linen, lavatories, urinal, bedpan, medical instruments) etc. ◆ Before moving from a contaminated body site to another body site during care of the same patient ◆ After contact with body fluids or excretions, mucous membrane, non-intact skin or wound dressing ◆ After removing sterile or non-sterile gloves
4. After touching a patient	◆ Helping a patient to move around, get washed ◆ Applying oxygen mask, giving physiotherapy, taking pulse, blood pressure, chest auscultation, abdominal palpation, recording ECG, etc. ◆ After removing sterile or non-sterile gloves
5. After touching patient surroundings	◆ After contact with inanimate surfaces and objects (including medical equipment) in the immediate vicinity of the patient, perfusion speed adjustment, monitoring alarm, holding a bed rail, leaning against a bed, clearing the bedside table, changing bed linen, with the patient out of the bed, etc. ◆ After removing sterile or non-sterile gloves

Adapted from the WHO *Guidelines on Hand Hygiene in Health Care*, 2009.

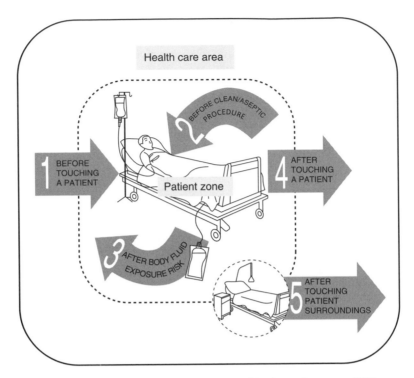

Fig. 8.2 Showing five moments of hand hygiene within the patient zone. With permission from Sax H, Allegranzi B. Uçay I, *et al.* 'My five moments for hand hygiene': a user-centered design approach to understand, train, monitor and report hand hygiene. *Journal of Hospital Infection* 2007; **67**(7):9–21.

and Figure 8.2. The '*patient zone*' is defined as the patient's intact skin and his/her immediate surroundings which are colonized/contaminated by the patient flora and the '*health care area*' as containing all other surfaces outside the patient zone.

For effective hand hygiene, the following criteria must be met: 1) using an *effective compound*, 2) enough *amount of product* available to cover hands, 3) use of *correct technique* to cover all areas, and 4) performing hand hygiene at the *right moment*.

The perfect hand hygiene technique has never been evaluated in prospective clinical trials. However, the proposed technique and steps recommended for hand hygiene (see Figure 8.3) allows effective hand disinfection as it covers all parts of the hand and can significantly improve bacterial killing. The last two steps are very important, i.e. wetting of the thumb and the fingertips as these parts of the hands are frequently touched during patient care activity and are most often missed during hand hygiene (Figure 8.4) by the HCWs. Nails should be kept short to allow thorough cleaning of the hands and to prevent tears in gloves. Artificial nails should be discouraged as they contribute to increased bacterial counts.

Hand hygiene compliance

Although hand washing is considered to be the most important single intervention for preventing HCAIs, studies have repeatedly shown poor compliance with hand hygiene

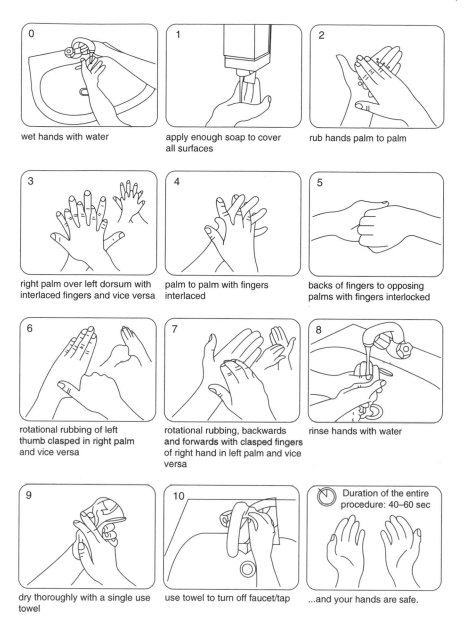

Fig. 8.3 Hand washing Technique. The recommended duration of the entire procedure for hand washing using soap and water is 40–60 seconds. Reproduced with permission from the World Health Organization. © World Health Organization 2009. All rights reserved.

by hospital personnel. Failure to comply is a complex problem that includes elements of lack of motivation and lack of knowledge about the importance of hand hygiene. It may also be due to real or perceived obstacles, such as understaffing, inconveniently located hand washing facilities, ready availability of the hand hygiene products, and an

FRONT   BACK

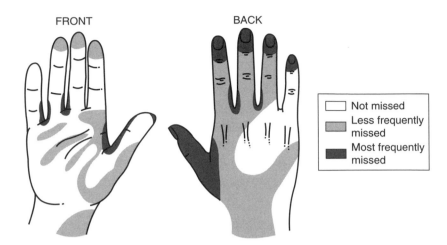

☐ Not missed

▨ Less frequently
   missed

■ Most frequently
   missed

Fig. 8.4 Parts of the hands most frequently missed during hand decontamination.

unacceptable hand washing product. One of the most important factors for compliance is that alcohol hand rub should be available at the *point of care.*

The acceptability of the agent in use is a crucial determinant of HCW compliance. Therefore it is an essential criterion for the selection of preparations for hand hygiene and is dependent upon general appreciation of the product, and its ease of use combined with its dermatological effects. All preparations used for hand hygiene must be acceptable to the user and should not damage the skin on repeated use. If staff do not accept the preparation, it will not be used. Therefore, it is recommended that a trial be undertaken before introduction of a new product in some areas to assess the acceptability by staff. A standardized and validated methodology is available from the WHO website (http://www.who.int/gpsc/en) which includes: 1) a protocol for evaluation of tolerability and acceptability of alcohol-based handrub in use or planned to be introduced, and 2) a protocol for evaluation and comparison of tolerability and acceptability of different alcohol-based hand rub products.

While the cost of hand hygiene products will continue to be an important issue for departments responsible for purchasing such products, the level of acceptance of products by HCWs is even more important. An inexpensive product with undesirable characteristics may discourage hand hygiene among HCWs and the resulting poor compliance will not be cost-effective.

A number of strategies have been suggested to improve compliance with hand hygiene. Long-term success will require development of multifaceted programmes, and sustained efforts at promoting compliance with hand hygiene. WHO has developed comprehensive tools to promote hand hygiene in health care facilities and these tools are available from the WHO website (http://www.who.int/).

Monitoring of consumption of hand hygiene products

Monitoring of consumption of hand hygiene products, e.g. consumption of the number of bars of soap used and/or amount of alcohol hand rub and liquid soap used in litres, as a measure of hand compliance is *not* effective as it lacks a denominator. In addition, in some countries (especially in the UK) hand hygiene products are also used by visitors and patients, therefore consumption measurement does *not* reflect how much it has been used by the clinical team. The consumption data are imprecise as resources are required to keep an accurate record of the products issued by the pharmacy or store to each ward/department and do not guarantee that the product which has been issued is *actually* used.

Observations of hand hygiene compliance

Hand hygiene compliance can be calculated using the following formula:

$$\text{Compliance of hand hygiene} = \frac{\text{No. of hand hygiene actions performed}}{\text{Required hand hygiene actions (opportunities)}} \times 100$$

Direct observation to monitor hand hygiene compliance is ideal but it is time-consuming, and requires skill and training. It is subject to various bias and confounding.

Bias

The method proposed by WHO states that hand hygiene observations should be open and the observer should declare his/her presence before commencing. It is important that observers should be trained using the WHO *Hand Hygiene Technical Reference Manual* and the *Hand Hygiene Training* film (http://www.who.int/gpsc/en). Hand hygiene observations should include all opportunities in the visual field and the observer's moves (if needed) to follow action. In addition to interobserver variation, hand hygiene observation is also subject to bias from HCWs (especially if s/he is doing her own ward/department) and the Hawthorne effect (where subjects improve or modify their behaviour in response to the fact that they are being 'observed') thus giving an increased compliance. However if the observational surveys are conducted regularly, this bias would be equally distributed among all observations and HCWs are likely to get used to the fact that they are being observed.

Confounding

Monitoring of hand hygiene compliance is also subject to confounding factors. For example:

- Time of day/night when the observation is done.
- Type of patients and health care setting.
- Intensity of care.
- High number of opportunities in short time.
- Professional categories of included HCWs.

Therefore it is essential that *timely feedback* must be given to the clinical area which should provide details on the type of setting (ward/department), professional categories, type of indications, and number of observations with percentage of compliance.

Issues related to alcohol-based preparations

Alcohols are flammable. Flashpoints of commonly used alcohol-based hand rubs range from 17.5–24.5°C, depending on the type and concentration of alcohol present. Therefore, it is important that alcohol-based hand rubs should be stored away from high temperatures or flames. After using hand rub, the hands should be completely dry before contacting electrical outlets or plugs. Consult the safety officer at your health care facility for specific guidelines.

Alcohol use is prohibited in some religions and the adoption of alcohol-based formulations for hand hygiene may cause difficulties for some HCWs mainly because of their concern about its absorption via the skin. In the Islamic tradition, which generally poses the toughest challenge to alcohol use, the Qur'an permits any substance that man can manufacture or develop to alleviate illness or contribute to better health, and this includes alcohol as a medical agent (Ahmed *et al*, 2006; Allegranzi *et al*, 2009).

Where there is thought to be a high risk of ingestion, consideration should be given to the labelling of the hand rubs with an emphasis on the sanitizing properties and with a warning of dangers associated with ingestion. Bottles containing smaller quantities should be used, if possible, and 500-mL containers should be secured. Health care facilities should have local guidance on how to deal with ingestion based on products available.

Skin reactions related to hand hygiene

Frequent and repeated use of soaps and other detergents are responsible for chronic dermatitis among HCWs and this can be reduced by the addition of humectants, i.e. ingredient(s) added to hand hygiene products to moisturize the skin. In addition, skin irritation is also found due to the presence of antimicrobial agents and other ingredients present in the soaps of the formulation.

A skin reaction to hand hygiene products may be increased by low relative humidity which most commonly occurs in winter months in the northern hemisphere. This is because in dry seasons, the lipid depletion from hands occurs more quickly, especially in an individual with dry skin. In tropical countries and during the summer months in temperate climates, the skin remains more moisturized than in cold, dry environments. Therefore, introduction of new products during dry and cold periods with low relative humidity should be avoided. In addition, HCWs with darker skin have significantly healthier skin and less skin irritation than those with lighter skin.

Two major types of skin reactions are associated with hand hygiene:

Irritant contact dermatitis is extremely common and is caused by frequent use of hand hygiene products. The damage to the skin is caused by denaturation of stratum corneum proteins, changes in intercellular lipids, and decreased stratum corneum water-binding capacity. This can be reduced by using moisturizing skin care products and by avoiding soap and water hand washing before or after an alcohol-based product is used.

Allergic contact dermatitis is very rare and is present as delayed type reactions or less commonly as immediate reactions (contact urticaria). The most common causes of contact allergies are fragrances and preservatives present in the hand hygiene products.

Exposure to irritating soaps and detergents can be minimized by promoting the use of alcohol-based hand rubs containing humectants. These products are well tolerated and are associated with a better skin condition when compared with either plain or antimicrobial soap.

Hand care

Hand care is important, because intact skin is a natural defence against infection. Damage to the skin also changes skin flora, resulting in more frequent colonization by staphylococci and Gram-negative bacilli. In addition, the irritant and drying effects of hand preparations have been identified as one of the reasons for lack of compliance with hand hygiene. The following points must be kept in mind to reduce skin irritation:

◆ Frequent hand washing leads to progressive depletion of surface lipids due to the action of lipid-emulsifying detergents resulting in deeper action of detergents into the superficial skin layers. Alcohols are responsible for depletion of the lipid barrier on the skin due to lipid-dissolving properties of alcohols which is inversely related to their concentration, and ethanol tends to be less irritating than n-propanol or isopropanol. Therefore hand preparations containing emollients and moisturizers should be used.

◆ Washing hands with soap and water immediately before or after using an alcohol-based product is not only unnecessary, but may lead to dermatitis (Kampf, 2003).

◆ Donning of gloves while hands are still wet (either from hand washing or applying alcohol hand products) is also *not* recommended as it increases the risk of skin irritation.

◆ To minimize chapping of hands, don't use hot water and *pat hands* dry with good quality towel paper rather than rubbing them.

◆ Apply an emollient hand cream regularly to protect skin from the drying effect of hand washing preparations.

◆ Since liquid soaps, hand lotions, ointments, or creams used by HCWs may contain ingredients that cause contact allergies, it is essential that HCWs should use products approved by the health care facility's Occupational Health Department.

◆ Cover cuts and abrasions with water-resistant occlusive dressings which should be changed as necessary.

◆ Frequent use of gloves also contributes to dermatitis due to allergy to latex proteins and shear forces associated with wearing or removing gloves (see 'Gloves', Chapter 9).

◆ Seek medical advice if you have skin problems such as exudative lesions or weeping dermatitis and avoid direct contact with patient care until the condition resolves as per advice of the Occupational Health Department.

Hand care products

Hand care products are used to help prevent excessive dryness. Some are also responsible for skin sensitization, therefore, only suitable hand creams or lotions should be used and the following points should be considered in their choice:

+ They should be supplied in small, individual-use containers that are not refilled.

+ Some types of hand creams and lotions may interact with antiseptics (e.g. chlorhexidine) and affect the integrity of gloves.

+ Aqueous-based hand creams should be used before wearing gloves as oil-based preparations may cause latex gloves to deteriorate (see 'Gloves', Chapter 9).

Key references and further reading

Ahmed QA, Memish ZA, Allegranzi B, *et al.* Muslim health-care workers and alcohol-based handrubs. *Lancet* 2006; **367**:1025–7.

Allegranzi B, Memish ZA, Donaldson L, *et al.* Religion and culture: potential undercurrents influencing hand hygiene promotion in healthcare. *American Journal of Infection Control* 2009; **37**:28–34.

Kampf G, Loffler H. Dermatological aspects of a successful introduction and continuation of alcohol-based hand rubs for hygienic hand disinfection. *Journal of Hospital Infection*, 2003; **55**:1–7.

Lee WS, Schwarz N. Washing away postdecisional dissonance. *Science* 2010; **328**:709.

Pittet D, Boyce JM .Hand hygiene and patient care: pursuing the Semmelweis legacy. *Lancet Infectious Diseases* 2001; **April**:9–20.

Pittet D, Allegranzi B, Sax H, *et al.* Evidence-based model for hand transmission during patient care and the role or improved practices. *Lancet Infectious Diseases* 2006; **6**:641–52.

Price PB: The bacteriology of normal skin: A new quantitative test applied to a study of the bacterial flora and the disinfectant action of mechanical cleansing. *Journal of Infectious Diseases* 1938; **63**:301–18.

Sax H, Allegraniz B. Uçay I, *et al.* 'My five moments for hand hygiene': a user-centered design approach to understand, train, monitor and report hand hygiene. *Journal of Hospital Infection* 2007; **67**(7):9–21.

WHO. *WHO Guidelines on Hand Hygiene in Health Care: First Global Patient Safety Challenge. Clean Care is Safer Care.* Geneva: World Health Organization, 2009.

Chapter 9

Personal protective equipment

> Some little bug is going
> to find you some day,
> some little bug will creep
> behind you some day.
>
> *Roy Atwell, 1878*

In 1890, William Halsted was using carbolic acid in the operating theatre, as introduced by Joseph Lister after the publication of germ theory. Since his nurse's hands were sensitive to carbolic acid, in order to prevent damage to her skin he asked the Goodyear Tyre & Rubber Company if they could make a rubber glove which could be dipped in carbolic acid. Subsequently, the first disposable latex medical gloves were manufactured in 1964 by Ansell who based the production on the technique for making condoms.

The primary aim of using personal protective equipment (PPE) in health care settings is to protect the skin and mucous membranes of HCWs from exposure to blood and/ or body fluid. It also prevents contamination of clothing and reduces the opportunity of spread of microorganisms from patients and/or fomites to other patients, staff, and environments. It is essential that PPE conforming to appropriate national/international standards should be used. The decision to use and select appropriate PPE must be based upon an assessment of the level of risk associated with contamination of skin, mucous membranes, and clothing by blood and/or body fluids from a specific patient care activity or intervention. *Do not assume* that staff will be able to put on and remove PPE without contaminating themselves or others. Therefore, education and *practical training* on how to don and remove PPE safely must be given to *all* members of staff, including senior medical and nursing staff. Figure 9.1 shows the correct sequence that should be followed when donning and removing PPE to minimize contamination. It is essential that all used PPE must be disposed of following local policy.

Gloves

If gloves are correctly used, they can perform the following functions:

- Provide a protective barrier and prevent contamination of the hands when touching blood and/or body fluids from a patient or fomites.
- Sterile gloves reduce the likelihood of transmission of microorganisms from the HCW's hands to the patient during sterile and invasive procedures.

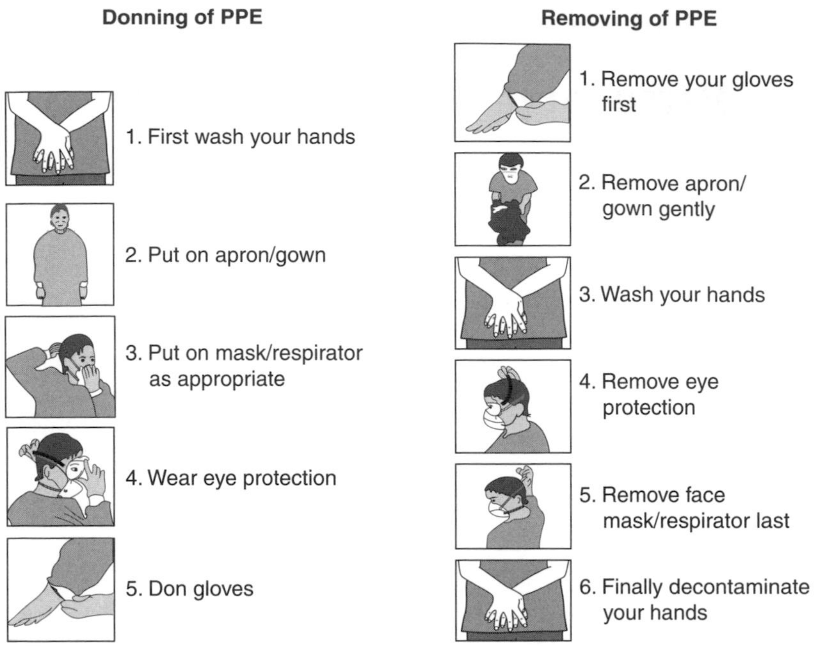

Donning of PPE

Removing of PPE

Donning of PPE	Removing of PPE
1. First wash your hands	1. Remove your gloves first
2. Put on apron/gown	2. Remove apron/ gown gently
3. Put on mask/respirator as appropriate	3. Wash your hands
4. Wear eye protection	4. Remove eye protection
5. Don gloves	5. Remove face mask/respirator last
	6. Finally decontaminate your hands

Fig. 9.1 Figure showing correct sequence of donning and removing PPE to minimize contamination. Adapted with modification from WHO *Infection prevention and control of epidemic-and pandemic-prone acute respiratory diseases in health care,* 2007.

Wearing of gloves provides a 'safe haven' for microorganisms, as it creates a moist, warm, and occlusive environment between the skin and the glove which supports microbial growth. Prolonged and inappropriate use of gloves (see Box 9.1) can be a hazard and has been associated with cross-infection and should be avoided. Once the task is finished, hands must be washed *immediately after removal* to prevent cross contamination.

In addition, gloves may have defects or tears after extended use and hands may be heavily contaminated if the proper method of removal is not followed after use. Therefore, it is important that *hands must always be decontaminated after removal of gloves* and gloves should *never* be viewed as a substitute for appropriate hand washing.

Gloves must be changed both *between patient contacts* and *between separate procedures* on the same patient. They should be removed carefully to avoid contamination of hands or other surfaces and be changed if torn or punctured. Gloved hands should neither be wiped with any form of alcoholic substance nor washed. Gloves contaminated with blood and/or body fluids must be treated as clinical waste and disposed of accordingly. Figure 9.2 shows how to don and remove single-use non-sterile gloves safely.

Glove materials

A number of materials are used in the manufacture of gloves. It is important that the most appropriate material for the purpose should be selected (see Table 9.1).

Box 9.1 Routine use of gloves is *not* recommended in the following situations (unless the patient is under contact precautions)

- For routine patient care activities, e.g. taking blood pressure, temperature, and pulse.
- Giving IV, IM, and SC injections.
- Giving oral medications (avoid contact of oral medications with hands).
- Serving food.
- During bathing and dressing the patient.
- Transporting patient.
- Caring for eyes and ears (without secretions).
- During maintenance of IV cannula (provided there is no presence of blood leakage); adequate hand disinfection would be sufficient.
- Wearing of gloves is not required for routine entry into isolation rooms if contact with the patient and/or environment is not anticipated.
- *Don't wear gloves* when using computer keyboard, telephone, writing in the patient's chart, collecting patient's dietary trays, and removing and replacing linen for patient's bed.

Adapted from WHO guidelines on hand hygiene in health care (WHO, 2009).

Latex gloves are the most widely used during surgery, especially when dexterity is required, as they are the most sensitive. Recently the quality of vinyl gloves has improved and providing the type chosen reaches the specified standards, they can be considered suitable for barrier protection. Polythene gloves are not suitable for clinical use due to their permeability and tendency to damage easily. Synthetic materials are

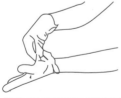 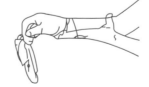 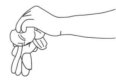

1. Pinch one glove at the wrist level to remove it, without touching the skin of the forearm, and peel away from the hand, thus allowing the glove to turn inside out.

2. Hold the removed glove in the gloved hand and slide the fingers of the ungloved hand inside between the glove and the wrist. Remove the second glove by rolling it down the hand and fold into the first glove.

3. Discard the removed gloves.

Fig. 9.2 Figure showing how to remove single-use non-sterile gloves. With permission from WHO. *WHO Guidelines on Hand Hygiene in Health Care: First Global Patient Safety Challenge. Clean Care is Safer Care.* Geneva: World Health Organization, 2009.

Table 9.1 Types of gloves and suggested uses

Glove type (materials)	Features and suggested use
Plastic/co-polymer	Cheap but fit poorly on hands and tear easily therefore they are *not recommended* as barrier precautions for infection control purposes
Non-sterile latex (natural rubber latex)	Strong and good fit but carry risk of sensitization due to latex. Non-sterile gloves should be used for procedures involving contact with blood and/or body fluids, excretions, and secretions or non-intact skin or mucous membranes where there is a risk of infection to the HCW
Sterile latex (natural rubber latex)	Strong and good fit but carry risk of sensitization due to latex. They are used when sterility is required, e.g. for sterile and aseptic procedures to prevent patients acquiring infection from HCWs. In addition, they also provide protection against blood and/or body fluids during surgical and invasive procedures
Vinyl (polyvinyl chloride)	Fit is not as good as latex gloves but less risk of sensitization. They are used for handling cytotoxic agents
Nitrile (nitrile-butadiene rubber)	More expensive than latex but less risk of sensitization. The material molecular structure is very similar to that of latex. They are not available as a surgical glove and can be used for individuals working with glutaraldehyde
Neoprene (polychloroprene)	More expensive than latex and are available as a surgical glove. They can be used for individuals who are sensitive to latex
Rubber	They are general-purpose heavy duty or household type gloves. They are used for environmental cleaning and decontamination procedures because they are robust and offer greater protection to the HCW. They should be washed in detergent and stored dry after each use. They should be replaced if punctured, torn, cracked, or showing signs of deterioration

generally more expensive than latex and due to certain properties may not be suitable for all purposes. The problem of patient or HCW sensitivity to latex proteins must be considered when deciding on glove materials.

Types of gloves

As with all items of PPE, the need for gloves and the selection of appropriate materials must be subject to careful assessment of the task to be carried out and its related risks. Having decided that gloves should be used, HCWs must make a choice between the use of sterile or non-sterile gloves depending on the tasks being undertaken. Table 9.2 summarizes the indications and the types of gloves used for various clinical activities.

Storage of gloves

Storage of glove boxes is important as once the box is open the exposed glove can be contaminated with microorganisms. In addition, gloves are much more susceptible to degradation by adverse storage conditions especially when the package is open and gloves are exposed. To preserve the integrity, it is essential that gloves are stored away

Table 9.2 Summary of the aims and indications for various clinical activities using sterile/non-sterile gloves

Type of gloves	Aims	Indications	Examples
Sterile gloves	To prevent transfer of microorganisms from HCWs to patients. In addition, they also provide protection against blood and/or body fluids during surgical and invasive procedures	For *all* surgical and aseptic procedures	◆ All surgical procedures ◆ Vaginal delivery ◆ Insertion of indwelling devices: CVC and urinary catheters, chest drain, etc. ◆ Performing lumber puncture, giving epidural, etc. ◆ Invasive radiological procedures ◆ Preparing total parenteral nutrition and chemotherapeutic agents
Non-sterile gloves	To protect HCWs from acquiring microorganisms from patients or contaminated environment	*Whenever* there is potential for touching blood and/or body fluids, secretions, excretions or contact with infectious and dangerous microorganisms *both* from direct and indirect contact either with patients, items/equipment or environment	Direct contact with blood and/or body fluids by: ◆ Contact with non-intact skin or mucous membranes e.g. per vaginal examination, oral care, emptying urinary bags, suctioning non-closed systems of endotracheal tubes ◆ Contact with potential presence of infectious and dangerous microorganisms both on intact and non-intact skin Indirect contact with blood and/or body fluids by: ◆ Handling and cleaning of contaminated items/equipment ◆ Handling of hospital waste ◆ Cleaning up spills of blood and body fluids

from sunlight, excessive heat, high humidity, and moisture. In addition, they must also be kept away from x-ray machines, high-intensity fluorescent light and ultraviolet light, and sources of ozone.

Integrity of gloves

It is important to note that lotions containing oils (including mineral, lanolin, coconut, palm, or jojoba), petroleum jelly, and other petroleum-based products break down chemical bonds of latex gloves thereby weakening their barrier properties. Water or glycerine-based lotions will not compromise the integrity of gloves and are acceptable if their use is considered necessary. If alcohol hand rub products are used on hands prior to donning of gloves, it is important that alcohol must be allowed to dry on hands as if liquid alcohol is present on hands, it may degrade the gloves.

Long fingernails and jewellery don't only harbour microorganisms but can also cause minor breaks which may not be visible to the naked eye. In addition, they may tear and rip gloves.

Latex allergy

With the advent of the HIV/AIDS epidemic in the mid 1980s, CDC introduced the term 'universal precautions' and recommended the use of gloves for all blood and body fluids. As a result, use of gloves increased substantially and has contributed to a rise in the incidence of latex allergy amongst HCWs.

Latex protein is a natural component of rubber which tends to produce an immediate hypersensitivity reaction (Type I) whilst other chemicals used in processing latex products can cause delayed hypersensitivity responses (Type IV). The usual route of exposure is the skin. To minimize the risk of allergy, latex gloves should have low levels of extractable proteins and residual accelerators. Evidence indicates that glove powder aerosolizes latex proteins causing the allergens to be inhaled by both the glove wearer and others in the immediate environment.

To minimize it, it is recommended that all latex gloves should contain low/no powder. Patients should be asked about a history of allergy to latex. Some health care facilities are creating a 'latex free' zone. In order to minimize latex allergy amongst HCWs, it is important that gloves should be worn only when necessary and be removed as soon as possible after the task is completed. HCWs who develop sensitivity or allergy to latex should be referred to the Occupational Health Department and should be advised to use other types of gloves, (see Table 9.1).

Aprons and gowns

Aprons

Single-use disposable plastic aprons are recommended for general use and should be worn when there is a risk that clothing or uniforms may become exposed to blood and/or body fluids (Table 9.3). Plastic aprons should be worn as single-use items for one procedure or episode of patient care only. Once the task is performed, they must be removed *immediately after use* by tearing the neck strap and waist tie and

Table 9.3 Assessment of apron and gown types against use

Apron/gown types	Aim	Suggested uses
Disposable plastic aprons	◆ To prevent contamination of uniform and clothing as they may spread microorganisms ◆ To prevent uniform from getting wet	◆ Whenever there is likelihood of splashing with blood and/or body fluids ◆ Contact with patients who are likely to contaminate uniform with pathogens or multiresistant microorganisms ◆ Carrying out procedures such as bathing patients, etc
Full length plastic aprons *or* disposable water impervious gowns	◆ To prevent contamination of uniform and clothing as they may spread microorganisms	◆ Whenever there is likelihood of splashing with large amount of blood and/or body fluids ◆ Likelihood of prolonged/extensive contact with patients who are likely to contaminate uniform with pathogens or multiresistant microorganisms
Sterile, water-impervious gowns	◆ To prevent spread of microorganisms from the HCW during aseptic/surgical procedures ◆ To prevent contamination of clothing and skin of wearer during surgery and aseptic procedures	◆ For use in surgical and aseptic procedures

gently rolling it inwards to minimize contamination of microorganisms during disposal. They must be removed before leaving the isolation room to prevent dispersal of micro-organisms in the environment (see Figure 9.3). Hands must be washed immediately after removing and bagging the soiled plastic aprons in the clinical waste bags.

Gowns

Clean, non-sterile gowns should be worn during procedures which are likely to expose HCWs to spraying or splashing of blood and/or body fluids (Table 9.3). Gowns should be *impermeable* and *water repellent* or have water-repellent panels in the areas most prone to exposure. If the gown is expected to become wet during the procedure and if a water-repellent gown is not available, a plastic apron should be worn over the gown. Once the task is performed, the gown must be removed *immediately* after use by *gently rolling it inwards* to reduce contamination of microorganisms during disposal. Soiled gowns should be placed in a clinical waste bag before leaving the room (see Figure 9.4). Heavily soiled gowns made of fabric should be placed in the leak-proof laundry bag.

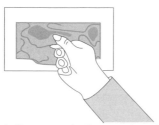

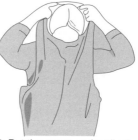

1. Remove a plastic apron from the dispenser.

2. Put the apron on by slipping the neck end over the head.

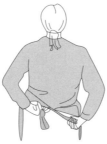

3. Secure the apron to the body by tying the waist ties.

How to safely remove plastic apron

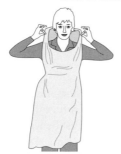

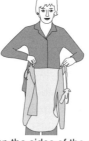

1. Grasp the sides of the apron at the top and pull to break the neck end gently and roll inwards.

2. Grasp the sides of the apron (at waist level) and pull to break the waist ties, and gently roll plastic apron inwards.

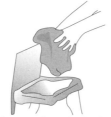

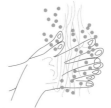

3. Remove from the body and discard into the waste bin.

4. Decontaminate the hands.

Fig. 9.3 Figure showing how to wear and remove a plastic apron.

How to wear protective gown

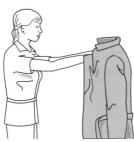

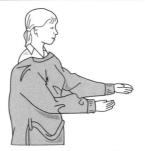

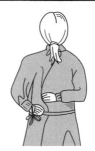

1. Select a gown and holding it by the neck, allow it to unfold downwards, open side in front of you.

2. Slip the hands through the cuffs and adjust to a comfortable fit by pulling inside the neck so that the gown sits comfortably on the neck and shoulders.

3. Tie the neck tapes and the waistbelt at the side of the garment using a bow.

How to remove a protective gown

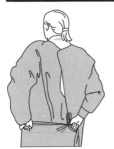

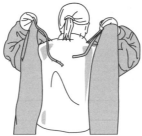

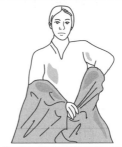

3. Untie the waistbelt.

2. Untie the neck-ties and undo the closure.

3. Remove first one then the other sleeve and slip the gown off.

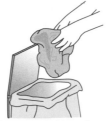

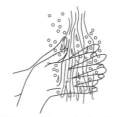

4. Handling by the inside surface only and holding away from the body, discard the gown into a waste bin.

5. Decontaminate the hands.

Fig. 9.4 Figure showing how to wear and remove a protective gown.

Protective eye/facewear

The aim of protective eyewear (glasses, goggles, or face-shields) is to help guard the mucous membranes of the eyes, nose, and mouth of the HCW from exposure to blood and/or body fluids that may be splashed, sprayed, or splattered into the face during clinical procedures. Protective eyewear must be worn during procedures that are likely to generate droplets or aerosols of blood and/or high-risk body fluids. They should comply with approved standards, must be close fitting, optically clear, anti-fog, distortion free, and shielded at the side. They can be integral with some surgical facemasks and this can be convenient when both are required.

Surgical face mask

The type of mask best suited to a particular situation depends on the body substances likely to be encountered and the nature of the activity. Wearing of masks during routine ward procedures such as wound dressing or invasive medical procedures is *not* necessary. Masks in conjunction with eyewear should be worn during procedures that are likely to generate aerosols or splashes of blood and/or body fluids to prevent contamination of mucous membranes of the mouth, nose, and eyes.

It is important to note that surgical masks provide protection against droplets nuclei because they are not designed to provide a close facial seal which is essential for protection of airborne particles of <5 μ. In addition they should also be changed as soon as practicably possible if they become visibly contaminated or moist.

Figure 9.5 shows how to wear and remove face masks properly. If the masks are used then they should:

- Be fitted according to the manufacturer's instructions.
- The front of the mask should not be touched by hands while being worn and must be removed by untying and handling *only by the ties* and *never* by the face-covering part which may be heavily contaminated with microorganisms.
- Not be worn loosely around the neck, but be removed and discarded as clinical waste as soon as practicable after use.

Respirators

The respirator provides protection against inhalation of very tiny (<5 microns in size) airborne particles to the HCWs. They should be close fitting and must filter particles of size of 1–5 μm. In the USA, it is recommended to use NIOSH-certified N95 particulate respirators. N series respirators provide protection against non-oil-based aerosols, including *Mycobacterium tuberculosis* and the '95' indicates that the mask material is capable of 95% efficient filtration of particles 0.3 μm in diameter. In Europe, use either FFP2 (= N95) or FFP3 (= N100). Masks must conform to BS EN 149: 2001 Standard. FFP is an abbreviation of 'filtering face piece' and the '3'denotes the filtration efficiency of the respirator. FFP3 masks can be used for up to 8 hours provided the integrity of the mask is not compromised.

The respirator must seal tightly to the face to prevent air entering from the sides. A good fit is only achievable where there is good mask-to-skin contact (Figure 9.6). FFP2 or FFP3 respiratory masks are unsuitable for HCWs with facial hair as it affects the seal between the mask and the face. Beards, sideburns, or even a visible growth of stubble will affect the face seal of such masks which rely on close contact between the face and the mask.

The efficiency lost to facial leakage is not indicated by a grading but on individual facial fit testing alone. Staff who may be required to wear an FFP3 mask *must be trained* in how to fit the mask to their face for maximum benefit. In the UK, fit testing is a legal requirement as is keeping a record of such testing. The mask should be replaced after

How to wear a Facemask

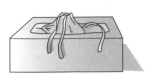

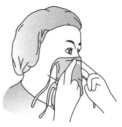

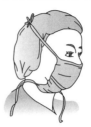

1. Select a facemask from the dispenser box.

2. Bring the mask to the face, placing the metal nosepiece over the bridge of the nose to ensure a close and comfortable fit.

3. Secure by tying the top set of strings behind the head.

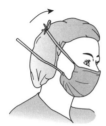

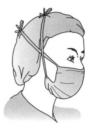

4. Pull the bottom of the mask to fit closely under the chin.

5. Secure by tying the bottom set of strings, high on the head above the first set.

How to remove a Facemask

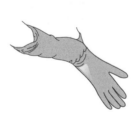

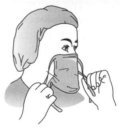

1. Remove gloves if worn and decontaminate the hands.

2. Untie the strings and remove the mask handling only by the strings.

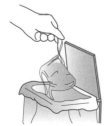

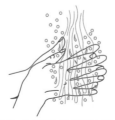

3. Dispose of the mask into the waste bin.

4. Decontaminate the hands.

Fig. 9.5 Figure showing how to wear and remove a face mask properly.

1. Noseclip is located in top panel. Preform the noseclip by gently bending at the centre of the panel. Hold respirator in one hand and pull out bottom panel to form a cup.

2. Turn respirator over to expose headbands.

3. Cup respirator under chin and pull the straps over the head.

4. Locate the lower strap below the ears and the upper strap across the crown of the head. Adjust top and bottom panels for a comfortable fit.

5. Using both hands, mould noseclip to the shape of the lower part of the nose. Pinching the nosepiece using only one hand may result in less effective respirator peformance.

6. The seal of the respirator on the face should be fit-checked prior to wearing in the work area.

Fig. 9.6 Figure showing how to wear a 3M respirator properly.

each use and changed if breathing becomes difficult or if the mask becomes damaged or obviously contaminated, or if a proper face fit cannot be maintained.

The choice of the measure is driven by the degree of protection deemed necessary, and secondary factors such as the acceptance of the mask (comfort) may also play a role in the choice. Some respirators with certified protection factors are sold with or without exhalation valves. Masks with such valves are much more comfortable to wear, especially in the long run, but provide no protection to the environment from the aerosol emissions of the wearer.

Fit testing

If a HCW fails the fit test then this should be repeated using the same mask and ensuring that the mask is fitted to the face correctly. If a HCW fails the fit test on two separate occasions then alternative masks/hoods are considered as one mask type will not fit everyone; in such cases purchase of additional types of masks is necessary for some staff. It is recommended that fit testing should be undertaken on a yearly basis.

Aerosol generating procedures

The FFP3 or N95 particulate respirators should be used when caring for patients with known/suspected open pulmonary or laryngeal tuberculosis. It should also be used when managing patients with highly infectious respiratory tract infection (e.g. SARS, pandemic or avian influenza) only when aerosol-generating procedures (AGPs) are performed. Where possible, AGPs should be avoided or alternative methods should be considered. When performing AGPs, only essential staff should be present. According to World Health Organization (WHO, 2009), the following are classified as AGPs:

Intubation and related procedures, e.g. manual ventilation, respiratory and airway suctioning (including tracheostomy care and open suctioning with invasive ventilation), cardiopulmonary resuscitation, bronchoscopy, collection of lower respiratory tract specimens (e.g. bronchial and tracheal aspirates), and autopsy procedures. In dental practice, it includes the use of hand pieces (especially air rotor) in the patient's mouth, and scaling using an ultrasonic or air scaler (but not hand scaling).

The following procedures are *not* classified as AGPs:

Mechanical ventilation or respiratory therapy treatment unless an AGP is being performed on an open system, closed suctioning with invasive ventilation, non-invasive positive pressure ventilation (BiPAP), bi-level positive airway pressure (BPAP), nasopharyngeal aspiration, and nebulisation (but this procedure should be performed in an area physically separate from other patients). Chest physiotherapy is not considered an AGP but a surgical mask should be worn by the patient if tolerated and HCWs should wear PPE as recommended for routine care (surgical mask) during the procedure.

Once the task is complete, the contaminated respirators should be disposed of immediately as clinical waste and not laid on any working surface. Hands should be decontaminated immediately after removing and disposing of respirators. It is also important that when a respirator is used, HCWs should not fall into a false sense of security and they must follow all other recommended IPC precautions. In the event of a break in infection control procedures, e.g. incorrectly worn FFP3 during an AGP, the member of staff should be reviewed by Occupational Health.

Key references and further reading

CDC/HICPAC. Guideline for isolation precautions: preventing transmission of infectious agents in healthcare settings 2007. *American Journal of Infection Control*, 2007; **35**(10):S65–S164.

Medical Devices Agency. *Latex Sensitization in the Health-care Setting (Use of Latex Gloves)*. (Device Bulletin No MDA DB 9601). London: Medical Devices Agency, 1996.

Pratt RJ, Pellowe CM, Wilson JA, *et al*. epic 2: National Evidence-based guidelines for preventing healthcare associated infections in NHS hospital in England. *Journal of Hospital Infection*; 2007; **65**(Suppl):S1–S64.

WHO. *WHO Guidelines on Hand Hygiene in Health Care: First Global Patient Safety Challenge. Clean Care is Safer Care*. Geneva: World Health Organization, 2009.

WHO. *Infection Prevention and Control of Epidemic-and Pandemic-prone Acute Respiratory Diseases in Health Care*. Geneva: World Health Organization, 2007.

WHO. *Infection Prevention and control during health care for confirmed, probable or suspected cases of pandemic (H1N1) 2009 virus infection and influenza like illness*. Geneva: World Health Organization, 2009.

Chapter 10

Control of multiresistant microorganisms

2000 BC – Here, eat this root
1000 AD – That root is heathen. Here, say this prayer
1850 AD – That prayer is superstition. Here, drink this potion
1920 AD – That potion is snake oil. Here, swallow this pill
1945 AD – That pill is ineffective. Here, take this penicillin
1955 AD – 'Oops' . . . bugs mutated. Here, take this tetracycline
1960–1999 – 39 more 'oops' . . . Here, take this more powerful antibiotic
2000 AD – The bugs have won! Here, eat this root.

Anonymous

Antibiotic stewardship

All species on this planet have an obvious goal—to get fitter and survive! Microbes are the simplest form of life, first appearing over 3.5 billion years, and are arguably the most adaptable organisms, inhabiting nearly every corner of the globe. They existed in the world before dinosaurs; while the dinosaurs are extinct, microbes have not only survived but have mutated and flourished with time. The main reason for their survival is that, unlike dinosaurs, they are extremely adaptable to the ever changing environment. As Charles Darwin puts it, 'it is not the strongest of the species that survive, nor the most intelligent, but the ones most responsive to change'.

Microbes, due to their adaptability, have not only survived the selective pressures exerted by the indiscriminate use of antimicrobial agents but have successfully adapted and evolved in to multidrug-resistant organisms (MDROs). It is important to note that indiscriminate use of antimicrobial agents is not only common in health care setting but is also common in veterinary practices where up to 50% of antibiotics are consumed.

A plethora of guidelines to control and promote rational use of antimicrobials has not curtailed the plague of antimicrobial resistance. For various reasons, non-compliance with guidelines, policies, and procedures is not uncommon. It is well acknowledged that mankind has not always complied perfectly with authority, reasons, or evidence. According to the book of Genesis, man was exiled from the Garden of Eden because of non-compliance with divine expectations. Therefore successful implementation of any guidelines is not an easy task.

Clinicians play a key role in controlling inappropriate use of antibiotics and should take responsibility for rational prescribing not only to prevent emergence of antibiotic-resistant microorganisms (MRSA, ESBL, VRE, etc.) but also to prevent *Clostridium difficile*-associated diarrhoea. It interesting that when meticillin was available in the 1960s, St George's Hospital, London used it for 'fogging' in the nursery air to eliminate staphylococcal infections in neonates (Elek et al., 1960). During the same time, meticillin was also sprayed on the surgical wards in Melbourne hospitals to prevent surgical site infections. The following strategies should be used in health care setting to promote appropriate use of antimicrobial agents:

◆ Educate clinical staff on appropriateness of prescribing preferably by a clinical microbiologist.

◆ Distribute approved guidelines to all medical staff preferably as a simplified pocket guide and keep a copy on the ward/department and make it easily available on the on intranet, if possible.

◆ Microbiology laboratories should introduce restricted reporting based on the local guideline to encourage use of narrow-spectrum antibiotics and antibiotics which are part of the antibiotic formulary.

◆ Prescribe antibiotics with good clinical reasons and not 'just in case' and the reasons for prescribing must be documented in the medical notes.

◆ If an antibiotic therapy is prescribed on an empirical basis, then it must be reviewed on a daily basis. Change to a narrow-spectrum antibiotic once the bacteriology results are available or stop if the infective cause is excluded.

◆ Prescribe narrow-spectrum antibiotics, where possible, with minimum duration. Consider introducing automatic stop date after 5 days unless specified otherwise in the clinical notes.

Antibiotic cycling refers to the rotation of antibiotics with similar spectrums of activity, with a return to the original antibiotic after a defined period of time. The basic premise of this intervention is that during periods when an antibiotic is out of rotation, resistance to those agents declines because of reduced selective pressure on those antibiotic classes. However, systematic review examining the efficacy of antibiotic cycling concluded that the current evidence is too weak to support the advocacy of this intervention as a means of reducing antibiotic resistance rates (Brown et al., 2005).

Antibiotic resistance

Types of antibiotic resistance

They are two types of resistance: 1) **intrinsic resistance** depends on the natural properties of bacteria and mechanisms of action, e.g. Gram-negative bacteria are naturally resistant to vancomycin and enterococci are resistant to cephalosporins, and 2) **acquired resistance** can be either through chromosomal mutation or by plasmid transfer. Plasmids are extra-chromosomal elements of bacterial DNA and, like the chromosome, carry genetic information about antibiotic resistance. Another means of resistance transfer is by means of minute mobile genetic (DNA) elements found on either chromosome or plasmid (*transposons*, which are often found on plasmids) which can move from plasmid to plasmid or to the chromosome. A transposon can mediate single or multiple resistances and can, after entering a bacterial cell, become incorporated in its plasmid or chromosome. It is not uncommon for more than one resistance mechanism to be present in a single bacterial strain.

Plasmid-mediated resistance is generally of greater clinical importance than chromosomal, since bacteria which have undergone chromosomal mutation are usually metabolically impaired and less well able to multiply than non-mutant members of the population.

Plasmid-mediated resistance is usually based on the synthesis of proteins which either act as enzymes or change the cell wall in such a way that the antibiotic can no longer penetrate. Plasmids can be transferred from one bacterial cell to another by conjugation, transduction, or by transformation.

Conjugation is the main method of transfer for Gram-negative bacteria in which genetic material is transferred between bacterial cells by direct cell-to-cell contact or by a bridge-like connection between two cells. It is regarded as the bacterial equivalent of *sexual mating* since it involves the exchange of genetic material by the *donor cell* which transfers a mobile genetic element (a plasmid or transposon) via pilius to the *recipient* cell that does not contain a similar element.

Transduction is the process by which DNA is introduced into another cell via a viral vector or bacteriophages (viruses that infect bacteria). When transduction happens, it goes through either the lytic cycle (lysis) of bacterial cell or the lysogenic cycle. If the lysogenic cycle is adopted, the phage chromosome is integrated into the bacterial chromosome, where it can remain dormant for many years.

Transformation occurs as result of uptake or incorporation of exogenous genetic (DNA) material from its surrounding after the destruction of a cell which is taken up through the cell membrane(s). It occurs most commonly in bacteria and in some species occurs naturally but it can be affected by artificial means.

Mechanisms of acquired antibiotic resistance

Mechanisms of acquired antibiotic resistance can mainly occur as a result of:

- Destruction or inactivation of antibiotics, e.g. beta-lactam antibiotics, chloramphenicol, and aminoglycosides.

- An alteration of antibiotic target site to reduce/eliminate binding of the antibiotic to the target, e.g. beta-lactam antibiotics, fusidic acid, glycopeptides, erythromycin.

- Impaired uptake of the antibiotic either due to reduction in the cell permeability or blockage of the mechanism by which the antibiotic enters the cell, e.g. beta-lactam antibiotics, chloramphenicol, and quinolones.

- Enhanced efflux of the antibiotic, e.g. tetracycline.

- Acquisition of a replacement for metabolites step inhibited by antibiotic, e.g. trimethoprim and sulphonamides.

Examples of *chromosomally mediated resistance* mechanisms included altered penicillin-binding protein (PBP) with reduced affinity for beta-lactam antibiotics (e.g. MRSA), mutations in DNA gyrase enzyme resulting in resistance to quinolones, and overproduction of dihydrofolate reductase enzyme found in isolates resistant to trimethoprim. Examples of *plasmid-mediated resistance mechanisms* are production of beta-lactamase enzymes that hydrolyse penicillins, production of extended spectrum beta-lactamases (ESBL) that can hydrolyse third-generation cephalosporins, and production of aminoglycoside-modifying enzymes and resistance to tetracycline due to energy-dependent efflux mechanisms.

Role of drugs and therapeutics committee

The drugs and therapeutics committee of the hospital plays a key role in the promotion of rational antibiotic prescribing. They should meet on a regular basis with following objectives:

- Formulate antibiotic guidelines based on the local antimicrobial resistance pattern and review guidelines on a regular basis. Send guidelines for wider consultation to the clinical staff to ensure ownership.
- Formulate guidelines for both hospital and community settings.
- Regularly review antibiotic utilization and cost data.
- Approve use of newer agents based on the clinical efficacy, cost, and side effect profile. Once approved, the use of new antimicrobial agents should be restricted to agreed clinical conditions and be prescribed only on the advice of a clinical microbiologist or infectious diseases physician.
- Monitor compliance with the guidelines and feedback data to the senior medical staff on a regular basis to influence prescribing habits. It is important to note that compliance data with the guidelines are generally collected by pharmacists will *not* provide information on the *appropriateness* of prescribing as they do not have the qualifications and expertise to assess whether patients had an infection or not.

If the resources are available, conduct **antibiotic ward rounds** at least once a week involving microbiologist, antimicrobial pharmacist, and a nominated clinical member (McCorry et al., 2010). The information from the antibiotic ward round must be fed back to the senior clinicians and senior management in a timely manner. During the antibiotic ward rounds, consider to review the following data:

- Does the patient really need antibiotic(s)?
- Is the reason for prescribing documented in the medical notes and supported by the clinical and other relevant information?
- Have the appropriate specimens been collected prior to starting antibiotic therapy?
- If the microbiology reports are available, was the antibiotic switched to a narrow-spectrum agent(s)?
- Is the dose, frequency, and route of administration appropriate?

- Is prescribing in accordance with local antibiotic guidelines?
- Is the selection of an antibiotic based on the previous/recent bacteriological reports?
- Is there any clear documentation of allergy to antibiotics?

Control of multidrug-resistant microorganisms

Beside parasites, viruses, and mycobacteria, the most clinically important multidrug-resistant bacterial infections encountered in health care setting are:

- Meticillin-resistant *Staphylococcus aureus* (MRSA).
- Multi-resistant species of coagulase negative staphylococci.
- Vancomycin-resistant enterococci (VRE).
- Penicillin resistant *Streptococcus pneumoniae* (PRP).
- Multidrug resistant Gram-negative bacilli (e.g. *Escherichia coli*, *Klebsiella* spp., *Enterobacter* spp., *Citrobacter* spp., *Serratia* spp., *Pseudomonas* spp., and *Acinetobacter* spp.).

Control of multidrug-resistant microorganisms is essential, as it has following impacts:

- The patient is less likely to respond to the first-line empirical antibiotic therapy.
- Restriction of use of narrow-spectrum agents which has a lesser incidence of *C. difficle* infections.
- Limited choice in selection of older 'tried and tested 'agents which are cheaper and their efficacy and side effect profiles are well known.
- Use of more expensive, newer agents with increasing cost. In addition, newer agents have restricted licensing conditions due to limited availability of clinical data on their efficacy and side effect profiles.
- Patients may have to stay longer in the hospital as some preparations are available only in IV formulation and some MDROs have higher morbidity.
- Increased costs of isolation precautions and cost of additional investigations due to extra length of stay.

The management approach depends on two factors: 1) endemicity of the resistant microorganisms in the health care facility, and 2) vulnerability of the patients in the wards/unit where they occur. It is important to ensure that a proper surveillance and monitoring system is in place for all MDROs. Risk factors for multidrug-resistant microorganisms are outlined in Box 10.1 and overall strategies for the prevention and control of MRDOs are outlined in Tables 10.1 and 10.2 which summarize the overall characteristics of the most commonly encountered MRDOs in health care setting worldwide.

Box 10.1 Risk factors for multidrug-resistant microorganisms

- Use of broad-spectrum antibiotics (esp. second- and third-generation cephalosporins and quinolones). Treatment with previous glycopeptide (e.g. vancomycin, teicoplanin) in VRE patients.
- Patients with severe underlying disease and who are chronically debilitated.
- Immmunocompromised and patients with extensive burns.
- Critically ill patients with prolong hospital stay, especially in ICU, oncology, transplant, and burns wards.
- Presence with indwelling devices, e.g. IV lines, urinary catheters, endotracheal intubation, surgical drains, PEG tubes, gastrostomy, and jejunostomy tube.
- Patients who have intra-abdominal, cardiothoracic, orthopaedic, vascular, and urological procedures/surgery.
- Contact with health care facilities (hospital or community long-term care facility) where MRDO is endemic and patients have spent more than 12 continuous hours in the past 12 months (PIDAC guideline, 2007).

Table 10.1 Strategies for the prevention and control of MRDOs

Key strategies	Action for the prevention and control of MRDOs
Implementation and monitoring of antibiotic stewardship programme	◆ Inappropriate and indiscriminate use of antibiotics exerts selective pressure and leads to emergence of MDROs. Therefore antibiotic stewardship programmes should be implemented both in hospitals and the community ◆ Use narrow-spectrum antibiotics, if possible. Avoid use of broad-spectrum antibiotics (esp. third-generation cephalosporins and quinolones). Judicious use of glycopeptides (e.g. vancomycin, teicoplanin) to prevent emergence of VRE
Identification of patients by active surveillance	◆ Active surveillance should be instituted at the time of admission to identify colonized/infected patients esp. from health care facilities and/or countries where MRDOs is endemic ◆ Active surveillance will help identify clusters/outbreaks of MDROs and assist IPC to investigate and take appropriate IPC measures to minimize spread and control outbreaks in health care facilities
Prompt isolation of patients and implementation of contact precautions	◆ Early identification by taking screening swabs and prompt isolation is an essential step in control of MDROs. This is essential esp. if the patients are being admitted to high-risk unit, i.e. ICU, NNU, burns, transplant unit, etc. The patients should be kept in isolation until the swab results are available ◆ On confirmation, application of contact precautions must be instituted immediately ◆ Hand hygiene is crucial to prevent cross-infection and this must be rigorously enforced. Hands must be washed after removing gloves and PPE ◆ Decolonization therapy should be used to reduce the bioburden of microorganisms and should be considered for patients with MRSA. However, for other MDROs, decolonization therapy is not effective and should not be used (see Table 10.2)

(continued)

Table 10.1 (*continued*) Strategies for the prevention and control of MRDOs

Key strategies	Action for the prevention and control of MRDOs
Prevent spread in health care facilities	◆ Restrict unnecessary movement of patients between wards/hospitals. If transfer is essential then receiving ward/department/hospital must be informed in advance so that patients are isolated in a side room with appropriate infection control precautions implemented on admission. On transfer/discharge of patients to other wards and/or health care facilities, it is the responsibility of the clinical team to communicate with the receiving ward/health care facilities so that appropriate measures are taken to prevent cross-infection and patients are isolated ◆ Consider early discharge of patient to home, if possible ◆ Tagging of patients' medical notes with MDROs must be done so that on readmission these patients should be isolated immediately in a side room ◆ Electronic database of patients may also be tagged so that there is an alert to a health care facility on readmission
Role of microbiology laboratory	◆ The microbiology laboratory must use internationally accepted methods for prompt and *accurate* identification and antibiotic susceptibility testing of microorganisms ◆ Keep up to date in the methods of detection resistance in MDROs and send isolates to reference laboratory for further confirmation, if required ◆ Microbiology laboratory should introduce restricted reporting based on the local guideline to encourage use of antibiotics which are narrow spectrum and in accordance with local guidelines based on the local resistance pattern ◆ Establish local laboratory surveillance system (e.g. WHO net) and feed data into the national surveillance system ◆ Surveillance of MDROs will help the IPC team to monitor epidemiological trends, and measuring the effectiveness of IPC interventions and help the hospital to develop antibiotic guidelines based on local antibiotic resistance patterns
Cleaning and decontamination of patient care items/equipment	◆ Consider use of single-use disposable items, if possible. Some patient care items should be dedicated (i.e. thermometers, tourniquet, and stethoscope) to single-patient use only. Other items can be discarded (if heavily soiled, or cannot be adequately decontaminated) or must thoroughly be cleaned and disinfected/sterilized as per local protocols
Cleaning and disinfection of environment	◆ Cleaning schedules should be increased to reduce the bioload of the microorganisms in the environment and appropriate disinfectant should be used in addition to detergent to decontaminate environment with special emphasis on cleaning of 'hand touch' surfaces
Education and training	◆ For any programme to be successful, education and training of health care personnel in appropriate infection prevention and control procedures, aseptic techniques for medical and nursing procedures, and antibiotic prescribing is essential

Table 10.2 Summary and characteristics of most commonly encountered MRDOs in health care setting

	Gram-positive		Gram-negative	
	MRSA	VRE	ESBL and *Pseudomonas spp.*	*Acinetobacter*
Pathogenicity	High/moderate	Low	High/moderate	Low
Human reservoirs of organisms	Nose and moist and hairy areas of the body area, e.g. groin and axillae	GI tract, anterior urethra, vagina, skin, and oropharynx	GI tract	Human skin, forearm, forehead and toe webs
Antibiotic selective pressure	Quinolones (e.g. ciprofloxacin, levofloxacin, moxifloxacin). Cephalosporins esp. 3rd-generation	Glycopeptides (e.g. vancomycin, teicoplanin)	2nd- and 3rd-generation cephalosporins, carbapenems, and aztreonam	Broad spectrum antibiotic esp. 3rd-generation cephalosporins and imipenem
Patients placement in a side ward	Yes esp. if the patient has skin conditions, URT with sneezing/cough and open wounds and draining lesions which cannot be covered	Yes esp. if the patient has diarrhoea	Yes esp. if the patient has diarrhoea or indwelling devices	Yes esp. in high risk area ICU, burns unit etc.
Isolation precautions	Contact	Contact	Contact	Contact

(continued)

Table 10.2 (*Continued*) Summary and characteristics of most commonly encountered MRDOs in health care setting

	Gram-positive		Gram-negative	
	MRSA	**VRE**	**ESBL and Pseudomonas spp.**	**Acinetobacter**
Screening swabs from hospitalized patients	Nose, perianal, or groin swab. Skin lesions, wounds, incisions, ulcers and exit sites of indwelling devices, if present. Umbilicus swab from newborn infants	Faeces or deep rectal swab or colostomy. Umbilicus swab from newborn infants	Faeces or deep rectal swab or colostomy. Umbilicus swab from newborn infants	Skin lesions, wounds, incisions, ulcers and exit sites of indwelling devices, if present. Umbilicus swab from newborn infants
	Colonize wounds, ulcers and medical device sites	Colonize wounds, ulcers and medical device sites	Colonize wounds, ulcers and medical device sites	Colonize wounds, ulcers and medical device sites esp. in ICU
Decolonization therapy available	Yes (selected cases only. see 'Decolonization therapy' section)	Not effective	Not effective	Not effective
Survival in the environment	7 days to 7 months	5 days to 4 months	Few hours to several months	3 days to 5 months esp. humid conditions
Comments	Staff with skin lesions, eczema, or superficial skin sepsis should be excluded from contact with the patient (esp. in high risk areas) as these HCWs are more likely to get colonized and may act as 'disperser'	Enterococci persist in the environment for a prolonged period	Enterobacteriaceae and Pseudomonas spp. survive in wet environments. Keep environment and items/equipment clean and dry	A. baumannii is the most commonly seen in ICU setting. Infections are more common in warm climates and in summer months. It is relatively resistant to drying and disinfectants. Once endemic, the organism is difficult to eradicate and has been called as 'Gram-negative MRSA'

Meticillin-resistant *Staphyloccocus aureus*

The name *Staphylococcus* originated from the Greek word *staphyle* [bunch of grapes] + *kokkos*, [berry]). The bacterium was discovered in 1881 by Sir Alexander Ogston who was a professor at the University of Aberdeen. *Staph. aureus* is carried by approximately 30% of healthy people in their nose and other moist and hairy areas of the body, e.g. groin and axillae; in addition, another third are occasional carriers. It is one of the most common pathogens, well known for causing skin and soft tissue infection, e.g. impetigo, folliculitis, cellulitis, abscesses. In addition, *Staph. aureus* may cause systemic infections such as pneumonia, osteomyelitis, septicaemia, endocarditis, and meningitis.

Meticillin-resistant *Staph. aureus* (MRSA: MIC to oxacillin/meticillin of ≥ 4 µg/mL) arose from meticillin-sensitive *Staph. aureus* (MSSA: MIC to oxacillin/meticillin of ≤ 2 µg/mL) by the acquisition of the *mec* A gene which is located on a genetically mobile chromosomal determinant termed staphylococcal cassette chromosome *mec* (SCC *mec*). *Mec* A gene encodes an additional penicillin-binding protein (PBP2a) which has low affinity for isoxazolyl-penicillins, such as meticillin. They are resistant to all of the beta-lactam classes of antibiotics (such as penicillins), penicillinase-resistant penicillins (e.g. Flucloxacillin, cloxacillin), and cephalosporins. In addition, vancomycin/glycopeptide-intermediate *Staph. aureus* (VISA/GISA) has been detected in some countries. In June 2002, the first clinical isolate of vancomycin resistant *Staph. aureus* (VRSA: MIC to vancomycin of ≥ 16 µg/mL) that contains the resistance genes Van-A or Van-B was isolated from the USA. It has been postulated that the transfer of the resistance occurred from a patient who was colonized with VRE.

MRSA is generally no more virulent than MSSA but they are resistant to flucloxacillin and other most commonly used anti-staphylococcal agents. However in recent years, this infection can be successfully treated with newer but more expensive agents. MRSA is usually associated with high morbidity and mortality in patients, especially in ICU and those patients who develop severe infections.

Despite vigorous attempts, eradication of MRSA over the last 30 years has not been very successful for the following reasons:

- Continued use of inappropriate/excessive use of broad-spectrum agents, especially quinolones (e.g. ciprofloxacin, levofloxacin) and cephalosporins.

- Continued failure to adhere to standard infection control practices, e.g. hand hygiene, use of aseptic non-touch technique, inadequate decontamination of items/equipment, and clinical environment.

- Overcrowding of wards with higher concentrations of long-term patients with multiple comorbidity.

- Increasing and inappropriate use of indwelling devices.

- Higher throughput of patients which can lead to inadequate decontamination of equipment and environment.

- Understaffing leading to break in implementation of infection control practices.

◆ Increased use of agency nursing/medical staff who are unfamiliar with local infection control procedures.

Community-associated MRSA

In recent years, community-associated MRSA (CA-MRSA) has emerged as a major pathogen. Infection with CA-MRSA presents most commonly as relatively minor skin and soft tissue infections, but severe invasive disease, including necrotizing pneumonia, necrotizing fasciitis, severe osteomyelitis, and a sepsis syndrome with increased mortality have also been described in children and adults.

Community strains of *Staph. aureus* (both MRSA and MSSA) also produce several toxins which are not commonly found in hospital strains notably *Panton-Valentine leukocidin* (PVL), which causes leukocyte destruction and tissue necrosis. In the USA, the predominant molecular genotypes that cause CA-MRSA infections are USA 300 and USA 400 while the hospital strains are predominantly molecular genotypes USA 100 and USA 200. In contrast, other countries (including the UK) report a variety of different clones circulating amongst the community. Guidance on the diagnosis and management of PVL-associated *Staph. aureus* infection is available from the UK Health Protection Agency web site (http://www.hpa.org.uk).

Control measures

Summary of infection control measures for MDROs including MRSA are outlined in Box 10.2. If it becomes apparent that the rate of MRSA is disproportionately high, then specific and locally appropriate preventative measures need to be developed and implemented.

Non-endemic situation

In health care facilities where the MRSA is non-endemic, efforts should be made to be eliminate MRSA using a 'search and destroy' approach (Dutch Infection Prevention Working Party, 2007). Rigorous application of IPC measures have been shown to be effective in containing or eliminating the problem, although this can be expensive. Elimination involves confining colonized/infected MRSA individuals once they are identified, and detecting other patients to whom the infection may have been transmitted (as for outbreak screening). This includes early discharge of colonized/infected patients.

Endemic situation

In health care facilities where the MRSA is endemic the object to prevent transmission by isolation/cohorting of known colonized/infected patients and implementation of effective IPC measures is recommended. In high-risk patients and clinical areas (ICU, NNU, burns unit, etc.), some form of ongoing screening programme is essential in identifying those colonized at admission. An alert system for readmission of these patients is also required to make this fully effective, because MRSA carriage can be very prolonged. The benefit of universal screening of all patients on a routine basis is less clear, and costs can be considerable.

Box 10.2 Summary of infection control measures for MDROs

◆ **Patient's placement:** the patient should be nursed in a single room with *en suite* toilet facilities, if possible. If the isolation facilities are not available the patients should be risk assessed and can be cohorted into bay/area. S/he should be advised that there is no risk to healthy relatives or others outside the hospital and should be given a fact sheet. As a general rule, infected/colonized patients should be seen towards the end of a ward round, if practical. The number of staff caring for the patient should be kept to a minimum.

◆ **Visitors:** visitors must report to the nurse-in-charge before entering the room. Number of visitors should be kept to a minimum and those who are susceptible are probably best advised not to visit a patient. This must, however, be balanced against the visitor's and patient's wish for contact.

◆ **Hand hygiene:** physically clean hands must be disinfected using an alcoholic hand rub. Alternatively, wash hands with soap (or antiseptic chlorhexidine/detergent) and water before and after contact with the patient or their immediate environment.

◆ **Personal protective equipment:** single-use disposable gloves must be worn when handling contaminated tissue, dressings, or linen. Hands must be washed *after* removing gloves. Single-use disposable plastic aprons must be worn for activities involving contact with the patient or his/her environment and should be discarded into a clinical waste bag before leaving the room. Non-permeable disposable gowns are required only for extensive physical contact with the patient. Masks should be used for procedures that may generate staphylococcus aerosols, e.g. sputum suction, chest physiotherapy, or procedures on patients with an exfoliative skin condition, and when performing dressings on patients with extensive burns or lesions.

◆ **Decontamination of item/equipment:** use dedicated equipment (e.g. stethoscope, sphygmomanometer, thermometer, and tourniquet). Any reusable disposal items must be disinfected/sterilized according to local policy.

◆ **Clinical waste:** all single-use items must be disposed of as clinical waste. Clinical waste bags must be sealed before leaving the room.

◆ **Laundry:** used linen must be handled *gently* at all times in order to prevent excessive dispersal of MRSA in the environment; they should be processed as 'infected linen 'according to the local policy. All linen must be put into the appropriate bag, sealed at the bedside, and removed directly to the dirty utility area or to the collection point. As fabric in contact with the person colonized/infected with MRSA/VRE can act as a source of infection, the following measures should be adopted to minimize the bioburden:

  • Bed linen must be changed daily.
  • Undergarments and nightwear should be changed daily.

Box 10.2 Summary of infection control measures for MDROs (*continued*)

- Towels and washcloths should be laundered after each use.
- Disposable washcloths should be used in hospitals.
- **Environmental cleaning:** the patient's room must be thoroughly cleaned and disinfected with appropriate detergent/disinfectant preparation on a daily basis. On discharge of patient, the room must be terminally cleaned and disinfected using appropriate disinfectant (e.g. freshly prepared hypochlorite solution 1000 ppm av Cl_2). Once the room is dry it can be used for other patients.

Health care workers

It is essential that HCWs adhere to the recommended infection control practice. Although HCWs can become colonized with MRSA, such workers are rarely the cause of MRSA outbreaks in acute care settings as the carriage is usually transient and usually occurs at the end of the shift. Therefore *routine screening* of MRSA is *not* recommended, however it should be considered if there epidemiological evidence linking HCWs for ongoing MRSA transmission.

Instances where the colonized HCWs are associated with increased risk of MRSA transmission to patients have occurred these are almost exclusively situations when HCWs have:

- Chronic skin conditions (e.g. contact dermatitis, eczema).
- Chronic otitis media, or
- Nasal colonization concurrently with viral respiratory infections resulting in increased shedding of MRSA.

Surgical operations

Infection with MRSA should be treated prior to surgery. Colonized patients who are undergoing surgical procedures should receive decolonization therapy prior to surgery (see Box 10.3). In elective cases, the decolonization therapy should start 5 days prior to surgery and on the day of operation the patients should be dressed in a theatre gown as close to the time of operation as is practical. The bed linen should be changed at this time and a further clean sheet placed over the patient's bedding immediately before leaving the ward for theatre. Vancomycin should be given as a surgical prophylaxis as per local protocol (see Chapter 15, Table 15.4).

Patients should be operated on at the end of the operation list where possible to allow time for decontamination procedures. Where this is not possible, as in cases of emergency surgery, theatre surfaces in close contact with the patient, such as the operating table, equipment, and trolley, should be thoroughly cleaned and decontaminated before being used for the next patient. Any infected or colonized lesions must be covered with an impermeable dressing during the operation and the adjacent areas treated with an appropriate antiseptic. Patients should be allowed to recover after surgery in the operating theatre or an area not occupied by other patients to avoid possible contamination of the usual recovery area.

Box 10.3 Decolonization therapy for MRSA

Treatment should be prescribed by a medical practitioner and should be continued for 5 days. For effective decolonization, it essential that towels, bed linen, and patients' clothing (including undergarments and night wear) must be washed and *changed daily* until the end of the treatment to reduce bioburden. The clothing should wash in the machine using a hot cycle which achieved at least at 60°C. Woollen clothes should be dry cleaned.

- **Nose:** apply 2% nasal mupirocin (*Bactroban Nasal*®) ointment three times a day for 5 days. A small amount of ointment (about the size of a matchstick head) should be placed on a cotton bud and applied to the anterior part of the inside of each nostril. The nostrils are closed by gently pressing the sides of the nose together; this will spread the ointment throughout the nares. Mupirocin ointment should be reserved for the treatment of MRSA only. A prolonged course (>7 days) or repeated courses (>two courses per hospital admission) should be avoided to prevent the emergence of mupirocin resistance. If a sample is taken to confirm eradication on MRSA, then it should be taken at least 2 days after completion of therapy.

- **Mupirocin resistant MRSA:** two types of mupirocin resistance have been identified, i.e. low- (MIC = 8–256 mg/L) and high-level resistance strains (MIC >512 mg/L). Success with low-level resistance strains is about 80% but with high-level resistance strains is only about 27%. Therefore high-level resistance strains can be treated with Naseptin® (0.5% neomycin and 0.1% chlorhexidine) nasal ointment four times a day for 10 days. Naseptin® is less successful then mupirocin in eradication of MRSA and re-colonization can occur very frequently. However it is useful in reducing the bioload of microorganisms in the nose. Naseptin® contains peanut oil and is contraindicated in persons with peanut allergy.

- **Throat:** chlorhexidine gluconate spray or gargle for pharyngeal carriage may be added but its efficacy is not known. Topical nasal applications are *not* effective in clearing throat or sputum colonization. Eradication of throat colonization by use of systematic antimicrobial therapy is not part of routine decolonization therapy but if considered essential, then this can be given on the advice of a medical practitioner on an individual patient basis. A combination of any two oral antibiotics from fusidic acid, rifampicin, trimethoprim, and doxycycline or co-trimoxazole can be prescribed for 7 days based on the antibiotic sensitivity testing.

- **Body bathing:**
  - *Shower:* the antiseptic body wash should be applied directly to the skin, paying particular attention to the hair, around the nostrils, under the arms, between the legs (groin, perineum, and buttock area), feet, and working downwards. The antiseptic body wash should *not* be diluted. Rinse from head to toe and dry the body with a clean towel. For an antiseptic to be effective, recommended contact time on skin must be followed (e.g. triclosan should be in contact with the skin for about 1 min and then thoroughly rinsed, and Octenisan® should be left on skin for 3 minutes and 2% chlorhexidine should be applied to the skin till it is dry). All antiseptic should be used with care in patients with dermatitis and broken skin and *must be discontinued* if skin irritation develops. Chlorhexidine is harsher than triclosan. Octenisan® is the only product licensed to be used in neonates.

> **Box 10.3 Decolonization therapy for MRSA (*continued*)**
>
> - For the *bath* add antiseptic concentrate to a bath full of water immediately prior to the patient entering the water.
> - *Body bathing or bed bathing:* patients confined to bed can be washed with an antiseptic solution. Wet the skin and apply the antiseptic preparation directly onto the skin using a disposable clean cloth; alternatively use pre-soaked antiseptic disposable towel. Wash and rinse from head to toe. Dry body with a clean towel.
> - **Colonized lesions:** dressing containing an antiseptic, e.g. sliver, povidone-iodine or chlorhexidine may be applied to the infected wound. Flamazine ointment can be applied topically. Mupirocin ointment should be applied three times a day to *small lesions* for 5 days in selected cases only.
> - **Antiseptic powder:** 1% chlorhexidine dusting powder can be used to treat carrier sites and should be applied to intact skin such as the perineum, buttocks, flexures, and axillae three times daily for 5 days.

Screening for MRSA

The value of 'universal' MRSA screening in the prevention and control of MRSA infections remains controversial as its cost-effectiveness has not been fully established. Currently, screening of MRSA is recommended in the following 'high risk group' of patients (Department of Health, 2007).

- Preoperative patients in certain surgical procedure, e.g. elective orthopaedics, cardiothoracic, vascular, and neurosurgery.
- Emergency orthopaedic and trauma admissions.
- Critical care, e.g. ICU, high-dependency, and neonatal units.
- Patients of renal units on dialysis.
- Other specified patient groups.
- All previously known MRSA-positive patients.
- All elective surgical patients.
- Oncology/chemotherapy inpatients.
- Patients admitted from high-risk health care facilities settings/countries where MRSA is endemic.

Clearance of MRSA

Surveillance specimens should be taken once the antibiotic/decolonization has been discontinued for at least 72 hours as the specimens may show a false negative result if the patient is on an antibiotic. Once the patient is positive for MRSA, swabs from the carrier and other sites should be taken *at least* 3 days after stopping the MRSA treatment protocol. Carriage of MRSA strains may persist for months or years and may reappear in an apparently 'clear or cured' patient. Certain body sites are more resistant to the eradication of MRSA, e.g. tracheostomy sites, deep pressure sores and wounds, chronic leg ulcers, rectal and perineal regions, and colostomy sites.

Laboratory identification

A swab moistened with sterile water should be used to sample carrier sites and lesions. The screening swabs should be taken from the nose, perineum/groin, operative and wound sites, abnormal or damaged skin, invasive devices, catheter urine samples, and sputum, if expectorating.

Direct culture methods: swab can be plated directly on to selective chromogenic agar. The result is usually available at 24 hours. However, the method is less sensitive than enrichment broth.

Broth enrichment culture: swabs are placed in enrichment broth and subsequently plated on to selective chromogenic agar. This method is more sensitive then the direct culture method but it can take up to 48 hours to get the confirmation.

Polymerase chain reaction (PCR): PCR is a rapid and extremely sensitive method. The result is usually available within 3 hours but it has has not been widely adopted. This is because the test is very expensive and has reduced sensitivity for samples other than nasal swabs. Although the specificity is high at 93–98%, this will still mean that the positive predictive value in a low-prevalence population will be low. It addition, the swab has to be inoculated on culture medium for final confirmation and antibiotic sensitivity testing, which is required for treatment of patients and typing which is essential for epidemiology purpose.

Decolonization therapy for MRSA

Decolonization treatment takes the form of body washes and shampoos, antibacterial nasal ointment or cream, and silver dressings to colonized wounds (see Box 10.3). Patients who have had three negative MRSA screens often become positive again even if there has been no further exposure to colonized individuals and MRSA can return, especially under the pressure of antibiotic exposure. In hospital, MRSA decolonization may reduce the bioload of MRSA from patients and thus decrease transmission to others and this is an important part of outbreak control measures. However, the initial success of decolonization is short-lived, with only half of successfully decolonized patients remaining MRSA-free 12 months later with an overall success rate of 32%. Of the factors examined, throat colonization, mupirocin resistance and age greater than 80 years were significantly associated with failure of decolonization (Gilpin et al., 2010).

The universal decolonization of *all positive* patients requires further evaluation as clearance of MRSA is not successfully achieved in the majority of patients. However, decolonization therapy should be considered in the following situations:

- When MRSA-positive patients are associated with ongoing transmission or in an outbreak situation.
- In colonized MRSA patients having a surgical procedure that has been identified as high risk for MRSA surgical site infection, e.g. orthopaedic, vascular, and other implant surgery.
- In certain patient populations in an attempt to reduce the risk of subsequent MRSA and meticillin susceptible *Staph. aureus* infections among colonized persons undergoing dialysis, patients with recurrent *Staph. aureus* infections, patients in intensive care, and patients undergoing targeted surgical procedures where evidence has shown benefit.

Ambulance transportation

The ambulance service should be notified in advance. Provided that standard Infection control precautions are followed there is no evidence that ambulance staff or their families are at risk from transporting patients with MRSA. Those who are no longer colonized or infected and those in whom the site/s of colonization or infection does not pose a risk of infection to others, may be transported without the need for any additional infection control precautions.

The following infection control measures should be taken for patients who are colonized or infected in one or more sites which cannot be covered with an occlusive dressing are liable to present a risk of cross-infection to other patients:

◆ The patient should be given clean clothing before transport.

◆ A disposable plastic apron should be worn for patient contact.

◆ Physically clean hands can be disinfected with an alcoholic hand rub after contact with the patient or the environment.

◆ The patient's contact area, e.g. chair and the stretcher, should be cleaned and disinfected with a large alcohol impregnated wipe or disinfectant solution after transport of an affected patient.

◆ Blankets and pillow cases should be placed in an appropriate bag for laundering according to local protocol.

◆ The vehicle should be thoroughly cleaned with detergent and disinfected with freshly prepared hypochlorite solution (1000 ppm av Cl_2). Fumigation and prolonged airing is not necessary. The vehicle may be used when all surfaces are dry.

Vancomycin-resistant enterococci

Enterococci are anaerobic Gram-positive cocci. The word 'enterococcus' originates from the Greek word *enteron* meaning 'the gut or intestine' and *kokkos* meaning 'a berry'. The first clinical strains of vancomycin or glycopeptide-resistant enterococci (VRE or GRE) were reported in 1988. Since then, the incidence of VRE (*Enterococcus faecium* or *Enterococcus faecalis*) has been rising steadily. VRE do not generally appear to be more virulent than sensitive strains and the majority of individuals who have VRE are colonized with it particularly in wounds, ulcers, and medical device sites in hospitalized patients. Because of its resistance patterns, they are more difficult to treat if infection occurs and they also have a high propensity to become endemic due to better survival in the environment.

Source of infection

E. faecium and *E. faecalis* are commensal bacteria in the gastrointestinal tract of healthy individuals. It can also be present in the anterior urethra, vagina, skin, and oropharynx. It is commonly found in patients who had been treated with broad-spectrum antibiotics and have received vancomycin. Most enterococcal infections have been attributed to endogenous sources. However, in an outbreak situation or when the organism is endemic in a health care facility, patient-to-patient cross-infection can occur either through direct or indirect contact via the hands of personnel or from contaminated patient-care items, equipment, and environmental surfaces.

Screening of patients

Routine screening for VRE is *not* recommended as the costs can be considerable and benefits are less clear. Based on the local surveillance, selective screening should be considered for high-risk patients in identifying colonized individuals. In an outbreak situation, screening swabs for culture from multiple body sites, i.e. stool or rectal swabs, perineal area, areas of broken skin (i.e. ulcer and wound), urine from catheterized patients, or colostomy site, should be taken to identify carriers. Since the most frequent site of colonization is the large bowel, a faecal sample is the most useful screening specimen. It is important to emphasize that stool carriage may persist for months or years and oral antibiotic therapy to eradicate the carriage is *not* successful.

Infection control measures

Infection control measures are summarized in Box 10.2. Dischare patients if s/he is clinically fit. Patients can remain colonized for a long time after discharge from hospital therefore an alert system for re-admission of these patients is required so that these patients can be promptly identified and placed in a single room with en suite toilet and isolation precautions. Patients with VRE and diarrhoea or incontinence pose a high risk of transmission to others and must be isolated in a single room.

Multi-resistant Gram negative bacteria

Emergence of multi-resistant Gram-negative (MRGN) bacteria poses a serious threat to patients as these strains are resistant not only to beta-lactam antibiotics but also other agents, including fluoroquinolones and aminoglycosides. It also poses problems to health care facilities as numerous outbreaks have been reported worldwide. The most common MRGN bacteria which are extensively resistant to antibiotic are:

1. **Enterobacteriaceae family**: *Escherichia coli*, *Klebsiella* spp. have both inducible and acquired beta-lactamases therefore accurate speciation of Enterobacteriaceae is essential: 'SCEMP' microorganisms, e.g. *Serratia* spp., *Citrobacter freundii*, *Enterobacter* spp., *Morganella morganii*, and *Providencia* spp. These organisms can develop resistance during treatment against third-generation cephalosporins (cefotaxime, ceftriaxone, and ceftazidime) due to the induction of chromosomal AmpC beta-lactamases.

2. **Non-fermenters**: *Pseudomonas aeruginosa*, *Acinetobacter baumannii*, *Stenotrophomonas maltophia*, etc.

Most of the MRGN bacteria exert resistance by producing various enzymes which are responsible for inactivating various classes of antibiotics leaving very limited options for treatment. Although newer agents are available, they are not as effective as older agents and their side effects and clinical efficacy for treatment of various infections is not fully evaluated.

Infection control precautions

MRGN infections are common both in hospital and community. Most of the patients from the community are colonized in the urinary tract and wound sites. Control of MRGN control measures are summarized in Box 10.2.

- ◆ Early identification by taking screening swabs and prompt isolation is essential, especially if the patients are being admitted to a high-risk unit, e.g. ICU, NNU, burns, transplant unit, and urology.

- ◆ Screening of patients who are being admitted from hospitals and/or from countries where MRGN is endemic is also an important part of control measures. These patients should be isolated until the screening swab results are available.

- ◆ Since Gram-negative bacteria mainly survive in wet environments, it is essential that the environment be kept clean and dry.

- ◆ Make sure that bedpan washer disinfector, or macerators are in good condition and in working order. If a bedpan washer disinfector breaks down, it should be repaired as an emergency.

- ◆ Bedpans and urinals should be disinfected using heat treatment, if possible, or disposable bedpans and urinals can be used, if available.

- ◆ Communal equipment (especially if wet) may act as a source for these organisms, therefore ward equipment must be stored dry. Soaking of instruments in disinfectant solution must be avoided.

- ◆ Urine drainage bags must be emptied by the tap, for which single-use disposable gloves should be used and hands must be washed after the procedure. A separate jug or container should be used for *each* patient when emptying urinary drainage bags.

Extended-spectrum beta-lactamases

Many soil microorganisms are capable of producing beta-lactamases as part of defence mechanisms to protect themselves. The first reports of extended-spectrum beta-lactamases (ESBLs) in Gram-negative bacilli came from Europe and were quickly followed by reports from the USA and are now recognized worldwide. These organisms have a propensity to spread from patient to patient and represent a major threat as several outbreaks have been reported worldwide due to spread of mobile genetic element plasmids or transposons and the dispersion of specific clones. ESBLs are generally acquired by horizontal gene transfer and confer resistance to various classes of antibiotics. Recent emergence of metallo-beta-lactamases has compromised the clinical utility of this class of antibiotics. In addition, resistance to carbapenems may also be induced as a result of increased production of either AmpC beta-lactamases coupled with increased efflux of the drug. Alternatively they could be acquired as in the NDM (New Delhi metallo-beta-lactamases) 1 carbapenamases. Most of the carbapenamases are either intrinsic to some species as in *Acinetobacter* and *Stenotrophomonas* while others are plasmid mediated.

Beta-lactamase enzymes can be broadly divided into: 1) serine beta-lactamases which use a serine amino acid in their active site to hydrolyse β-lactams, and 2) metallo-beta-lactamases, which use Zn^{++} cations to disrupt the beta-lactam ring. Classification of selected beta-lactamase of Gram-negative bacteria are summarized in Table 10.3.

Table 10.3 Classification of selected beta-lactamases of Gram negative bacteria

Beta-lactamase	Type of enzymes	Comments
Broad-spectrum These enzymes hydrolyse penicillins and 'early' cephalosporins only	TEM1–2, SHV-1 Most commonly found in *Klebsiella pneumoniae* and *E. coli*	Usually plasmid-mediated except SHV-1 which is mainly chromosomal in *K. pneumonia*. Inhibited by clavulanic acid or tazobactam
Extended-spectrum These enzymes hydrolyse penicillins and cephalosporins but not cephamycins (cefoxitin) or carbapenems	TEM-3, SHV-2, CTX-M-15	Usually plasmid-mediated
Amp C-related In contrast to ESBLs, they usually hydrolyse cephamycins (cefoxitin) and coxyimino-cephalosporins except 4th-generation cephalosporin (cefepime)	Amp C cephalosporinases. Enterobacteriaceae, *Pseudomons* spp. and *A. baumannii*	Chromosomal Amp C. Enzyme production can be inducible or constitutive
Carbapenemases (Carbapenem-hydrolysing beta-lactamases e.g. meropenem, ertapanem, imipenem) Resistant to all beta-lactams except monobactams (aztreonam)	VIM-l, NDM-1	Often plasmid-mediated
Resistant to carbapenems and monobactams	OXA class	Chromosomal and/or plasmid mediated

Non-fermenters Gram-negative bacteria

Acinetobacter baumannii

Acinetobacter spp. are non-motile, non-fermentative, oxidase-negative, aerobic Gram-negative coccobacilli. There are over 30 species and the organism is found in soil, sewage, and water and is occasionally a cause of food spoilage. Various species colonize the human skin and they may be readily recovered from the forearm, forehead, and toe webs of healthy volunteers. There are differences in the spectrum of diseases associated with *A. baumannii* and non-*A. baumannii* species, with the former being responsible for most infection associated with humans and transmission is mainly restricted to hospital settings often with patient-to-patient transmission.

A. baumannii is not a ubiquitous microorganism and its natural habitat remains to be defined. However, it is has become a major cause of hospital-acquired infections because of its remarkable ability to survive and spread in the hospital environment and to rapidly acquire resistance determinants to a wide range of antibiotics. It is an organism of low pathogenicity and risk of transmission of *A. baumannii* is higher in the ICU than on wards as most of these patients have multiple risk factors. Once it is acquired, the organism is carried for prolonged periods. *A. baumannii* is increasingly being seen in hospitals during outbreaks in dry environments as bed linen, mattresses, pillows, fans, and cupboard surfaces and in wet environments, on plastic tubing, pressure monitors, sinks, ventilators, cleaning cloths, and face flannels. The organisms may persist in the environment of hospital units that harboured colonized patients long after these have been discharged. *A. baumannii* infections are more common in warm climates and in the summer months in temperate countries, but there appears to be little difference in human skin carriage between temperate and tropical climates. Most *Acinetobacter* spp. associated with hospital infection are relatively resistant to drying and disinfectants and epidemic strains of *A. baumannii* survive equally as well in high relative humidity. Once endemic, *A. baumannii* is difficult to eradicate therefore repeated deep/internal cleaning of all equipment and whole ICU is required until the environment is clear of the organisms.

Pseudomonas aeruginosa

P. aeruginosa is a true opportunistic pathogen and is responsible for causing a variety of infections in clinical settings in both immunocompetent (e.g. folliculitis resulting from bathing in hot tubs) and immunocompromised hosts. However, in most cases, *P. aeruginosa* infections occur in patients who have been compromised in some way, e.g. diabetic patients. It causes malignant external otitis, and it colonizes and infects the lower respiratory tract in patients with cystic fibrosis. In hospitalized patients, particularly those who are intubated and undergoing mechanical ventilation in the ICU, *P. aeruginosa* is a prominent cause of ventilator-associated pneumonia and also figures prominently in infections of indwelling devices, such as urinary catheters.

Stenotrophomonas maltophilia

Stenotrophomonas maltophilia (previously known as *Pseudomonas maltophilia* or *Xanthomonas maltophilia*) is a non-fermentative, motile, oxidase-negative, aerobic Gram-negative bacillus. It is found widespread in the environment in water, soil, plants, animal sources, and sewage. Transmission of infection is associated with nosocomial sources including hospital water and contaminated disinfectant solutions.

Currently little is known about the virulence factors but it is an organism of limited pathogenicity and causes infection in patient who have multiple risk factors (see Box 10.1). However, infection is common in severely compromised patients with significant morbidity and mortality, particularly patients with risk factors (see Box 10.1) underlying malignancy and/transplantation and profound neutropenia as the major predisposing factors.

In addition to treatment to other broad-spectrum antibiotic, prior therapy with carbapenems (especially imipenem) has been identified as a major predisposing factor. Since this organism is very resistant to various antibiotics, treatment with co-trimoxazole is usually considered as a first-line agent as it is the most potent agent available.

Key references and further reading

Antibiotic stewardship and multidrug resistant organisms

Brown EM, Nathwani D. Antibiotic cycling or rotation: a systematic review of the evidence of efficacy. *Journal of Antimicrobial Chemotherapy* 2005; 55:6–9.

CDC. *Management of Multidrug-Resistant Organisms in Healthcare Settings, 2006.* Atlanta, GA: CDC, 2006.

Elek SD, Fleming RC. A new technique for the control of hospital cross-infection. *Lancet* 1960; **ii**:569–71.

IDSA and SHEA. Guidelines for Developing an Institutional Program to Enhance Antimicrobial Stewardship. *Clinical Infectious Diseases* 2007; **44**:159–77.

McCorry A, Damani N, Rajendran R, *et al.* Reducing the use of 'high-risk' antibiotics through implementation of an antibiotic stewardship programme. *British Journal of Clinical Pharmacy* 2010; **2**:341–4.

PIDAC Guideline. *Best Practices for Infection Prevention and Control of Resistant Staphylococcus aureus and* Enterococci *in all health care settings, 2007.* Canada: Provincial Infectious Diseases Advisory Committee, 2007.

SHEA Guidelines. SHEA guidelines for preventing nosocomial transmission of multidrug-resistant strains of *Staphylococcus aureus* and *Enterococcus. Infection Control and Hospital Epidemiology* 2003; **24**:362–86.

WHO. *Infections control programmes to control antimicrobial resistance* (WHO/CDS/CSR/DRS/2001.7). Geneva: World Health Organization, 2001.

Meticillin-resistant *Staph. aureus*/Vancomycin-resistant enterococci

Albrich WC, Harbarth S. Health-care workers: source, vector, or victim of MRSA? *Lancet Infectious Disease* 2008; **8**:289–301.

APIC. *Guide to the Elimination of Methicillin-Resistant Staphylococcus aureus (MRSA) Transmission in Hospital settings,* 2nd edn. Washington, DC: Association for Professionals in Infection Control & Epidemiology, 2010.

BSAC/HIS/ICNA working Party. Guidelines for the Control and prevention of meticillin-resistant *Staphylococcus aureus* in healthcare facilities by the joint BSAC/HIS/ICNA working party on MRSA. *Journal of Hospital Infection* 2006; **63**(suppl 1):S1–S44.

CDC. *Management of Multidrug-Resistant Organisms in Healthcare Settings, 2006.* Atlanta: CDC, 2006.

DeLeo FR, Otto M, Kreiswirth BN, *et al.* Community-associated meticillin-resistant *Staphylococcus aureus. Lancet* 2010; **375**:1557–68.

Department of Health. *Screening for meticillin-resistant Staphylococcus aureus (MRSA) colonisation. A strategy for NHS trusts: a summary of best practice.* London: Department of Health, 2007.

Dutch Infection Prevention Working Party. *Hospital guidelines for control of MRSA, 2007.* Available at: http://www.wip.nl/.

Gilpin DF, Small S, Bakkshi S, *et al.* Efficacy of a standard meticillin-resistant *Staphylococcus aureus* decolonisation protocol in routine clinical practice. *Journal of Hospital Infection* 2010; **75**:93–8.

Health Protection Agency. *Guidance on the diagnosis and management of PVL-associated Staphylococcus aureus infections (PVL-SA) in England.* London: Health Protection Agency, 2008.

HIS Working Party Report. Guidelines for the control of glycopeptide resistant enterococci (GRE) in hospital. *Journal of Hospital Infection*; 2006; **62**:6–21.

Institute of Health Improvement. *Infection Prevention Bundle: Reduce Methicillin-Resistant Staphylococcus aureus (MRSA) Infection, 2007.* Available at: http://www.ihi.org/ihi.

Loveday HP, Pellowe C, Jones S, *et al.* A systematic review of the evidence for interventions for the prevention and control of methicillin-resistant *Staphylococcus aureus* (1996–2004): report to the joint MRSA working party (subgroup A). *Journal of Hospital Infection* 2006; **63**(suppl 1):S45–S70.

Patel R. Clinical impact of vancomycin-resistant enterococci. *Journal of Antimicrobial Chemotherapy* 2003; **51**(Suppl. S3):iii13–iii21.

Ridwan B, Mascini E, van der Reijden N, *et al.* What action should be taken to prevent the spread of vancomycin-resistant enterococci in European Hospitals? *British Medical Journal* 2002; **324**:666–8.

SHEA/IDSA Practice Recommendation: Strategies to prevent Transmission of Methicillin-Resistant *Staphylococcus aureus* in Acute Care Hospitals. *Infection Control and Hospital Epidemiology* 2008; **29**(Suppl 1):S62–S80.

Multi-resistant Gram negative bacteria

Anthony D, Harris AD, McGregor JC, *et al.* What infection control interventions should be undertaken to control multidrug-resistant Gram-negative bacteria? *Clinical Infectious Diseases* 2006; **43**:857–6.

CDC. Guidance for control of infections with carbapenem-resistant or carbapenemase-producing enterobacteriaceae in acute care facilities. *Morbidity and Mortality Weekly Report* 2009; **58**(10):256–60.

Karageorgopoulo DE, Falagas ME. Control and treatment of multi-resistant *Acinetobacter baumannii* infections. *Lancet infectious Diseases* 2008; **8**:751–62.

Kumarasamy KK, Toleman MA, Walsh TR, *et al.* Emergence of a new antibiotic resistance mechanism in India, Pakistan, and the UK: a molecular, biological, and epidemiological study. *Lancet infectious Diseases* 2010; **10**:597–602.

Chapter 11

Special pathogens

A mighty creature is the germ,
Though smaller than a pachyderm.
His customary dwelling place
Is deep inside the human race.
His childish pride he often pleases
By giving people strange diseases.
Do you, my poppet, feel infirm-?
You probably contain a germ.

Ogden Nash

Clostridium difficile-associated diarrhoea

Clostridium difficile is an anaerobic, Gram-positive bacterium that was first identified and characterized in 1935. The word *difficile* originated from the Latin word meaning 'difficult' as the organism was difficult to isolate. *C. difficile* was accorded little interest until 1978 when several reports identified its association with pseudomembranous enterocolitis. Infection with *C. difficile* has now become the most frequent cause of hospital-acquired diarrhoea. In recent years, the epidemiology of *C. difficile* has changed dramatically, with increases noted in the incidence of the disease internationally, and reports of *C. difficile* outbreaks within health care facilities in North America and Europe involving more severe disease caused by the emergence of the 027 hypervirulent epidemic strain.

Risk factors

Up to 5% of healthy adults carry *C. difficile* in their gut without symptoms. Asymptomatic colonization is common in up to two-thirds of infants. Colonization is markedly increased in patients beyond the age of 65 years. However the carriage can be as high as 20% in residents of long-term health care facilities and up to 14% of hospitalized elderly patients on acute medical wards are colonized with *C. difficile*. Risk factors for development of *C. difficile*-associated diarrhoea are summarized in Box 11.1.

Box 11.1 Risk factors for development of C. *difficile*-associated diarrhoea

- Exposure to especially high-risk antibiotics e.g. quinolones (e.g. ciprofloxacin, moxifloxacin and levofloxacin), 2nd- and 3rd-generation cephalosporins (cefuroxime, cefotaxime, ceftriaxone, ceftazidime etc.), clindamycin, and co-amoxiclav.
- Advanced age (>65 years), i.e. common in elderly, debilitated patients with comorbidities; outbreaks being more common in geriatric and long-stay wards.
- Poor host response (defects in phagocytic and humoral host defence).
- Admission from nursing home and health care facilities where C. *difficile* infection is endemic.
- Prolonged hospital stay.
- Malignancy (especially haematological malignancy).
- Gastric acid suppressant medications.
- Gastrointestinal and transplant surgery.
- Immunosuppression.
- Admission to ICU.
- Nasogastric intubation.
- Inflammatory bowel disease.
- Exposure to C. *difficile* from infected roommate/environment.
- Exposure to virulent 027 strain of C. *difficile*.
- Enteral (post-pyloric) tube-feeding (20% tube-fed vs. 9% non-tube fed). In addition, diet formula is rich in amino acids and short-chain fatty acids, which provides a good medium for growth of C. *difficile*.

Pathogenesis

C. *difficile* is spread via the faecal–oral route. The bacteria are ingested either as the vegetative form or as spores. After ingestion, the spores survive and traverse the acidic stomach. When they pass the small intestine, spores germinate into the vegetative form.

C. *difficile* then reproduces and multiplies in the intestinal crypts, releasing toxins A and B. Toxin A attracts neutrophils and monocytes, and toxin B degrades the colonic epithelial cells, leading to colitis, pseudomembrane formation, and profuse watery diarrhoea.

In past few years, health care facilities in North America and Europe have seen more severe disease caused by the emergence of a hypervirulent epidemic (BI/NAP1/027/toxin type III) strain. 027 hypervirulent strain has been found to produce 16-fold higher concentrations of toxin A and 23-fold higher concentrations of toxin B *in vitro*. In addition this strain also produces a binary toxin, the role of which is not yet clear.

Clinical features

The main symptom is diarrhoea which usually starts 5–10 days (range from a few days to 2 months) after commencing antibiotic therapy. It ranges from mild to severe foul-smelling diarrhoea containing blood/mucus, with fever, leucocytosis, and abdominal pain. Patients with *C. difficile* diarrhoea have a characteristic smell like a horse stable. In the majority of patients, the illness is mild and full recovery is usual. Elderly patients may become seriously ill with dehydration. Occasionally, patients may develop a severe form of the disease called pseudomembranous colitis. Complications include pancolitis, toxic megacolon, perforation, or endotoxin shock.

Laboratory diagnosis

Screening and treatment of asymptomatic patients is not necessary. Only *watery or loose stools* should be tested for *C. difficile* toxin. They should be transported as soon as possible and stored at 2–8°C until tested due to toxin inactivation. Once the diagnosis has been confirmed, *repeat specimens for clearance should not be taken* unless there is a relapse following treatment. This is because it is not uncommon for the faeces to remain toxin-positive for some time after the start of treatment even when the patient's symptoms have settled.

Persistently positive test results at the end of treatment are not predictive of a *C. difficile* relapse, and a positive test result in an asymptomatic patient may result in unnecessary treatment with antimicrobials, which can increase the patient's risk of developing *C. difficile* infection in the future.

C. difficile infection should be suspected in patients with diarrhoea and/or abdominal pain with recent exposure to antibiotics and have other risk factors (see Box 11.1). The diagnosis is usually confirmed with a laboratory-based assay. Current rapid tests for diagnosis of *C. difficile* infection have problems with both poor sensitivity and specificity and in order to overcome this problem, *two tests* are recommended to confirm the diagnosis.

- **Cytotoxicity assay:** the cell cytotoxicity assay (detects the cytopathic effect of toxin B on cultured cell lines), is considered the gold-standard clinical laboratory assay for the diagnosis; however, this facility is not available in most diagnostic *C. difficile* laboratories and has a prolonged turn-around time of up to 72 hours.
- **Enzyme immunoassays:** EIA tests to detect toxins A and/or B have become the most widely used laboratory-based methods because of their low cost, ease of use, and rapid turn-around time. If EIA kits are used, it is essential that that the test kit which uses *both toxin A and B* must be tested. The main disadvantage of this assay is it lacks both sensitivity and specificity compared to cell cytotoxicity assays.
- **Polymerase chain reaction:** PCR testing appears to be rapid, sensitive, and specific and is extremely useful for quick confirmatory testing and also confirms hypervirulent 027 strain.
- **Glutamate dehydrogenase:** GDH is a protein produced by *both* toxigenic and non-toxigenic *C. difficile* but also cross-reacts with other bacterial strains therefore it is *not specific* for *C. difficile*. It can be used as initial screen as the test result are available within 2 hours and some studies have reported a good negative predictive value. It *must not* be used on its own as a single test and positive results must be confirmed by an additional test for toxin A+B by ELISA, PCR, or other method to confirm the diagnosis.

- **Stool culture:** routine stool culture for detection of *C. difficile* is *not* recommended because it is slow and labour intensive and detects both toxigenic and non-toxigenic strain of *C. difficile*. However, stool culture are required in an outbreak situation for epidemiological investigations and are necessary for ribotyping.

Prevention strategies

Current strategies to prevent *C. difficile* infections are based on the implementation of a 'care bundle' (see 'Care bundle approach', Chapter 1) developed by the UK Department of Health and are summarized in Box 11.2.

Infection control measures

C. difficile is normally fastidious in its vegetative state but it is capable of sporulating when environmental conditions no longer support its continued growth. The capacity to form spores enables the organism to persist and survive in the environment for months. Environmental contamination can be heavy, especially if the diarrhoea is severe or accompanied by incontinence. Asymptomatic patients after infection may continue to shed organisms in their stools and serve as a source of contamination. The following infection control precautions should be taken:

- Promptly diagnosis and isolate all patients with *C. difficile* in a single room with en suite toilet facilities as soon as possible (preferably within 2 hours) or cohort all symptomatic patients. In a cohort area, mixing of patients carrying 027 strain and non-027 should be avoided.

- To prevent spread, transfer of patients between wards/units and health care facilities should be restricted unless considered essential.

- Hands can become contaminated by direct contact with patients colonized/infected with *C. difficile* or contact with environmental surfaces. Therefore, strict hand washing with soap and water before and after contact with patients and environmental surfaces is the most effective control measure to prevent cross-infection.

Box 11.2 *C. difficile* care bundle

- **Antibiotic prescribing**: stop antibiotic, if possible or change to low-risk narrow-spectrum agents.
- **Early diagnosis** to identify cases and start treatment to control symptoms.
- **Prompt isolation** of patients as soon as possible in a single room with en suite toilet.
- **Implement infection control precautions.**
- **Clean and disinfect environment.**
- **Decontaminate/sterilize patient care items/equipment.**

Adapted from Department of Health. *High Impact Intervention No 7. Care Bundle. To reduce the risk of Clostridium difficile.* London: Department of Health, 2007.

Alcohol hand disinfectants are effective against vegetative form but not effective against *C. difficile* spores, therefore disinfection of hands with soap and water is recommended to remove spores from contaminated hands.

♦ Use of non-sterile single-use gloves and a plastic apron for patient care activity. Hands must be washed *after* removing gloves.

♦ The recommended approach to reduce the environmental bioload of *C. difficile* microorganisms is meticulous cleaning and decontamination of the surfaces. The patient's immediate environment and other areas where spores may accumulate (e.g. sluice, commodes, toilets, bedpans, sinks, hand-touch surfaces in the patient's bathroom) and other soiled areas must be *thoroughly and frequently cleaned* and then *disinfected* using a 1000 ppm of freshly prepared hypochlorite solution.

♦ Separate cleaning equipment must be reserved for this purpose. Mop heads should be disposable or laundered after each use and single-use disposable cloths must be used.

♦ Patients can remain colonized for a long time after discharge from hospital. If the patient is discharged or transferred to another hospital or long-stay health care facility, appropriate personnel at the receiving health care facility must be informed.

Management

Management of *C. difficile* enterocolitis focuses on the following strategies:

♦ **Review antibiotic prescribing**: firstly, the antibiotic therapy that has mediated the change in the patient's gut microflora should be discontinued, if possible, or changed to an antibiotic which has less of an association with *C. difficile* infection.

♦ **Avoid antiperistaltic medication:** diarrhoea is the response of the infected host to expel pathogens/toxins responsible for enterocolitis. Use of opiates and antiperistaltic drugs results in the retention of pathogen/toxin, probably worsens enterocolitis-associated necrosis of the colonic mucosa, and increases the risk of toxic megacolon.

♦ **Rehydration of patients:** loss of fluid and electrolytes *must be* replaced using the IV route until diarrhoea has ceased and effective oral intake has resumed. In severe cases, patients' nutritional status should be assessed by the dietician.

♦ **Antibiotic therapy**: specific antibiotic therapy to treat *C. difficile* should be initiated. Oral metronidazole is administered 400 mg 8-hourly for 10–14 days, which should be given as the first choice for mild-to-moderate disease. Vancomycin should not be prescribed as a first-line therapy because of cost and problem of emergence of vancomycin-resistant enterococci. If metronidazole is not effective then oral vancomycin 125 mg 6-hourly for 10–14 days should be prescribed and this should be also considered as first-line therapy in severe disease. Since oral vancomycin is *not* absorbed, monitoring is not necessary. The majority of patients improve within 2–4 days. However, clinical relapse can occur in 15–25% of cases usually within 1–3 weeks.

- **Biotherapy**: biotherapy using *Lactobacillus* spp. or *Saccharomyces boulardii* (brewers' yeast) has been used with variable success. *S. boulardii* should not be used in patients with GI malignancy due to risk of developing fungaemia and in patients with a central line to avoid colonization of central venous catheters.

- **Intracolonic vancomycin**: in severe cases, consider giving intracolonic vancomycin (500 mg in 100–500 mL saline 4–12-hourly). This is given as retention enema using 18 gauge Foley catheter with 30-mL balloon inserted per rectum and then instilling vancomycin. The catheter is then clamped for 60 min, deflated and removed. This therapy should be given with or without IV metronidazole 500 mg intravenously every 8 hours and is the regimen of choice for the treatment of severe, complicated *C. difficile* infections (Dept. of Health, 2009).

It is important to remember that **monitoring severity of disease** by the number of stools passed each day by patients using Bristol stool chart may be an *unreliable indicator* of severity of disease; other parameters must also be monitored on a daily basis to assess the severity, e.g. increasing white blood cell count and serum creatinine and/or evidence of severe colitis by abdominal signs or by radiological examination.

Gastrointestinal infections

Worldwide, 1.7 million deaths occur from diarrhoeal diseases annually. Although diarrhoea and vomiting may be caused by infectious and non-infectious agents all cases of gastroenteritis should be regarded as infectious unless good evidence suggests otherwise. Refer to Table 11.1 for various infective causes of gastroenteritis.

Diarrhoea is defined as three or more loose/watery bowel movements that take up the shape of their container (which are unusual or different for the patient) in a 24-hour period. Infected individuals with gastroenteritis are classified into four risk groups that pose an increased risk of spreading infection (see Box 11.3). It is particularly important to assess infected people who belong to one of the four groups of persons for whom special action should be considered. A liquid stool is more likely than a formed stool to contaminate hands and the environment, and is consequently at greater risk of spreading faecal pathogens. Formed stools voided by asymptomatic infected people, or people who have recovered from illness, may contain pathogens and are less likely to transmit infection provided good personal hygiene can be achieved.

Viral gastroenteritis

Clinical and epidemiological features of gastroenteritis viruses are summarized in Table 11.2. Outbreaks of gastroenteritis caused by viruses are more common in health care settings, cruise ships, hotels and restaurants, day care centres and nurseries. Compared to bacteria, the viruses have a much lower infective dose, with many viral infections being largely asymptomatic or subclinical in healthy adults. Contamination of fomites from enteric viruses can also originate from aerosolized vomit which can spread over a very wide area resulting in contamination of both the environment and people in the vicinity. If strict hand hygiene is not performed, virus particles can be

Table 11.1 Microorganisms, incubation periods, pathogenesis, clinical features, treatment, infective dose and sources of infection of various pathogens responsible for gastrointestinal infections

Organisms	Incubation period	Microbiology and pathogenesis	Clinical features and treatment	Infective dose and mode of transmission	Comments
Bacillus spp.	1–6 h (emetic syndrome) 6–24 h (diarrhoeal syndrome)	Enterotoxins formed in food or in gut from growth of B. cereus	Nausea and vomiting Diarrhoea and abdominal pain; both self-limited to <1 day	Ingestion of contaminated food, especially reheated rice dishes	Reheated fried rice causes vomiting or diarrhoea
Campylobacter spp.	1–10 days (usually 2–5 days) After 1–6 h; mainly vomiting After 8–16 h; mainly diarrhoea	Organisms grow in jejunum and ileum Invasion and enterotoxin production uncertain	Fever, diarrhoea and fresh blood in stool, especially in children Vomiting is uncommon and is usually self-limited Give erythromycin or cirpofloxacin can be prescribed in severe cases with invasion Usually self-limiting; recovery in 5–8 days	500 microorganisms Ingestion or handling of contaminated food or water Person-to-person transmission can occur if hygiene is poor	Campylobacter does not multiply on food and food borne outbreaks are rarely recognized
Vibrio cholerae	4–72 h	Organisms grow in gut and produce toxin. Enterotoxin causes hypersecretion in small intestine	Abrupt onset of liquid diarrhoea in endemic area Needs prompt replacement of fluids and electrolytes IV or orally Tetracycline shortens excretion of vibrios	10^6–10^9 Ingestion or handling of contaminated food or water	Cause profuse watery diarrhoea with 'rice water' stool

(continued)

Table 11.1 (continued) Microorganisms, incubation periods, pathogenesis, clinical features, treatment, infective dose and sources of infection of various pathogens responsible for gastrointestinal infections.

Organisms	Incubation period	Microbiology and pathogenesis	Clinical features and treatment	Infective dose and mode of transmission	Comments
Clostridium botulinum	2 h to 8 days; usually 12–36 h	Clostridia grow in foods and produce toxin. Toxin absorbed from gut blocks acetylcholine at neuromuscular junction	Slurred speech, double vision, difficulty in swallowing, ptosis and respiratory paralysis Treatment requires clear airway, ventilation, and IV polyvalent antitoxin Mortality rate high	10^4–10^5 Ingestion of food contaminated with toxin	
Clostridium difficile	5–10 days; can be up to 2 months	Carriage of C. difficile in population can be up to 5%; higher in patients who have been in health care facility where C. difficile is endemic	Abrupt onset of foul smelling diarrhoea. Toxin can be detected in stool. Enterotoxin causes epithelial necrosis in colon which can lead to pseudomembranous colitis and toxic mega colon and death; common with 027 strain Treat with metrinodazole or vancomycin, if symptomatic	Can be endogenous. Person-to-person transmission by faecal-oral route and by environmental and hand contamination Outbreaks common in hospital and long-term health care facilities	Associated with use of broad-spectrum antibiotic especially cephalosporins and quinolones (see C.difficile-associated diarrhoea, p. 183)
Clostridium perfringens	4–24 h (usually 8–12 h)	Many C. perfringens in cultures of food and faeces of patients Enterotoxin produced in food and in gut causes hyper-secretion in small intestine	Abrupt onset of profuse diarrhoea and vomiting occasionally and abdominal pain Recovery usual without treatment in 1–4 days	Ingestion of contaminated food especially cooked meat and poultry dishes subjected to inadequate temperature control after cooking or cooling and inadequate reheating before consumption	Clostridia grow in re-warmed meat dishes and produce an enterotoxin

Cryptosporidium spp.	1–14 days (mean 7 days)	Parasitic infection. Oocysts present in humans and animals	Watery or mucoid diarrhoea. Excretion of oocysts continue in the stool for few weeks after infection	Ingestion of contaminated food or water, faecal–oral spread from cases and animals	Outbreaks have been associated with public and private water supply, swimming pools. Also associated with farm visits to feed and handle lambs and calves
Cyclosporiasis	7–11 days (mean 1 week)	Caused by protozoa Cyclospora cayentanensis	Watery or mucoid diarrhoea. Self limiting without treatment	Human GIT act as reservoir	Ingestion of contaminated food or water, particularly softer fruits and leafy vegetables, i.e. food which are difficult to wash
Amoebic dysentery	Usually 2–4 weeks	Caused by amoeba Entamoeba histolytica	Bloody diarrhoea	Human GIT act as reservoir. Faecal–oral spread	Water borne or via contaminated raw or undercooked foods
Giardia lamblia	3–25 days; median 7–10 days		Diarrhoea and abdominal pains. Often cause flatulence and steatorrhoea with pale, foul smelling, greasy stools	Faecal–oral spread. Ingestion of contaminated water	Person-to-person transmission can occur
Hepatitis A	15–50 days		Fever, malaise, jaundice. Young children are commonly asymptomatic	Ingestion of contaminated food or water. Faecal–oral spread	Period of infectivity starts 2 weeks before the onset of jaundice and maximum just before the onset of jaundice

(continued)

Table 11.1 (*continued*) Microorganisms, incubation periods, pathogenesis, clinical features, treatment, infective dose and sources of infection of various pathogens responsible for gastrointestinal infections.

Organisms	Incubation period	Microbiology and pathogenesis	Clinical features and treatment	Infective dose and mode of transmission	Comments
Escherichia coli	1–8 day; usually 3–4 days	*E. coli* 0157 is associated Enterotoxin causes hypersecretion in small intestine Some strain invade gut mucosa	Usually abrupt onset of diarrhoea; vomiting rare In adults, 'traveller's diarrhoea' is usually self-limited to 1–3 days 0157: diarrhoea, abdominal pain and blood. Treatment with antibiotic is usually not recommended for infection caused by *E. coli* 0157 Haemolytic uraemic syndrome can occur especially in young children	Faecal–oral spread. Person-to-person spread common	Commonest serotype of *E. coli* in UK is 0157: H7. Also associated with 'open' farm visits and ingestion of contaminated food especially beef and other meat products, e.g. undercooked beef burger
Listeriosis	1 day to 3 months	Caused by *Listeria monocytognes*	Septicaemia, meningitis in immunocompromised	Contaminated food, e.g. dairy products, meat based products, seafood and vegetable based products	Found in GIT tract of animals and birds

Organism	Incubation period	Pathogenesis	Infective dose / Clinical features	Transmission	Comments
Shigellosis	12 h to 7 days; usually 1–3 days	Organisms grow in superficial gut epithelium and gut lumen and produce toxin. Organisms invade epithelial cells; blood, mucus, and polymorphonuclear neutrophils in stools.	Abrupt onset of diarrhoea, often with blood and pus in stools, cramps, tenesmus and lethargy. Often mild and self-limited. Therapy depends on sensitivity testing, but the ciprofloxacin can be given in severe cases; do not give opioids	10–100 Person-to-person by faecal-oral and by contaminated environment	Highly infectious due to low infective dose
Salmonella typhi/ paratyphi	3 days to 1 month; usually 8–14 days		10–100 Enteric fever. Prolonged carriage is common	Ingestion of food contaminated by excreter/carrier	Prolonged carriage is common
Salmonellosis (excluding typhoid and paratyphoid)	6–72 h; usually 12–36 h	Organisms grow in gut. Do not produce toxin. Superficial infection of gut, little invasion	10^5–10^6 Gradual or abrupt onset of diarrhoea and low-grade fever. No antimicrobials unless systemic dissemination is suspected, in which case give a fluoroquinolone	Ingestion of food contaminated from its animal source	Over 2000 serotypes; most common in UK are *S. enteritidis* and *S. typhimurium*

(continued)

Table 11.1 (*continued*) Microorganisms, incubation periods, pathogenesis, clinical features, treatment, infective dose and sources of infection of various pathogens responsible for gastrointestinal infections.

Organisms	Incubation period	Microbiology and pathogenesis	Clinical features and treatment	Infective dose and mode of transmission	Comments
Staphylococcus aureus	1–8 h; usually 2–4 h, rarely up to 18 h	Infective dose: 10^6 staphylococci grow in meats and in dairy and bakery products and produce enterotoxin. Enterotoxin acts on receptors in gut that transmit impulses to medullary centres	Abrupt onset, intense vomiting and abdominal pain for up to 24h, regular recovery in 24–48h Occurs in persons eating the same food No treatment usually necessary except to restore fluids and electrolytes	Ingestion of food contaminated with toxin Source of infection can be from skin sepsis or skin/nasal flora in food handler	
Non-cholera vibrios	4–30 h		Diarrhoea and abdominal pain	Ingestion of contaminated food particularly shellfish	
Enteroviruses	12 h to 10 days; commonly 3–5 days		Diarrhoea and vomiting are not characteristically caused by these viruses	Faecal–oral and close contact Virus found in the upper respiratory tract	
Rotavirus	24–72 h		Diarrhoea and vomiting	Person-to-person by faecal–oral and by contaminated environment	Children are at particular risk

Organism	Incubation	Symptoms	Mechanism	Source/transmission
Noroviruses Norwalk-like viruses, small round structured viruses	10–50 h; usually 24–48 h	Vomiting (predominates) and diarrhoea		From cases (including first 48 h post recovery) by faecal–oral, transmission through ingestion/ inhalation of vomit and via fomites (particularly toilets and wash hand basins)
Yersinia enterocolitica	3–7 days	Severe abdominal pain, diarrhoea, fever. PMNs and blood in stool; polyarthritis, erythema nodosum in children / Gastroenteritis or mesenteric adenitis; occasional bacteraemia / If severe, give tetracycline or gentamicin	Enterotoxin produced.	Food-borne Ingestion of contaminated food. Fecal–oral transmission
Vibrio parahaemolyticus	6–96 h	Abrupt onset of diarrhoea in groups consuming the same food, especially crabs and other seafood. Recovery is usually complete in 1–3 days / Food and stool cultures are positive	Organisms grow in seafood and in gut and produce toxin or invade / Hypersecretion in small intestine; stools may be bloody	

Adapted with modification from Motarjemi, Y, van Schothorst, M. *HACCP Hazard Analysis and Critical Control Point Principles and Practice. Teachers Handbook*. Geneva: World Health Organization, 1999. WHO/SDE/PHE/FOS/99.3.

Box 11.3 Risk groups for gastroenteritis

Risk groups	Criteria	Comments
Group A	Any person of doubtful personal hygiene or with unsatisfactory toilet, hand-washing or hand drying facilities at home, work or school	People not in the these risk groups (A to D) present a minimal risk of spreading gastrointestinal illness and may return to any form of work from 48 h after they have recovered clinically and their stools have returned to normal consistency. In certain circumstances, food handlers will need to be temporarily excluded from work or restricted to non-food handling duties to reduce the risk of spreading infection via food. The decision to exclude or restrict any food handler should be based on individual risk assessment. With certain exceptions (refer to HPA Guideline) most notably infections with Vero cytotoxin-producing *E. coli* and typhoid/paratyphoid, microbiological clearance is unnecessary.
Group B	Children who attend pre-school groups or nursery	
Group C	People whose work involves preparing or serving unwrapped foods not subjected to further heating	
Group D	Clinical and social care staff in high-risk care facilities who have direct contact with susceptible patients or persons in whom a gastrointestinal infection would have particularly serious consequences	

Adapted from PHLS Advisory Committee on Gastrointestinal Infections. Preventing person to person spread following gastrointestinal infection: guidance to public health physician and environmental offices. *Communicable Disease and Public Health* 2004; 7(4):362–84.

Table 11.2 Clinical and epidemiological features of gastroenteritis viruses

Virus	Incubation period	Infectious dose*	Transmissibility in close contacts	Duration of viral shedding	Duration of infectivity	Survival in environment
Adenovirus serotypes 40 and 41	5–7 days	Not known	Moderate	5–7 days	5–7 days	7 days–3 months
Astrovirus	3–4 days	<100	Moderate	2–3 days	2–4 days	7–90 days
Calicivirus	24–48 h	10–100	High	1–2 days	2–4 days	8 h–7 days
Rotavirus	24–48 h	<100	High	4–7 days	4–7 days	6–60 days
Norovirus	15–50 h	10–100	High	1–2 days	2–4 days	8 h–7 days

*No. of virus particles to cause infection.

transferred from fomites to hands and then into the mouth. In addition, viruses aerosolized from flushing the toilet can remain airborne long enough to contaminate surfaces and items present in the bathroom. Therefore, it is advisable that the lid of the toilet should be closed *before* flushing.

Enteric viruses have been detected in carpets, curtains, and lockers, which can serve as a reservoir. In addition, norovirus, adenovirus, and rotavirus have all been isolated from naturally-contaminated fomites. Surfaces contaminated (e.g. knives or sinks) by virus-infected individuals during food preparation have been documented to be the source of several food-borne outbreaks. Adenovirus has been isolated on drinking glasses from bars and coffee shops, and rotavirus was detected on up to 30% of fomites in day care centres. Spread of all infectious diseases, both enteric and respiratory, is very common amongst children in nursery and day care centres. It has been observed that a small child puts his fingers in his mouth once every 3 min, and in children up to 6 years an average hand-to-mouth frequency of 9.5 contacts per hour.

Norovirus gastroenteritis

Norovirus belongs to the family of *Caliciviridae* viruses. It is a non-enveloped, small, round structured virus (27–32 nm diameter) and can account for greater than 90% of non-bacterial causes of gastroenteritis in health care settings. It has at least four norovirus genogroups (GI, GII, GIII, and GIV) which in turn are divided into at least 20 genetic clusters. Clinical findings associated with norovirus infection include a short incubation period, variable symptoms of upper (vomiting occurs in 50% of cases) and/or lower gastroenteritis (diarrhoea), and low-grade fever (38.3–38.9°C/101–102°F). Although outbreaks can occur throughout the year, most outbreaks in the Northern hemisphere occur during winter and spring hence the term *winter vomiting disease*. Microbiological and epidemiological features of norovirus that promote epidemics are:

♦ Large human reservoir with widespread host susceptibility. Strain-specific protective immunity lasts only up to 6 months. Infection from one strain does not confer immunity from other strain. The average attack rate (no. of people who get infected) is about 50% of those exposed. No vaccine or antiviral agent available.

- Multiple routes of transmission: faecal–oral, food and water-borne, aerosol from vomits contact with contaminated environment.

- Shorter incubation period and very low infective dose as only 10–100 particles are needed to cause infection. During peak shedding, it has been estimated that approximately 5 billion infectious doses contained in each gram of faeces and 30 mL of vomit may contain up to 30,000,000 virus particles. Quick resolutions of symptoms which usually last for 12–72 hours, but prolonged viral shedding of virus does persist (especially in immunocompromised individuals) many continue to contaminate the environment even when the outbreak is over.

- Prolong survival of virus, i.e. up to a week on the imamate surfaces and up to 10 days on foods in a refrigerator.

Diagnosis: ELISAs can be used as an outbreak screening assay test, as during an outbreak situation quicker diagnosis is needed, which should then be confirmed by RT-PCR. To achieve greater 90% sensitivity in an outbreak, collect six stool (and/or vomit) specimens to establish a diagnosis. The diagnostic rate in hotel/restaurant/ nursing home outbreaks is much higher than the diagnostic rate health care setting.

See Box 11.4 for infection prevention and control measures for norovirus (viral) gastroenteritis.

Box 11.4 Summary of infection prevention and control measures for norovirus (viral) gastroenteritis

Patient placement: isolate patient(s) in a single room with an en suite toilet if possible; more than one patient can be placed in a designated (cohort) area. In an outbreak situation, when the attack rate is high, apply contact infection control precautions to all patients in the ward. Use of anti-emetic should be considered to minimize vomiting.

Transfer of patients: avoid patient movement to unaffected wards/unit and health care facilities unless medically urgent. If the patient is clinically well, they can be discharged to their own home. Transfer of patients from an outbreak ward to other health care facilities (including nursing and residential homes) should be postponed until the patients are *asymptomatic* for at least 48–72 hours and *exposed patients* in the same bay have not developed symptoms within 72 hours to ensure that they are beyond incubation period. If the transfer of a patient is considered essential, then the receiving facility *must* be informed of the need for transfer and the patient should be isolated in the side ward with contact infection control precautions.

Visitors: visitors should be advised of the risk of infection and measures to protect themselves should they wish to visit. It is recommended, where visitors have any signs or symptoms of gastroenteritis, that they are requested not to visit the ward. The transmissible nature of the infection should be explained to them and they should be advised as to the reasons why they should not visit. A notice should be displayed during outbreaks advising visitors.

Staff: affected staff must not work for 48–72 hours until they are symptom free.

Diagnosis: collect at least six stool specimen in an outbreak.

Box 11.4 Summary of infection prevention and control measures for norovirus (viral) gastroenteritis (*continued*)

Closure of ward: as a part of control measures, it may become necessary to suspend admission of new patients until the outbreak is over.

De-clutter the ward: in order to aid cleaning, and reduce the bioload of virus on surfaces, all unnecessary items from locker-tops and tables must be removed. Water jugs and glasses used for patients must be covered. Remove exposed fruits and other edible items.

Hand hygiene: wash hands for *at least* 40 seconds after contact with an affected patient or their environment, and after removing gloves and plastic apron. Alcohol hand rub (>70% ethanol applied for 30 seconds) can be used on physically clean hands and be used as an adjunct in between hand washing with soap and water but should not be considered a substitute for hand washing.

Personal protective equipment: wear single use non-sterile gloves and a plastic apron for contact with secretions and excretions (e.g. handling bed pans, vomit bowls and urinals), handling the patient's clothes and bedding, and contact with the patient or their immediate environment. Always wash hands after removing gloves and plastic apron.

Clean and decontaminate all items and equipment which are used for more than one patient. Bed pans must be disinfected in the bed pan washer or use a macerator for single use disposal bed pans. Ensure that the bed pan washer and macerator are in working condition and sluice is clean, dry, and tidy. Non-disposable bed pans should be stored inverted.

Environmental cleaning: the frequency of routine cleaning and disinfection of ward/unit should be reviewed and increased with special emphasise on toilet, sluice area and hand touch surfaces. Use freshly-prepared hypochlorite solution 1000 ppm av Cl_2 to disinfect the environment. Carpets and soft furnishings that cannot be disinfected using chemical methods should be washed thoroughly with hot water and detergent, or preferably steam cleaned. Any spillage or contamination with faeces and vomit should be dealt with immediately.

Communal toilet facilities: toilet seats, flush handles, wash-hand basin taps, and toilet door handles *must be cleaned* and disinfected (e.g. with 1000 ppm of hypochlorite solution) more frequently depending on the level of use. After use, toilet seats lid *must* be covered when flushing the toilet to minimize environmental contamination.

Laundry: all laundry must be segregated and processed as infectious linen (see Chapter 18). In the home setting, soiled clothing should be washed separately from other clothes in a domestic washing machine using a high-temperature wash cycle. Soaking in disinfectant before washing is not necessary. The outside of the washing machine should be wiped down with warm water and detergent after soiled linen is loaded. Thorough hand washing is required after handling soiled linen or clothing.

Opening of ward: the ward should not be re-opened until at least 48–72 h after the last case of gastroenteritis has fully recovered. Before opening, the ward must be thoroughly cleaned and disinfected and all beds and curtains changed before re-opening the ward to new admissions.

Blood-borne viral infections

It has been estimated that about half a billion or one in 12 individuals of the global world population are living with chronic viral hepatitis B or C with an estimated mortality of 1.5 million a year. Because most individuals are asymptomatic, from an infection control perspective, it poses a great challenge. The discussion in this section will be confined to hepatitis B, C, and HIV as they are the most common infections encountered in the health care setting. In the health care setting, the risk of acquiring blood-borne infection is proportional to the *prevalence of infection* in the population served and the *chance of inoculation accidents* occurring during procedures.

The risk of infection following percutaneous exposure to the blood from an infectious source from hepatitis B patients is estimated to be between 5–30% and for hepatitis C infection is between 3–10%. The average risk for HIV infection after a percutaneous needle stick injury with HIV-infected blood is estimated to be 0.3% and the risk associated with mucous membrane exposure is estimated to be about 0.09%. However, all these estimates are generalizations and the volume of inoculum and the viral load in the source patient have a major effect on the risk in any individual incident. Immunization is an effective means of protection against hepatitis B virus but must not be used as a substitute for good infection control practice as the vaccine is not available against hepatitis C, HIV, and other viruses transmitted through the blood-borne route.

Viral hepatitis

To date, six types of viral hepatitis have been identified. Hepatitis B, C, D, and G are transmitted by the blood-borne route and hepatitis A and E are transmitted by the faecal–oral route and will not be discussed.

Hepatitis B

Hepatitis B virus (HBV) is a member of the Hepadnaviridae family of DNA viruses. The mean incubation period of acute HBV infection is 75 days but it may range from 45–180 days. After exposure to the virus, most infected adults recover completely from the acute illness; however, in-apparent infections are common, particularly among children and children are more likely to develop chronic infection. A small, and variable, proportion of individuals do not clear hepatitis B surface antigen (HBsAg), which is found circulating in blood during the latter part of the incubation period and in the acute phase of HBV (see Figure 11.1). They become chronic hepatitis B cases, (i.e. individuals who shed HBsAg into the circulation for more than 6 months) following acute infection. Some of these develop chronic active hepatitis, cirrhosis or hepatocellular carcinoma. The likelihood of a patient developing chronic hepatitis is inversely related to age at the time of infection.

Chronic infection occurs in at least 90% of cases following neonatal infection, 25% of children aged 1–10 years, and 5% or less in adults. Of these, 5–10% have persistent 'e' antigenaemia (HBeAg+ve), which correlates with a high level of viral replication and heightened infectivity; these are regarded as high-grade infections. Such high-grade infections are generally associated with HBV DNA levels of greater than 10,000 genomes/mL in serum. A patient who is in the early prodromal or acute phase of

---

Box 11.5 General infection control measures to protect against blood-borne viruses

- Apply standard infection control precautions (see Chapter 7, Table 7.1). Wash hand before and after contact with patient, after contact with blood and body fluids, and after removing gloves. Change gloves between patients.

- Use protective clothing as appropriate, including protection of the mucous membrane of the eyes, mouth, and nose from blood and body fluid splashes. Avoid wearing open footwear in situations where blood may be spilt, or where sharp instruments or needles are handled.

- Avoid sharps usage wherever possible and consider the use of alternative instruments, cutting diathermy, and laser. Where sharps usage is essential, exercise particular care in handling and disposal, following approved procedures and using approved sharps disposal containers.

- For all clinical procedures, cover existing wounds, skin lesions, and all breaks in exposed skin with waterproof dressings or with gloves if hands extensively affected.

- HCWs with chronic skin disease (e.g. eczema) should avoid invasive procedures, which involve sharp instruments or needles when their skin lesions are active, or if there are extensive breaks in the skin surface. A non-intact skin surface provides a potential route for BBV transmission, and blood-skin contact is common through glove puncture that may go unnoticed.

- Clear up spillage of blood and other body fluids promptly and disinfect surfaces (see Chapter 6, Box 6.5).

---

hepatitis B should also be considered as high grade. Most carriers, however, are 'e' antigen negative and can be classified as low grade with regard to transmission of infection. However, carriers of HBV who are negative for 'e' antigen can occasionally transmit infection. Some of these low-grade carriers have been associated with the presence of a viral mutation, which stops the synthesis of 'e' antigen but still allows production of infectious virus. Refer to Table 11.3 for interpretation of hepatitis B serological markers in immunocompetent individuals.

Hepatitis C

Hepatitis C virus (HCV) belongs to the Flaviviridae family. Incubation periods range from 20 days to 13 weeks. The acute phase of HCV infection is usually asymptomatic or mild and patients are usually unaware of the infection. Patients may complain of fatigue but a few have a history of acute hepatitis or jaundice. If it proceeds to chronic disease, progression is usually indolent and the most common complaint is fatigue. Up to 80% of people who are anti-HCV positive may continue to carry the virus, which may cause slow ongoing liver damage (Figure 11.2). It is thought that 10–20% of individuals with chronic hepatitis C will go on to develop cirrhosis over 20–40 years and a significant proportion of those with cirrhosis go on to develop liver cancer.

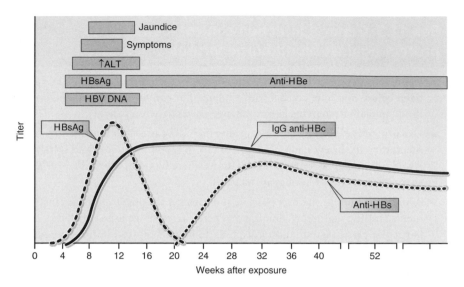

Fig. 11.1 The typical course of acute type B hepatitis. HBsAg: hepatitis B surface antigen; anti-HBs; antibody to HbsAg; HBeAg: hepatitis B 'e' antigen; anti-HBe: antibody to HBeAg; anti-HBc: antibody to hepatitis B core antigen; ALT: alanine aminotransferase.

Diagnosis of HCV is based on an enzyme immunoassay that detects antibodies to hepatitis C virus (anti-HCV). In general, the diagnosis is confirmed by use of a supplemental recombinant immunoblot assay (RIBA) or a second ELISA. However, detection and confirmation of antibodies to HCV alone does not distinguish between individuals who have been previously exposed to the virus and those who continue to have viraemia. Most antibody-confirmed patients are potentially infectious, as confirmed by use of a PCR-based test. The PCR test directly detects viral RNA and indicates if there is circulating virus.

Hepatitis D and G

Hepatitis D virus (HDV), previously known as the 'delta agent' is a defective virus that requires the presence and the helper activity of HBV to allow it to replicate. HDV virus can be co-transmitted with hepatitis B infection or can superinfect chronic HBV carriers. The mean incubation period is 35 days and transmission is mainly through parenteral routes. Hepatitis caused by HDV is usually severe and individuals with double infection, HBV and HDV, usually develop more rapidly progressive disease and cirrhosis at an earlier age than those with HBV infection alone. Hepatitis G is a flavivirus that can be transmitted parenterally. At present, the epidemiology and clinical correlation of HGV infection are not well characterized but the virus does not appear to be a significant cause of liver disease.

HIV infection

HIV is a member of the retrovirus family and responsible for HIV infections and cases of acquired immunodeficiency syndrome (AIDS). It was first isolated in 1983. Two genetically distinct types, HIV 1 and HIV 2, have been recognized. HIV 2, isolated in 1986, is prevalent only in certain West African countries. The term HIV used in these guidelines covers both types of virus.

Table 11.3 Interpretation of the common patterns of serological markers of HBV infection

HBsAg	Anti-HBc total	Anti-HBc IgM	HBe-Ag	Anti-HBe	Comments
Negative	Not tested	Not tested	Not tested	Not tested	Not infected
Negative	Positive	Not tested	Not tested	Not tested	The presence of antiHBc (usually with anti-HBs) indicates a *past infection* and *natural immunity* to hepatitis B
Positive	Negative	Negative	Positive	Negative	Suggests *early acute infection* with hepatitis B High infectivity High risk of transmission to the baby; give HB vaccine and HBIG at birth
Positive	Positive	Positive (high level)	Positive	Positive *or* Negative	Confirms *early acute infection* with hepatitis B High infectivity High risk of transmission to the baby; give HB vaccine and HBIG at birth
Positive	Positive	Positive (low level) *or* Negative	Positive	Negative	Consistent with *chronic infection* with hepatitis B High infectivity High risk of transmission to the baby; give HB vaccine and HBIG at birth
Positive	Positive	Negative	Negative	Positive	Consistent with *chronic infection* with hepatitis B Risk of transmission to the baby; give HB vaccine at birth
Positive	Positive	Negative	Positive *or* Negative	Positive *or* Negative	Consistent with *chronic infection* with hepatitis B Risk of transmission to the baby; give HB vaccine at birth. Baby may also require HBIG based on the clinical evaluation

HB = hepatitis B; HBIG = hepatitis B immunoglobulin.

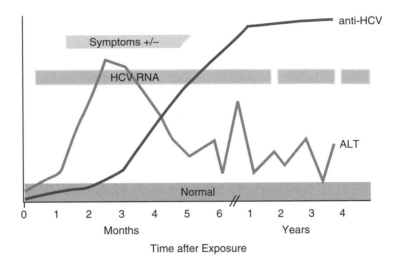

Fig. 11.2 Typical course of chronic hepatitis C infection.

Clinical features

After exposure to HIV most individuals develop antibodies within 3 months. During the acute phase (i.e. around the time when antibody first appears), there may be a self-limiting illness resembling glandular fever (infectious mononucleosis), with lymphadenopathy and rash. Later in the course of infection, non-specific illness (including fever, night sweats, and lymphadenopathy) is associated with progressive immune dysfunction. When AIDS develops fully it is characterized by the appearance of opportunistic infections and tumours.

Infection with yeast, *Candida* spp., may cause persistent and severe thrush in the mouth and oesophagus and there may be reactivation of common latent herpes viruses. Invasion of the lungs by *Pneumocystis jiroveci* often gives rise to a pneumonitis

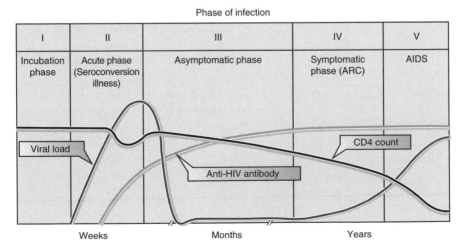

Fig. 11.3 Typical course of HIV infection.

with shortness of breath and diffuse shadowing sometimes seen on a chest x-ray. Some individuals may be infected with *Mycobacterium* spp., i.e. *M. tuberculosis, M. avium-intracellulare*. Many other infections may supervene including cytomegalovirus, hepatitis B, and protozoa such as *Toxoplasma* in the brain or *Giardia* and *Cryptosporidium* in the bowel. Some patients develop Kaposi's sarcoma, an unusual tumour of the skin. This appears as characteristic discrete purple patches, often affecting the extremities, although internal organs may also be involved. Still others develop lymphoma, often in the brain.

Laboratory diagnosis

Testing for HIV virus should be undertaken on the basis of clinical assessment. The provision of patient confidentiality, privacy, and informed consent for testing is essential. The individual requiring an HIV test should be offered appropriate discussion prior to testing, which should address the specific needs of the individual.

HIV serology: the gold standard for HIV screening assays are fourth-generation assays that simultaneously detect antigen and antibody and compared to third-generation assays (antibody only) considerably reduce the 'window period' between inoculation and test becoming positive. Positive specimens are then confirmed by a series of other tests to assure the specificity of the result. The 'window period' is usually between 10–30 days but may last several months in some cases. During this 'window period', the HIV antibody test will be negative; therefore a negative test is not an absolute exclusion of HIV infection.

HIV viral load: patients vary in their level of viraemia. HIV viral load tests assess the level of viral replication and provide useful prognostic information, which is independent of the information provided by CD4 counts (see below). Rapid progressors tend to have persistently high viral load whereas slow or non-progressors have low viral load. In the early stages of infection (including the 'window' period) the concentration of HIV in the bloodstream is very high. During this period the antibody test is negative, although tests for HIV RNA are positive. After the resolution of the seroconversion illness, the HIV viral load decreases due to the host immune responses and stabilizes at a lower level. As immunodeficiency progresses and AIDS develop the HIV viral load rises again (see Figure 11.3) .Viral load is also influenced by antiretroviral therapy. Most patients on combination antiretroviral therapy have a low HIV viral load.

CD4 lymphocyte count: several laboratory markers are available to provide prognostic information and guide decisions on starting and changing therapy. The most widely used marker is the CD4 lymphocyte count. Risk of progression to an AIDS opportunistic infection or malignancy is high with the CD4 count being lower than 200cells/mm^3. While CD4 count measures immune dysfunction, it does not provide a measure of how actively HIV is replicating in the body and therefore viral load is done to access the infectivity.

Routes of transmission

Blood-borne viruses (BBV) are transmitted through transfer of blood or 'high-risk' body fluids containing virus and may occur by:

♦ Unprotected penetrative sexual intercourse with an infected person (between men or between a man and a woman).

- ◆ Skin puncture by sharps contaminated with blood, i.e.
    - • Sharing used needles and syringes among IV drug users.
    - • Receipt of tattoos, ear piercing, communal hair cutting, acupuncture, dental treatment, electrolysis, etc.
- ◆ Inoculation/sharp injuries to HCW from an infected individual.
- ◆ Childbirth from an infected mother to her baby (intrauterine and peripartum) or through breastfeeding.
- ◆ Via infected blood transfusion, blood products, donations of semen, skin grafts, and organ transplants from someone who is infected.
- ◆ Transmission through contamination of open wounds and skin lesions, e.g. eczema, may also occur, splashing the mucous membrane of the eye, nose or mouth and through human bites when blood is drawn.

Blood is not the only concern, as various other 'high-risk' body fluids, i.e. cerebrospinal, peritoneal, pleural, pericardial, amniotic and synovial fluid, semen, vaginal secretions, and any other body fluids containing visible blood, and all tissues, organs and parts of bodies which are unfixed, are also hazardous. Exposure to 'low-risk' body fluids such as urine, faeces, nasal secretions, tears, saliva (except in relation to dentistry), sputum, and vomitus present a minimal risk of BBV infection unless contaminated with blood; although they may be hazardous for other reasons as they may contain other pathogenic microorganisms. When blood is mentioned, it should be taken to include blood and 'high-risk' body fluids unless otherwise stated.

Precautions during surgical procedures

Since the patient's infective status is not always known, each surgical procedure should be considered as a potential source of infection. It is essential that the operating team must demonstrate their knowledge of potential risks by ensuring that a 'confine and contain' approach is implemented for every procedure and must be immunized against HBV.

Preoperative testing of a patient for infectious agents should be on the basis of clinical indication, and medical practitioners should exercise their professional judgement. In the case of elective surgery, any testing considered relevant should be completed before admission. Discretion and patient confidentiality must be maintained in all circumstances. Surgery lists should be scheduled on the basis of clinical urgency, and in such a way as to allow ample time for adequate infection control procedures to take place.

In addition to the standard infection control precautions, the patient known to have BBV infection may require the following additional precautions for surgical operation:

- ◆ The lead surgeon is responsible for ensuring that all members of the team know of the infection hazards and that appropriate measures are followed.
- ◆ The surgical team must be limited to essential members of trained staff only.
- ◆ It may help theatre decontamination if such cases are last on the list, but this is not essential.

- Depilatory creams should be used for essential hair removal.

- Unnecessary equipment should be removed from the theatre in order to reduce the amount of decontamination required after the operation. Disposable items should be used wherever possible. If any item is not disposable it must be decontaminated by the sterile supply department (SSD). Special equipment reserved for these patients is not essential.

- Before any surgical procedure, the surgeon and scrub nurse should decide on the routine for passage of sharp instruments during the procedure. This may entail the designation of a *'neutral zone'*. The surgeon must avoid placing his/her less dexterous hand in potential danger. Sharp instruments should not be passed by hand. A specified puncture-resistant sharps tray must be used for the transfer of all sharp instruments. Only one sharp must be in the tray at any one time. If two surgeons are operating simultaneously, then each surgeon needs his/her own sharps tray.

- Disposable drapes should be used and the mattress should be protected by a plastic sheet.

- Diathermy and suction devices should be placed on the opposite side of the table to the surgeon, thereby ensuring the assistant does not reach across the table between the surgeon and nurse.

- Variations in operative technique, such as a non-touch approach, the avoidance of passing sharp instruments from nurse to surgeon and vice versa, and new techniques of cutting (e.g. with lasers), or of wound closure that obviate the use of sharp instruments and lessen the risk of inoculation are recommended. Needles must never be picked up with the fingers, nor the fingers used to expose and increase access for the passage of a suture in deep tissues.

- Where practical, blunt needles should be used to close the abdomen. When suturing, forceps or a needle holder should be used to pick up the needle and draw it through the tissue. Where practical, suture needles should be cut off before knots are tied to prevent needlestick injury. Surgeons may use a sterile thimble on the index finger of the less dexterous hand for protection when suturing. Wire sutures should be avoided where possible because of the high injury rate to the surgeon. After a surgical procedure, the skin should be closed with staples whenever possible. Hand-held straight needles should not be used.

- Hands of assisting HCWs must not be used to retract the wound on viscera during surgery. Self-retaining retractors should be used, or a swab on a stick, instead of fingers. Certain instruments should be avoided unless essential to the procedure, for example, sharp wound retractors such as rake retractors and skin hooks.

- Closed wound drainage systems should be used, where appropriate. Wound dressings with an impervious outer covering that will contain wound exudates should be used. If drainage is considered necessary, closed rather than open wound drainage is recommended. Blood should be cleaned off the patient's skin as far as possible at the end of the operation using suitable antiseptic/detergents solution.

- Where practical, used instruments should be washed mechanically using an ultrasonic washer rather than by hand. Surgical instruments and other tools used in operations should be put in a robust puncture-resistant container, labelled 'Danger of Infection' and returned to the SSD. Instruments for reuse should, as soon as possible after use, be immersed in warm water and detergent to prevent congealing or solidifying of blood and fatty materials, and must be thoroughly cleaned in the designated clean-up area before sterilization.

◆ Infectious waste excluding sharps must be placed in an appropriate colour coded infectious waste plastic bag, sealed, and removed from the operating room. Disposal of infectious waste must comply with local regulations.

◆ Needles and syringes, and disposable sharp instruments must be discarded into approved sharps boxes. The sharps container must be closed securely when three-quarters full. Scalpel blades and needles and all other non-reusable sharps should be placed in a designated puncture-proof sharps container, which should comply with local or international standard.

◆ Used linen and theatre clothing should be placed in a water soluble bag which is then placed in a second plastic bag and marked as 'Infected linen'. It should be handled in accordance with local policy.

◆ Blood and other body fluid spills should be disinfected and cleaned up immediately using sodium hypochlorite (1% or 10,000ppm available chlorine) or other appropriate disinfectant, in accordance with the local protocol.

◆ **Cleaning of operating theatre:** adequate time must be provided at the end of each case to allow for thorough cleaning of the operating theatre and the appropriate disposal of clinical waste. All surfaces (operating table, instrument table, equipment used, and the floor) should be carefully cleaned using warm water and detergent. Walls and other surfaces do not require cleaning unless contaminated with blood. Large volumes of fluid should be used for cleaning and gloves and a plastic apron should be worn by the operator. Appropriate disinfectant, (e.g. sodium hypochlorite 1000 ppm available chlorine) may be used after removal of gross soil. Surfaces should be cleaned and dried after applying disinfectants. Thorough rinsing is necessary to minimize damage to surfaces from the disinfectants.

Personal protective equipment

Gowns: all staff in the theatre should wear a disposable plastic apron under their gowns. A water-impermeable gown should be worn if gross contamination with blood or body fluids is likely. Where waterproof aprons are worn for procedures in which there is likely to be considerable dissemination of blood, it is essential that the aprons are of sufficient length to overlap with protective footwear. This is especially important for procedures carried out in the lithotomy position, since it is common for blood accumulating in the worker's lap to be channelled down into the boots. Caps should cover the hair completely.

Mask: the surgical team should each wear a mask and two pairs of gloves and skin lesions must be covered with waterproof dressings. Double sterile gloving, i.e. a double glove with the larger size glove on the inside is recommended for all surgeons involved in operating room procedures. If a glove is torn or a needlestick or other injury occurs, the gloves should be removed and hands washed when safety permits and new gloves put on promptly.

Eye protection: spectacles or goggles should be worn by those taking part in the operation to avoid conjunctival contamination or splashing.

Footwear: fenestrated footwear must never be worn in situations where sharps are handled. For tasks involving likely dissemination of blood it is recommended that Wellington boots or calf-length plastic boots are worn rather than shoes or clogs. Contaminated footwear must be adequately decontaminated after use with appropriate precautions for those undertaking it.

Protection of the newborn

Hepatitis B infection

The risk of perinatal transmission is up to 90% in mothers who are HBV e-antigen (HBeAg) positive and approximately 10% in women with antibody to e antigen (Anti-HBe). Infection can result in an acute or chronic infection. A chronic infection with HBV may result in cirrhosis of the liver and liver cancer therefore screening of mothers to identify HBV status is crucial to prevent both acute and chronic infection in babies. In high prevalence areas, hepatitis B immunization should be given to all pregnant women to prevent perinatal transmission from mother to baby. In other countries, those providing antenatal care will need to take steps to identify infected mothers during pregnancy and make arrangements to ensure that babies born to these mothers receive a complete course of immunization against hepatitis B infection. This is best done by screening women early in pregnancy. Where this has not been done, it should be possible to detect carrier mothers at the time of delivery. The transmission of infection from mother to baby can be successfully prevented by giving a vaccination to the baby within 24 hours of delivery, and at 1, 2, and 12 months, which will confer active immunity. In babies born to women with a higher risk of transmission, the addition of hepatitis B-specific immune globulin (HBIG) gives passive protection and can help reduce the risk further. With this strategy, transmission can be prevented in over 90% of babies exposed to maternal infection. The arrangements for the supply of hepatitis B vaccine and HBIG should be made well in advance. The newborn should be given 200 IU HBIG at birth or as soon as possible (within 24 hours of delivery). In addition, the first dose of vaccine should be given at birth or as soon as possible at a different site. The complete course of hepatitis B immunization regimen consists of a three-dose series of vaccine, with the first dose at the time of birth, the second dose 1 month later, and the third dose at 6 months after the first dose. The vaccine should normally be given intramuscularly and the anterolateral thigh is the preferred site in infants.

Hepatitis C infection: currently, there is no therapy available for the prevention of HCV infection in neonates born to mothers infected with HCV.

HIV infection: in order to prevent HIV infection in neonates, appropriate antiretroviral therapy can be given to both the mother before birth and to the neonate at birth to reduce the risk of HIV transmission. It is usually appropriate to advice against breastfeeding where the mother is known to be HIV positive.

Tuberculosis

Tuberculosis (TB) is a disease of antiquity and evidence of infection has been seen in the spines of Egyptian mummies. It was called the 'white plague' because of the waxen, pale countenance of individuals in the terminal stages of pulmonary TB. The disease is portrayed in art, literature, and music, e.g. the operas La Boheme and La Traviata depict TB. Many artists themselves suffered from fatal illness, e.g. Shelley, Keats, Voltaire, Chekhov, Franz Kafka, and George Orwell. It was thought that TB produce spells of euphoria, exacerbated sexual desire, and was imagined to be an aphrodisiac and to confer extraordinary powers of seduction. It made women more beautiful and men more creative as 'the toxins of tuberculosis have facilitated the creative personalities in many notable instances' (Jacobson, 1970).

TB remains one of the most devastating infectious diseases with more than 9 million cases worldwide and is responsible for 1.7 million deaths annually. It has been estimated that about one-third of the world population are currently infected with TB. Currently HIV infection is fuelling an epidemic of TB especially in sub-Saharan Africa.

Microbiology

TB is an infection caused by bacterium of the *Mycobacterium tuberculosis* complex (*M. tuberculosis, M. bovis, M. africanum*). *M. tuberculosis* and *M. africanum* are acquired primarily from humans and *M. bovis* primarily from cattle. It is usually a pulmonary disease; extrapulmonay TB is much less common, but infection may occur in any organ or tissue including lymph nodes, meninges, pleura, pericardium, kidneys, bones, joints, larynx, skin, peritoneum, intestines, and eyes. Most **non-mycobacteria tuberculous species** are saprophytic and can cause infection in mainly immunosuppressed patients. They are commonly found in water systems; older water systems have higher colonization rates. Higher colonization of *M. avium* and *M. xenopi* are found in hot water while *M. kansasii* are found in cold water.

Pseudo-infection/outbreaks can be caused by contamination of the sputum. Therefore tap water *must not* be used by the microbiology laboratory to perform a Ziehl–Neelsen (ZN) stain to avoid false diagnosis. Environmental mycobacteria frequently exist within biofilms which not only support its growth but also protect microorganisms from the effect of disinfectant. As a result, if the AER endoscopic machine is not maintained, contamination of bronchoscopes can occur (especially with *M. chelonae* which can be present in the rinse water) which subsequently contaminates bronchial washings leading to misdiagnosis of TB.

Treatment

In the UK, pulmonary TB is treated for a total of 6 months in two phases. *Initial phase*: combination of four drugs using isoniazid, rifampicin, pyrazinamide, and ethambutol for the first 2 months. *Continuation phase*: combination of two drugs isoniazid and rifampicin for a further 4 months.

The treatment of TB is complex and lengthy. Inadequate treatment and non-compliance with medication are the main causes of relapse and of the emergence of drug-resistant organisms. Therefore, the treatment should be *supervised by a medical practitioner* with expertise in the management of TB. Compliance with treatment must be monitored. If there is any doubt, measures such as pill counts, prescription checks, or urine tests may be used. Individual plans for non-compliant patients may involve arrangements for directly observed therapy. Most patients with TB can be treated at home; a few require hospital admission for severe illness, adverse effects of chemotherapy, or for social reasons.

Multiresistant tuberculosis

Definitions

Multidrug-resistant tuberculosis (MDR-TB) is resistant to at least isoniazid and rifampicin while **extensively drug-resistant tuberculosis** (XDR-TB) is resistant to at least isoniazid and rifampicin and *also* to any fluoroquinolones and at least one of three second-line injectable agents (Amikacin, capreomycin, or kanamycin).

Risk factors for M/XDR-TB

The risk factors for M/XDR-TB are: 1) history of previous drug treatment for TB (usually incomplete treatment or non-compliant patient), 2) known recent contact with a person with drug resistant TB, and 3) patients infected with HIV. In addition to above, additional risk factors for M/XDR-TB in the UK also include younger male patients (25–44 years), especially who were born outside the UK (especially in a country with high prevalence of M/XDR-TB) and those who are resident in the London area.

It is important that the patients with M/XDR-TB should be managed at facilities with expertise in such management. These patients should be isolated in a negative pressure ventilation room and their movement and contact around the facility must be minimized. In HIV-positive individuals, XDR-TB has been associated with very high mortality.

Clinical manifestations

The incubation period from exposure to demonstrable primary lesion or significant tuberculin reaction is in the range of 4–12 weeks. Early clinical symptoms include fatigue, weight loss, fever, cough, and night sweats. In more advanced disease, hoarseness, cough with blood-stained sputum, and chest pain are common.

Many initial infections with *M. tuberculosis* or related species are asymptomatic as activated macrophages control the spread and growth of the microorganisms. As a result pulmonary lesions heal spontaneously and form areas of fibrosis or calcification called 'Ghon lesions'. A Ghon lesion combination with hilar adenopathy is called a 'Ranke complex'. *M. tuberculosis* grows best in the region with high oxygen tension, including the kidneys, long bone epiphyses, and vertebral bodies. In the lung it most commonly infects the apices because these regions of the lungs have the highest oxygen content, and blood transport and oxygen extraction from the alveoli are less efficient in this region.

Of those people presumed infected, there is a 10–15% chance of developing clinical disease at some point in their lives. The risk of progressive pulmonary or extrapulmonary

Box 11.6 Summary of infection control for patients with tuberculosis

Patient placement

- All patients with suspected/confirmed pulmonary TB *must* be isolated in a single room with airborne infection control precautions. The door must be kept closed.

- No patient with suspected/confirmed respiratory TB should be admitted to an open ward, especially one where immunocompromised patients (e.g. HIV infected, transplant or oncology) are nursed and cough inducing procedure *must not* be performed in an open bay/ward.

- Isolate all patients with M/XDR-TB in a negative pressure ventilation room until three negative AAFB results of sputum are available. The door should be kept closed.

- Advise the patients about the cough etiquette by asking patient to cover their mouth and nose with tissue and turn away from others while coughing or sneezing. A box of tissues should be provided and used tissues should be disposed of as clinical waste.

- When the patient is required to leave a TB isolation room, they should wear a surgical mask to cover their mouth if they are coughing or cannot reliably cover their mouth.

Diagnosis

- Send three (preferably early morning) sputum specimens to the laboratory for diagnosis.

- If the facilities are available, perform PCR on the smear positive sample to confirm diagnosis of MTB and for rifampicin resistance gene as the results are available on the same day.

Infection control precautions

- Implement airborne transmission precautions (see Chapter 7, Table 7.1). Consider early discharge of patients, if possible.

- Contact with staff and visitors should be kept to a *minimum* without compromising patient care.

- HCWs should wear a FFP3/N95 respirator when entering the room and during bronchoscopy, prolonged care of a high-dependency patient, during cough-inducing procedures, physiotherapy, or lung surgery with high-speed devices and other aerosol generating procedures (see Chapter 9, p. 158) or when performing the last offices.

- Marked crockery and separate washing up facilities are *not* necessary, and no special precautions are needed for bed linen, books or other personal property as the transmission route is airborne.

Box 11.6 Summary of infection control for patients with tuberculosis (*continued*)

Visitors

- Visitors must be limited to those who have already been in close contact with the patient before the illness. All children with TB and their visitors should be segregated from other patients until the contacts have been screened and pronounced non-infectious.

Duration of isolation

- For *fully sensitive* strain of MTB, the AFFB smear will usually be negative (non-infectious) after two weeks of standard anti-TB chemotherapy. However, isolation of patient *must continue* for all patients with M/XDR-TB in a negative pressure ventilation room until three AAFB sputum results are negative. In *all cases*, advice from the IPC team *must* be sought before moving the patient in to an open ward. Infection caused by atypical *Mycobacterium* spp. should be regarded as non-infectious and may be nursed in a general ward.

Terminal cleaning of room:

- When a patient is discharged home, the room should be terminally cleaned. Fumigation of the room is *not* necessary.

TB is greatest in the first year or two after infection with the greatest risk in the first 6–12 months; about half of these occur in the first 5 years after infection. In cases where a long period elapses between infection and development of disease, dormant bacilli are thought to remain in either the lung or other sites (latent infection), which can 'reactivate' in favourable circumstances e.g. older age or other events that weaken the individual's immunity (see Host susceptibility, p. 216).

Diagnosis of tuberculosis

Chest x-ray: a posterior–anterior chest x-ray should be taken. If chest x-ray is suggestive of TB, further diagnostic investigations should be followed.

Ziehl–Neelsen stain: ZN stain is used to look for AFFB in the specimen and can be done on sputum, urine, pus, and tissue biopsies and has advantages of simplicity and gives rapid results. However, it has only a 60% sensitivity compared to sputum culture. In addition, microscopy for AFFB requires 5000–10,000 bacilli/mL of sample while culture, though slow, is more sensitive, requiring only 10–100 bacilli/mL.

Three sputum specimens are required as release of the microorganism is intermittent. Out of three specimens *at least* one early morning specimen is required as this specimen has the highest yield due to high concentration of microorganisms.

Polymerase chain reaction: PCR examination of direct smears of clinical specimens for acid-fast bacilli is rapid and can effectively detect as few as 10 organisms in a clinical specimen. The major benefits of this rapid diagnostic test are improved patient care, reduced medical costs, and more effective use of isolation rooms. The PCR can not only quickly confirm the diagnosis *M. tuberculosis* in a few hours but also help to exclude the diagnosis of MRD-TB if the PCR is negative for rifampicin resistant gene.

Culture method: definite diagnosis is achieved by culturing the TB bacterium in liquid and solid culture medium; however, it takes time because conventional bacteria grows quicker and gives results within 24 hours. *M. tuberculosis* takes 24 hours to replicate and about a month to produce visible growth on solid media and therefore full identification and sensitivity testing against anti-tuberculosis drugs takes 6–8 weeks.

Interferon-gamma test: interferon-gamma tests (IGTs) are commercially available (QuantiFERON-TB Gold® and T-SPOT®) and have been developed using the TB antigens. The test involves taking a blood sample. The test is not only helpful for the diagnosis of MTB, but also useful if someone has been exposed to MTB and may have latent infection. IGTs showed little evidence of being affected by prior BCG vaccination, and showed stronger correlation with exposure categories than the Mantoux tests. Consideration should be given to use IGTs for people ages 5 years and older in an outbreak situation when large numbers of people may need to be screened.

Tuberculin skin test: Mantoux test is a tuberculin skin test (TST) and involves intradermal injection of purified protein derivative (PPD) from *M. tuberculosis* (MTB). It is routinely used not only to identify subjects infected with MTB, but also to assess cell-mediated immune response against MTB in order to guide decisions about chemoprophylaxis and treatment.

Most of the individuals infected with MTB develop a delayed-type hypersensitivity response in 2–4 weeks after infection. The tuberculin tests had the advantage of being cheap and relatively easy to perform. However, it has certain disadvantages as the test results have to be interpreted within a certain timescale, and some patients who do not return, or delay returning, will have either no result or a possibly inaccurate one. In addition, false positive results can occur because of the sensitizing effect on the immune system of either prior BCG vaccination or exposure to the opportunist environmental mycobacteria. False negative results can occur due to impaired immunity, particularly co-infection with HIV, but also treatments such as cytotoxics, or immunosuppressive agents. Extensive pulmonary or miliary TB can itself also temporarily depress the immunity, and can lead to a paradoxically negative Mantoux result. There is an increase the likelihood of false negative results if the individuals have received MMR vaccines in the previous 4 weeks. In addition, it is essential that TST should be *read by a trained* health care professional.

Mode of transmission

TB is usually transmitted by exposure to airborne droplet nuclei (approx. 1–5 microns in diameter, containing 1 to 10 bacilli). It is produced by people with 'open' pulmonary TB (AFFB positive from sputum) when bacilli are released when they are coughing, sneezing, or singing. Once discharged, the aerosolized droplets containing tuberculi bacilli remain afloat and viable in the environment for a prolonged period of time. When inhaled, these tuberculi bacilli can settle in the alveoli of lungs, where they may result in TB infection.

Sputum smear positive is thought to be six to ten times more contagious than a smear negative case and laryngeal TB cases are four to five times more contagious than smear positive pulmonary cases. Patients whose bronchial washings are smear-positive should be managed as if non-infectious unless the sputum is also smear-positive or becomes soon after bronchoscopy or they are on a ward with immunocompromised patients, or they are known or suspected of having M/XDR-TB. Infections caused by atypical mycobacteria are *not* infectious.

Transmission from infants and children younger than 10 years of age with pulmonary TB are *much less* contagious because their pulmonary lesions are small and cavitary disease is rare, they have reduced ability to expectorate, and few bacilli are expulsed due to low microorganism load.

Infection by direct contact with mucous membranes or skin lesions is extremely rare. Extrapulmonary TB is generally *not* communicable apart from exceptionally rare circumstances where there is a draining abscess. Bovine TB may result from drinking unpasteurized infected milk or by aerosol transmission from infected animals to farmers or animal handlers.

Duration of infectivity

The person is considered infectious and can transmit infection as long as sputum smear is positive ('open case') for *M. tuberculosis* by ZN staining methods. Effective treatment with antimicrobial chemotherapy usually eliminates communicability within 2 weeks provided that strain if fully susceptible and therefore patient should remain in isolation for *at least* 2 weeks. However, in some cases, especially in the case of multi-drug resistant tuberculosis, inadequate treatment or non-compliance with treatment, the patient may remain sputum-positive or be sputum-positive intermittently for a lengthy period of time and this must be guided by smear (AAFB) result from the microbiology laboratory. Cases of extrapulmonary TB are typically non-infectious and contact investigations should be aimed at identifying a source of infection in those with greatest exposure to the case.

Risk of acquisition

The degree of communicability to the other individuals depends on: 1) duration of exposure, 2) opportunities from exposure, 3) number of bacilli discharged from the patient, 4) host susceptibility, 5) virulence of the bacilli. These factors should be taken into consideration during contact tracing (see 'Contact tracing', below).

Duration of exposure

The likelihood of transmission *of M. tuberculosis* increases with the intensity, frequency, and duration of exposure to a case. Usually it takes many hours or days to transmit an infectious dose, but casual/short exposures may lead to transmission if the case is infectious and environmental air conditions are favourable. Exposure duration of less than eight hours is generally considered not to be significant and current UK and USA guidelines recommend cumulative contact of 8 hours or more require investigation of contact.

Indoor environment

Transmission is rarely thought to occur outdoors. Risk of transmission is greatest where there is prolonged, close contact with a case in an indoor environment. This is due to small volumes of shared indoor air, limited ventilation of the airspace with outdoor air and recirculation of air in closed circulation heating or air conditioning systems. In addition, indoor environments that are poorly ventilated, dark or damp, can lead to increased concentration and survival of *M. tuberculosis* in the environment.

Host susceptibility

- TB is also common in individuals who have a poor socioeconomic background, are malnourished, homeless, in prison, and are chronic alcohol misusers and/or drug users.

- The risk of developing disease is much greater in infants and children *under 5 years* of age because they have a less developed immune system than adults and they are more likely to develop active and more serious disease. The incubation period is usually short in this age group. Therefore, children under 5 years of age should be assigned a *high priority* for contact investigation.

- People living with patient diagnosed with TB or who have close contact with people with active TB.

- In countries where the TB prevalence is low, higher incidence is also found in individuals who have arrived or returned from high-prevalence countries within the last 5 years.

- For individuals with latent infection, the risk of reactivation is increased in immunocompromised individuals who are on prolonged courses of steroid use (i.e. equivalent to 15 mg prednisolone daily for at least 1 month), patients receiving TNF-α antagonists (e.g. infliximab and etanercept), anti-rejection drugs such as ciclosporin, various cytotoxic treatments and azathioprine.

- Patients who have comorbidity states affecting the immune system, for example, chronic renal disease, many haematological and solid cancers, and diabetes mellitus.

- TB patients who are HIV-infected with low CD4 T-cell counts frequently have chest x-ray findings that are not typical of pulmonary TB. Atypical radiographic findings increase the potential for delayed diagnosis which increases transmission.

- **HIV infected and tuberculosis** patients should *not* be mixed. In settings where other patients may be infected with HIV or otherwise immunocompromised, suspected or confirmed cases of pulmonary TB should be considered as potentially infectious on every admission until proven otherwise, and segregated accordingly. Patients with potentially infectious TB should be segregated from other immunocompromised patients by admission to a single room with en suite toilet facility in a separate ward or to a negative pressure ventilation room, if available. For all patients in a HIV ward, aerosol generating procedures such as bronchoscopy, sputum induction, or nebulizer treatment should *never be performed in an open ward or bay*.

- **Tuberculosis in children**: it is very difficult to diagnose TB in children, mainly because of the difficulty in obtaining sputum specimens. Gastric lavage can be done occasionally but it is a messy procedure and does not give reliable results. In addition, because IGT tests rely on a fully developed immune system negative

IGT could *not* completely exclude infection in children. Most paediatricians would choose to treat a high-risk child if they had a positive Mantoux test and negative IGT. All children with TB and their visitors should be segregated from other patients until their contacts have been screened and pronounced non-infectious. It is possible that one of the visitors may have been the source of the child's infection and hence be a risk to other patients if the child is in an open ward.

Contact tracing

It is essential that cases of TB must be notified to the appropriate authority (CCDC in the UK) to ensure that contact tracing is carried out in the community. Initial notification should be as soon as possible, by telephone followed by written communication. Contacts tracing should only be considered in the case of smear positive or open pulmonary TB and in the first instance should be limited to close contacts of index case and individuals with impaired host susceptibility (see p. 216). If initial investigation reveals a number of contacts with evidence of TB, consideration should be given to widening the circle of contacts that may be offered screening (Refer to the NICE web site: www.nice.org.uk/ for the most up-to-date guidance). The person responsible for local contact tracing should be named both in the hospital and community policy.

Immunocompetent individuals: all household contacts, i.e. all individual sharing bedroom, kitchen, bathroom, or sitting room with an open case. In addition, all adult contacts with a cumulative total exposure of 8 hours or more in a restricted area equivalent to a domestic room which may include girlfriend, boyfriend, close friends, sexual partners, frequent visitors to the home, etc.

Susceptible individuals: a reduced cumulative total exposure time of 4 hours or more may need to be considered for vulnerable contacts exposed in a restricted area e.g. children aged less than 5 years and immunocompromised individuals (see 'Host susceptibility') either due to disease or therapies (HPSC, 2010).

Health care workers: HCWs and individuals exposed during medical procedures when *no* appropriate PPE were used and no recommended infection control was followed, e.g. mouth-to-mouth resuscitation, bronchoscopy, sputum induction, or autopsy. Also staff who had prolonged care of patient in a high-dependency patient or repeated chest physiotherapy should be considered as close contacts. All members of staff should be seen in the OHD and have their occupational health notes reviewed to ascertain whether they have had a Heaf test, history of BCG vaccination and BCG scar. Enquiries should be made as to any current illness or treatment that might result in their immune system being compromised leading to a false negative Heaf test. Those who do not require further investigation should be advised of the possible symptoms of TB and the importance of reporting such symptoms promptly.

Patients: if an individual on an open ward is diagnosed as having infectious TB, the risk of other patients being infected is likely to be small depending on the immune status of the patient. However, the decisions about appropriate action should take into account the degree of infectivity, the length of time before the infectious individual is isolated, the proximity of contact, and whether other patients are unusually susceptible to infection (see 'Host susceptibility'). If the exposure of another patient is sufficiently extensive to be equivalent to a household contact, or the exposed patient is known to be particularly susceptible to infection, they should be managed in the same way as a household respiratory contact. In general, patients in the same bay (rather than the whole ward) should be regarded as 'at risk', but only if the index case was coughing and was present in the bay for 8 hours or more before isolation. It is sufficient to document the possible exposure in the patient's records and the patient's medical practitioner must also be informed.

TB cases on aircraft: contact tracing of infectious (or potentially infectious) cases of TB on aircraft should be limited to flights which were at least 8 hours in duration and took place during the previous 3 months. The following criteria should also be used when determining the infectiousness of a case at the time of travel: 1) presence of cavitations on chest x-ray, 2) presence of symptoms at the time of the flight, and 3) documented transmission to close contacts of the index case is a passenger.

The contact details of passengers sitting in the same row and the two rows ahead and behind (from one side of the aircraft to the other because of ventilation patterns) of the index patient should be obtained. Inform contacts of possible exposure and advise screening of these contacts and of cabin crew who serviced the section in which the TB case was seated. If the index case is an aircraft is a crew member, contact tracing of passengers should not routinely take place. Contact tracing of other members of staff is appropriate which is in accordance with the usual principles for screening workplace colleagues. For detail please refer to WHO's *Guidelines for prevention and control of Tuberculosis and air travel* (2007).

Infectious TB in a health care worker: if the HCW has been at work while infectious (open case of pulmonary TB), it is essential to identify all patients, staff, and visitors who may have had significant contact and manage as per contact tracing procedures.

Respiratory viral infections

Worldwide, approximately 1.5 million deaths occur from respiratory infections of which an estimated 60% of infections are caused by viruses. Several different viruses cause respiratory infections, including influenza virus (A and B), human parainfluenza virus, respiratory syncytial virus (RSV), human coronavirus (SARS), rhinovirus, and adenovirus (serotypes 4 and 7).

Most respiratory viruses spread faster from person-to-person because they are spread by contact, droplet, and airborne routes. For example, it has been estimated that sneezing and coughing, which expel an estimated 10^7 infectious virus particles per millilitre of nasal fluid and can travel over 3 metres at 20 miles per second. Coughing and sneezing cause heavy contamination of surrounding fomites where the majority of viruses remain viable and then spread by contact via contaminated hands. Since viruses are obligate parasites, the level of viral infectivity on fomites therefore can only decrease over time. In general, UV exposure and pH have minimal effects on viral survival in indoor environments.

Studies have demonstrated that RSV, influenza virus, parainfluenza virus, and rhinovirus can survive on hands for significant periods of time and that these viruses can be transferred from hands and fingers to fomites and back again. Contaminated hands then frequently come into contact with the mouth, nasopharynx, and eyes which act as portal of entry where viruses can gain entry into the host systems to cause

infection. In addition, most viruses which cause respiratory illness have short incubation periods (1–8 days) and have greater infectivity due to lower infective dose. As a
consequence, rapid spread of viral disease is very common in crowded indoor establishments, including schools, day care facilities, nursing homes, offices, and health
care facilities.

Host susceptibility to viruses is influenced by previous contact with the virus and
the condition of the host immune system at the time of infection. Groups at increased
risk of complications are individuals suffering from chronic respiratory and/or heart
disease, chronic renal failure, diabetes, asplenia/splenic dysfunction, and frail elderly
individuals with comorbidity.

Influenza

The word 'influenza' originated before the discovery of germ theory, from the belief
that the disease was caused by the 'evil influence of star'. Influenza viruses are small
(80—120 nm diameter), contain RNA and are enveloped. There are three types: A, B,
and C. Type A is further classified according to the properties of the surface proteins
hemagglutinin (H) and neuraminidase (N). All A subtypes are found in aquatic birds,
which are the natural reservoir but only a few subtypes circulate in humans and other
mammals. Type B and C influenza have only one subtype and are restricted to
humans.

Influenza A is generally considered to be clinically more severe than influenza B and
influenza C and causes only a mild illness confined to the upper respiratory tract.
In the UK, 5000–10,000 deaths are associated with influenza A and B epidemics every
year; globally, influenza is responsible for 250,000 and 500,000 deaths every year.
In April 2009, a novel influenza virus (Hl Nl) originating from swine was identified in
humans in Mexico and the USA and subsequently spread to other parts of the world.
As a result, on 11 June, 2009, WHO officially declared the outbreak to be a pandemic.
Pandemics occur when a novel influenza virus emerges and spreads in the human
population against which there is little or no pre-existing immunity.

Antigenic alterations

Antigenic alterations occur frequently in influenza H or N antigenic sites and are the
mechanism for virus adaptation to the host and survival. When these antigenic
variations are relatively small, they are referred to as *antigenic drift*, and when they are
large, they are referred to as *antigenic shift*.

Antigenic drift occurs frequently, usually every year to every few years, and includes
minor antigenic changes in the H or N antigenic sites due to accumulated amino acid
changes. The virus responds to the selective pressure of the host and generates different
antigenic variants that avoid antibody neutralization against infection each year.

Antigenic shift refers to a major change in the H or N antigens that infect the
host—a new virus to which a susceptible host population has no immunity. The
mechanism for this change may be caused by a reassortment or recombination of
the eight gene segments, such as recombining gene segments from avian and human
influenza isolates that produce a new H and N combination, by adaptation via
an intermediate host, such as a pig, or by direct introduction of one species-specific

influenza virus to another species such as from a bird to a human. Influenza pandemics may occur as a result of antigenic shifts or antigenic drifts if the mutation of the virus leads to efficient human-to-human transmission.

Protective immunity to influenza is conferred by production of antibodies against infection. The ability of influenza to cause re-infections is related to the genetic mutability of the virus. In every replication round, mutant viruses are generated, some of which have a growth advantage because they can partially evade host immune responses and as a result the influenza vaccine composition has to be changed each year.

Infectivity

Patients should be considered potentially infectious from 1 day before to 7 days following illness onset or until symptoms resolve. Children, patients with lower respiratory tract infections, elderly, and immunocompromised patients might be infectious for up to 10 days or longer. This is due to low cytotoxic T-lymphocyte activity which is responsible for viral clearance and recovery from infection. Cytotoxic T-lymphocyte activity declines in the elderly as well as in immunocompromised individuals so that viral shedding could persist longer in them than that of seasonal human influenza which is usually between 1 and 4 days.

People with influenza-like illness should remain at home until at least 24 hours after they are free of fever (37.8°C), or signs of a fever without the use of fever-reducing medications. The use of facemasks and respirators in the community are not recommended, except for persons at increased risk of severe illness from influenza. Patients who are ill should avoid gatherings and stay at home for 7 days after the onset of illness or at least 24 hours after symptoms have resolved.

Clinical symptoms

Influenza A and B illness in humans ranges from subclinical or mild upper respiratory tract symptoms. The most common presenting symptoms are cough, high temperature, joint pain, and general malaise. The rapid onset and short incubation period (about 48 hours) are characteristic, though incubation can last up to 4 days. Individuals at greatest risk of complications are those with pre-existing cardiac and respiratory disease, the elderly, and those with impaired immunity (see above) in which the respiratory tract symptoms can cause more severe illness including laryngotracheitis and pneumonia or, less commonly, death from respiratory system failure. Therefore vaccination against influenza is recommended for high-risk groups, such as children and the elderly, or in people who have asthma, diabetes, heart disease, or are immunocompromised. In addition, HCWs should be immunized against influenza for their protection and for the protection of other HCWs and vulnerable patients and to prevent outbreaks in the health care setting.

Treatment

Oseltamivir (Tamiflu®) is a prodrug that is hydrolysed by the liver to its active metabolite. The drug acts by blocking the activity of the neuraminidase, and thus prevents new viral particles from being released by infected cells. The therapeutic oral dosage for infection in adults is 75 mg taken twice daily for 5 days, starting within 48 hours of the initial symptoms to capture the early phase of viral replication. For chemoprophylaxis, the recommended dosage is 75 mg taken once daily for 10 days after exposure.

Zanamivir (Relenza®) is administered by inhalation with a dry powder inhaler. About 90% of the absorbed dose is excreted unchanged in the urine. The therapeutic dose is 10 mg inhaled twice daily for 5 days starting within 48 hours of the initial symptoms. For chemoprophylaxis, the dose is 10 mg inhaled once daily for 10 days after exposure. Zanamivir is not recommended for treatment for patients with chronic airway disease or asthma as it can induce bronchospasm; use of oseltamivir is preferred over zanamivir during pregnancy.

Amantadine: the antiviral drugs amantadine and rimantadine block a viral ion channel (M2 protein) and prevent the virus from infecting cells. These drugs are sometimes effective against influenza A if given early in the infection but are always ineffective against influenza B because this virus does not possess M2 molecules. Resistance to amantadine has occurred due to the easy availability of these as part of over-the-counter cold remedies in some countries.

Respiratory syncytial virus

Respiratory syncytial virus (RSV) can cause bronchiolitis and pneumonia, mainly in infants and young children. It occurs in annual epidemics with a peak during the winter months, generally from October to April. Respiratory failure secondary to bronchiolitis may occur, especially in children with severe underlying cardiopulmonary conditions, children receiving chemotherapy for malignancy, and premature infants. Susceptible patients should therefore be isolated during peak seasons to protect them and isolated upon hospital admission.

Nasopharyngeal secretions should be sampled on all patients symptomatic for RSV. All suspected cases should be cared for in a designated area with both contact and droplet precautions until the test results are known. Remember, a negative RSV test does not always exclude diagnosis of RSV.

Transmission

Transmission can occur during close contact when the susceptible person's respiratory tract is exposed to the infected droplet nuclei or there is inoculation of the mucous membranes or conjunctivae. In the health care setting it can also spread indirectly from patients via contaminated secretions or fomites. The virus can persist on hands for up to 1 hour and on environmental surfaces for several hours.

Incubation period

The incubation period ranges from 2–8 days. However, 4–6 days is more common. The period of infectivity is from approximately 3 days prior to the onset of symptoms until the cessation of upper respiratory symptoms (usually <8 days) but viral shedding may occur for longer, especially in young infants where shedding may continue for as long as 3–4 weeks.

Infection control precautions

A variety of measures need to be instituted to control and prevent the spread of nosocomial RSV. These include:

- All children with suspected bronchiolitis must be isolated in a single room at the time of admission with full infection control precautions.

- When a single room is not available, the patient may be cohorted in a room/area with other patient(s) with an active infection.

- Screen all symptomatic patients for RSV by using rapid diagnostic techniques during the peak season. Place the patient on *contact and droplet precautions* until the test result is known.

- All babies should be cared for by a designated team of staff. Staff who nurse these children should ideally not have contact with other ill babies, those who are immunocompromised, or have a heart or lung defect. For those staff who must have contact with other children in the ward, e.g. medical staff, the contact should be at the end of the ward round, if possible.

- The child and parents must remain in the room in so far as this is possible.

- Physically clean hands can be decontaminated using alcohol hand rub after contact with a patient or after touching respiratory secretions or the environment, whether or not gloves are worn.

- Single-use disposable plastic aprons must be worn while in contact with the patient or their immediate environment. Plastic aprons and gloves should be changed between patients and after touching contaminated objects. Hands must also be disinfected after removing plastic aprons and gloves.

- Dedicated equipment such as stethoscopes, pulse oximeters, and electronic thermometers should be cohorted with patients who have RSV.

- All equipment must be properly stored in a cupboard, in a dispensing box or covered. For advice please contact the Infection Prevention and Control Nurse.

- Equipment may be removed to the dirty utility area for cleaning only by a person trained in the correct techniques.

- All medical equipment and other items, e.g. cots, prams, toys, must be adequately decontaminated with an appropriate disinfectant before further use.

- Environmental cleaning must be performed by properly trained staff using a detergent/hypochlorite (1000 ppm av Cl_2) solution.

- Staff with respiratory illness should report to the Occupational Health Service to be evaluated for fitness to work.

- Exclude visitors who show signs and symptoms of respiratory infection.

- An information pamphlet should be given to patients' families explaining the need for these precautions.

- Limit the number of visitors. Instruct family members/visitors to wash hands when coming and going from rooms. Instruct family members/visitors with

RSV-infected children not to visit other hospitalized children or common areas within the hospital. Place appropriate signs at the entrance to paediatrics wards instructing visitors with respiratory symptoms not to visit.

Legionnaires' disease

The first recorded outbreak of Legionnaires' disease occurred in 1976 in Philadelphia during an American Legion Convention and the following year the bacterium was named as *Legionella*. Legionellosis is a collective term describing infection produced by *Legionella* spp. whereas Legionnaires' disease is a multisystem illness with pneumonia. So far 48 species of *Legionella* have been recognized but *Legionella pneumophila* is responsible for 90% of infections; most of the infections are caused by serogroup 1. The incubation period of Legionnaires' disease is 2–10 days.

Clinical features

Legionellosis is an acute bacterial pneumonia characterized initially by anorexia, malaise, myalgia, and headache. Within a day, there is usually a rapidly rising fever associated with chills. A non-productive cough, abdominal pain, and diarrhoea are common. Chest radiograph may show patchy or focal areas of consolidation that may progress to bilateral involvement. Severe infections may lead to respiratory failure and death. The case-fatality rate has been as high as 40% in hospitalized cases. **Pontiac fever** is a clinical syndrome which may represent reaction to inhaled *Legionella* antigen rather than bacterial invasion. An incubation period is 5–72 hours. It is not associated with pneumonia or death and patients recover spontaneously within 2–5 days without treatment.

Risk factors

Legionellosis may occur as sporadic cases or outbreaks, and infections are more frequently reported in summer and autumn months. The incidence of infection increases with increasing age (i.e. persons >50 years of age) and smoker are at the highest risk. Males are affected more commonly than females. As expected, immunosuppressed patients (e.g. transplant patients, cancer patients, patients receiving corticosteroid therapy), and immunocompromised patients (e.g. surgical patients, patients with underlying chronic lung disease, dialysis patients, diabetes mellitus) are more susceptible to infections.

Source of infection

Airborne transmission in water aerosols is the major route of transmission infection. The reservoir and source of infection for Legionnaires' disease are hot and cold water systems, air-conditioning and wet cooling system towers, evaporative condensers, humidifiers, whirlpool and natural spas, and decorative fountains/sprinkler systems. In several hospital outbreaks, patients were considered to be infected through exposure to contaminated aerosols generated by cooling towers, showers, faucets, respiratory therapy devices (e.g. humidifiers, and nebulizers) and room-air humidifiers. *Person-to-person transmission has not been documented.*

Diagnosis

The diagnosis of legionellosis purely by clinical criteria can be difficult and reliance is therefore placed on laboratory tests which include isolation of the causative organism on special media and demonstration by direct immunofluorescence (IF) stain of involved tissue or respiratory secretions (see Box 11.7). It can also be diagnosed by detection of antigens of *L. pneumophila* in urine by RIA or by serology showing four-fold or greater rise in IFA titre between an acute (blood specimen take at the onset of illness) and convalescent phase serum sample taken between 3–6 weeks *after* the initials symptoms.

Box 11.7 Case definitions for Legionnaires' disease

Confirmed case: any person meeting the clinical diagnosis of pneumonia and the laboratory evidence of *one or more* of the following laboratory test:

* **Culture**: isolation of any *Legionella* spp. from respiratory secretions or any sterile site.

* **Urinary antigen**: detection of *L. pneumophila* antigen in urine. This test detect *only L. pneumophila* serogroup 1.

* **Serology**: *Legionella pneumophila* serogroup 1-specific antibody response.

Probable case: any person meeting the clinical diagnosis of pneumonia criteria and at least one positive laboratory test for a probable case **or** an epidemiological criteria (see below).

* **Culture**: detection of *L. pneumophila* antigen in respiratory secretions or lung tissue by direct fluorescent antibody staining using monoclonal-antibody derived reagents.

* Detection of *Legionella* spp. nucleic acid in a clinical specimen.

* **Serology** *L. pneumophila* non-serogroup 1 or other *Legionella* spp.-specific antibody response.

* *L. pneumophila* serogroup 1, other serogroups or other *Legionella* spp.; single high titre in specific serum antibody*.

Epidemiological criteria

At least *one* of the following two epidemiological links:

* Environmental exposure.

* Exposure to the same common source.

* UK, Health Protection Agency uses a single titre of 1:128 or 1:64 in an outbreak.
Source: European Working Group for Legionella Infection. *European guidelines for control and prevention of travel-associated Legionnaires' disease.* London: European Working Group for Legionella infection, 2005.

Prevention

Respiratory tract infections from *Legionella* spp. are exclusively acquired from the environmental source by inhalation of infected aerosols. Since, the highest concentrations of *Legionella* spp. are found in cooling towers and water systems, its instillation should be should be avoided where possible. If the construction of new cooling towers in the health care facility is planned, it is important that they must be sited and directed away as far as practicable from patient and public areas. Drift must be directed *away* from the air-intake system and drift eliminators should be installed.

Adequate maintenance of wet cooling towers and water systems is essential and must be carried out in accordance with written policy based on national and international guidelines. A written record must be kept of detailed maintenance, including environmental test results. Cooling towers should be mechanically cleaned to remove scale and sediment at regular intervals and appropriate biocides should be used on a regular basis to prevent the growth of slime-forming organisms. Cooling towers should be drained when not in use.

Since *Legionella* is a very widespread organism, prevention must therefore focus on reducing the risk of the organism being aerosolized. The prime aim is to avoid creating conditions favourable for the organisms to multiply in water and be disseminated in air through droplets and aerosols. This can be achieved by ensuring that *adequate maintenance of potential reservoirs of infection*, such as cooling towers, hot water and air conditioning systems, spa baths, humidifiers, and respiratory therapy equipment. Tap water *must not* be used in respiratory therapy devices, e.g. humidifiers and nebulizers.

It is important to highlight that the following factors *enhance* colonization and growth of *Legionella* in water environments:

◆ Temperatures of 25–42°C (77–107.6°F).

◆ Presence of organic matter.

◆ Stagnation of water.

◆ Scale and sediment.

◆ Presence of certain free-living aquatic amoebae that can support intracellular growth of *Legionella*.

Therefore it is essential that health care facilities should either maintain potable water at the outlet at 51°C (>124°F) or lower than 20°C (<68°F) or chlorinate heated water to achieve 1–2 mg/L (1–2 ppm) of free residual chlorine at the tap. Maintenance of hot water system temperatures at 50°C (122°F) may reduce the risk of transmission. Decontamination of implicated sources by chlorination and/or superheating of the water supply have been shown to be effective.

In recent years, increased use of alcohol hand rubs to disinfect hands has decreased usage of water in many hospitals and as a result, reduced exposure of water to disinfectant has resulted in increased *Legionella* colonization rates in water system. This can be reversed by periodic flushing of the water outlets (20 min once per month) to increase disinfectant exposure (Risa et al., 2007). It is important to note that if the hospital units that have been closed for any reason (renovation, etc.) are also vulnerable to colonization and it is essential that *before* opening of these wards/units, all lines must be flushed and cultured for *Legionella* spp. and units should not house any patients until culture result are available (Lin et al., 2011).

Surveillance and notification

Hospital surveillance should detect health care-associated Legionnaires' disease. Isolated cases may be difficult to investigate. All laboratories confirmed cases of legionellosis should be reported to appropriate personnel as per local policy. This is to ensure that appropriate control measures are taken and that the source of *Legionella* spp. is removed. In the community, cases must be reported to the appropriate local health department (CCDC in the UK). Steps in an epidemiological investigation for legionellosis include:

- ◆ Review medical and microbiological records.
- ◆ Initiate active surveillance to identify all recent or ongoing cases.
- ◆ Develop a line listing of cases by time, place, and person.
- ◆ Determine the type of epidemiological investigation, i.e. case–control or cohort study.
- ◆ Assess risk factors among potential environmental exposures, e.g. showers, cooling towers, respiratory therapy equipment.
- ◆ Gather and analyse epidemiological information.
- ◆ Collect water samples from environmental sources implicated by epidemiological investigation.
- ◆ Subtype strains of *Legionella* spp. cultured from both patients and environmental sources.
- ◆ Review autopsy records and include autopsy specimens in diagnostic testing.

Since *Legionella* is present in the water supply, routine culturing of water in the absence of proven or suspected hospital transmission is generally not recommended and effort must be focused to *control the processes* to prevent the growth of micro-organisms by regular maintenance of the system as per recommended best practice guidelines. However, in the recent years, culture of *Legionella* is recommended in certain countries especially in the units and wards housing high-risk patients and readers are advised to follow the most recent national guidelines. WHO recommends that drinking water cultures for *Legionella* be performed every 3 months, to verify the efficacy of disinfection (WHO, 2007). The UK Department of Health has recently updated there guidelines for control of *Legionella* (Health Technical Memorandum 04-01, 2010).

It is important to note that maintenance of water systems is essential not only to control *Legionella* but also to ensure that other pathogens which can cause infections in susceptible individual e.g. *Pseudomonas aeruginosa*, *Stenotrophomonas maltophilia*, *Aspergillus* spp., and *Cryptosporidium* spp. which can also colonize water and disinfectant use to control *Legionella* spp. may also lead to suppression of these other water-borne pathogens.

Meningococcal infections

Meningococcal disease is caused by *Neisseria meningitidis* or meningococci. They are Gram-negative diplococci which are divided into antigenically distinct groups. The commonest groups are B, C, A, Y, and W135. The nasopharyngeal carriage rate of all meningococci in the general population is about 10%, although rates vary with age and up to 25% of young adults may be carriers.

N. *meningitidis* cause meningitis and septicaemia. Septicaemia without meningitis has the highest case fatality of 15–20% or more, whereas in meningitis alone, the fatality rate is around 3–5%. Most cases are a combination of septicaemia and meningitis. The disease can affect any age group, but the young are the most vulnerable. Cases occur in all months of the year but the incidence is highest in winter.

Transmission

Person-to-person transmission is mainly by droplets spread from the upper respiratory tract. There is no reservoir other than humans and the organism dies quickly outside the host. The incubation period is 2–10 days but most invasive disease normally develops within 7 days of acquisition. Therefore, for practical purposes a 1-week period is considered sufficient to identify close contacts for prophylaxis.

The onset of disease varies from with mild prodromal symptoms to fulminant infection with meningitis and septicaemia. Early symptoms and signs are usually malaise, pyrexia, and vomiting. Headache, photophobia, drowsiness or confusion, joint pains, and a typical haemorrhagic rash of meningococcal septicaemia may develop. In its early stages, the rash may be non-specific. The rash, which may be petechial or purpuric, *does not blanche* and this can be confirmed readily by gentle pressure with a glass slide, etc., when the rash can be seen to persist. Patients may present in coma. In young infants particularly, the onset may be insidious and the classical signs are absent. The diagnosis should be suspected in the presence of vomiting, pyrexia, and irritability, and, if still patent, raised anterior fontanelle tension.

Emergency action

Urgent admission to the hospital is a priority in view of the potentially rapid clinical progression of meningococcal disease. Early treatment with benzyl penicillin is recommended and may save life. Therefore, all GPs should carry benzyl penicillin in their emergency bags and give it while arranging the transfer of the case to the hospital. The only contraindication is a history of penicillin anaphylaxis. In these instances chloramphenicol (1.2 g for adult; 25 mg/kg for children under age of 12 years) may be given by injection. Immediate dose of benzyl penicillin for suspected cases are:

- Adults and children (10 years or over): 1200 mg.
- Children aged 1–9 years: 600 mg.
- Children aged less than 1 year: 300 mg.

This dose should be given as *soon as possible*, ideally by IV injection. IM injection is likely to be less effective in shocked patients, due to reduced perfusion, but can be used if a vein cannot be found.

Management in hospital

On arrival in the hospital of a suspected case, doctors should take blood for culture and other appropriate investigations give benzyl penicillin (or suitable alternative) *immediately* if this has not already been done. All patients with known or suspected meningitis must be isolated in a single room at the time of admission. The patient should be isolated for a *minimum of 24 hours* after the start of appropriate antibiotic and a full course of chemoprophylaxis has been given unless the patient has been treated with ceftriaxone.

Laboratory investigations

- **Blood culture**: blood for culture in all cases.
- **Cerebrospinal fluid**: lumbar puncture should be performed if there are no clinical contraindications and this decision should be based on clinical assessment and not on CT (cranial computed tomography) scan as CT scan is unreliable for identifying raised intracranial pressure. *Do not* perform a lumbar puncture if the CT scan shows radiological evidence of raised intracranial pressure (NICE, 2010).
- Send CSF for direct microscopy and culture. CSF should be submitted to the laboratory to hold for PCR for *N. meningitidis* and *S. pneumoniae,* but only perform the PCR if the CSF culture is negative.
- **PCR testing**: CSF and blood (EDTA specimen) should be taken on admission for PCR testing. Remember that a negative blood PCR test result for *N. meningitidis* does not rule out meningococcal disease.
- Other laboratory investigations (CRP, white blood cell count, etc.) should be done as clinically indicated.
- Since nasopharyngeal (taken from mouth) swabs are less affected by prior antibiotic therapy, they can be taken as a part of investigation of invasive disease and afford the possibility of identifying a strain esp. in the event of an outbreak/cluster of cases. The overall yields from these swabs are about 40–50%. Aspirate from a normally sterile site, skin rash aspirate or biopsy culture can be taken as appropriate.

Notification

In most countries, meningococcal infections are notifiable diseases. Notification to appropriate local authorities is important to ensure prompt follow-up of close contacts. Close contacts should be offered chemoprophylaxis and immunization where appropriate, which can be offered up to 4 weeks after the index case became ill.

Management of contacts

After a single case

Chemoprophylaxis should be offered to all close contacts (defined as people who had close, prolonged contact with the case) as soon as possible, i.e. within 24 hour after the diagnosis of the index case. Prophylaxis is recommended to the contacts of confirmed or probable cases 7 days before the case became ill. Contacts of possible cases do not need prophylaxis unless or until further evidence emerges that changes the diagnostic category to confirmed or probable. It is recommended in the following situations:

+ **Household**: immediate family and close contacts, i.e. people sleeping in the same house, boy/girlfriends, and mouth-kissing contacts of the index case.

+ **Index case**: index case should receive prophylaxis (unless they have already been treated with ceftriaxone) as soon as they are able to take oral medication.

+ **Health care worker**: HCWs are advised to reduce the possibility of exposure to large particle droplets nuclei (by wearing surgical masks and using closed suction) when carrying out airway management procedures (i.e. endotracheal intubations/management, or close examination of oropharynx), *on all patients with suspected meningococcal septicaemia or meningitis.* Chemoprophylaxis is recommended *only* for those HCW who were in direct contact with respiratory secretions (i.e. mouth or nose is directly exposed to large particle droplets/secretions) and have not used appropriate barrier precautions. This type of exposure will only occur among staffs who are working close to the face of the case without wearing a surgical mask. In practice, this implies a clear perception of facial contact with droplet secretions and is unlikely to occur unless undertaking airway management or being coughed at, directly in the face. General medical or nursing care of cases is *not* an indication for prophylaxis.

Cluster of cases

A cluster is defined as two or more cases of meningococcal disease in the same pre-school group, school, or college/university within a 4-week period. If two possible cases attend the same institution, whatever the interval between cases, prophylaxis to household or institutional contacts is not indicated. If two confirmed cases caused by different serogroups attend the same institution, they should be regarded as two sporadic cases, whatever the interval between them. Only household contacts of each case should be offered prophylaxis.

If two confirmed or probable cases who attend the same preschool group or school arise within a 4-week period and are, or could be, caused by the same serogroup, wider public health action in the institution is usually indicated.

The principle of managing such clusters is to attempt to define a group at high risk of acquiring meningococcal infection and disease, and to target that group for public health action. The target group should be a discrete group that contains the cases and makes sense to staff and parents, e.g. children and staff of the same preschool group, children of the same school year, children who share a common social activity, or a group of friends.

It is important to emphasize that chemoprophylaxis is effective in reducing the nasopharyngeal carriage rates after treatment but does not completely eliminate transmission between household members. Contacts should be reminded of the persisting risk of disease, whether or not prophylaxis is given, and of the need to contact their general practitioner urgently if they develop any symptoms suggestive of meningococcal disease.

Chemoprophylaxis

Chemoprophylaxis should be offered to all close contacts (defined as people who have had *close, prolonged contact* with the case) as soon as possible, i.e. within 24 hours after the diagnosis of the index case. It is recommended in the following situations:

Although penicillin and cefotaxime are the drugs of choice for the treatment of meningococcal infection, they have *no effect* on the elimination of nasopharyngeal carriage of the organism and are therefore not indicated for prophylaxis. Rifampicin, ciprofloxacin, and ceftriaxone are effective in reducing the nasopharyngeal carriage rate and are therefore recommended for chemoprophylaxis. *Prophylaxis of the index case is not required if patient has been treated with ceftriaxone.*

Rifampicin: in the absence of contraindications, rifampicin can be used in all age groups. It should preferably be taken at least 30 min before a meal or 2 hours after a meal to ensure rapid and complete absorption. Dosage of rifampicin is as follows:

◆ Adults: 600 mg every 12 hour for 2 days.

◆ Children: (over 1 year) 10 mg/kg every 12 hours for 2 days (up to a maximum of 600 mg per dose).

◆ (3 month to 1 year) 5 mg/kg every 12 hours for 2 days.

Rifampicin is contraindicated in the presence of jaundice or known hypersensitivity to rifampicin. Interactions with other drugs such as anticoagulants and anticonvulsants should be considered. It also interferes with hormonal contraceptives (Family Planning Association advice for a 'missed' pill should be provided if rifampicin is prescribed to an oral contraceptive user) and causes red colouration of urine, sputum, and tears (soft contact lenses may be permanently stained). Other side effects include itching, skin rashes, and GI reactions may also occur. These side effects should be explained to the patients and the information should be supplied with the prescription. Rifampicin is *not* recommended in pregnancy or for lactating women.

Rifampicin is effective in reducing the nasopharyngeal carriage rates by 80–90% 1 week after treatment and therefore may be expected to reduce, but *not* completely eliminate, transmission between household members. Contacts should be reminded of the persisting risk of disease, whether or not prophylaxis is given and of the need to contact their GP urgently if they develop any symptoms suggestive of meningococcal disease.

Ciprofloxacin: Ciprofloxacin is recommended for use in all age groups (apart from babies under one month of age) and in pregnancy. It has advantages over rifampicin in that it is given as a single dose therefore avoiding problem with compliance, it does not interact with oral contraceptives, and is more readily available in community pharmacies. (UK Health Protection Agency, 2011). The following doses are recommended for prophylaxis.

Adults and children: > 12 years 500 mg stat

Children: 5–12 years 250 mg stat

Children: 1 month–4 years 125 mg stat

It is contraindicated in cases of known ciprofloxacin hypersensitivity. It has an unpredictable effect on epilepsy but may be preferable to rifampicin if the patient is on treatment with phenytoin.

Ceftriaxone: although no drug is considered to be safe in pregnancy, all pregnant women who are contacts should be counselled carefully about risks and benefits and the option to give prophylaxis should be discussed. Ceftriaxone can be given in pregnancy. Ceftriaxone dose is:

◆ Adults: a single dose of 250 mg IM injection.

◆ Children: a single dose of 125 mg IM injection (from 6–12 weeks).

Ceftriaxone is contraindicated in patients with a history of hypersensitivity to cephalosporins. It is not recommended for premature infants and full term infants during the first 6 weeks of life.

Immunization of contacts

Close contacts of cases of meningococcal meningitis have a considerably increased risk of developing the disease in the subsequent months, despite appropriate chemo-prophylaxis. Therefore, immediate family or close contacts of cases of group A or group C meningitis should be given meningococcal vaccine in addition to chemo-prophylaxis. The latter should be given first and the decision to offer vaccine should be made when the results of serotyping are available. Vaccine should *not* be given to contacts of group B cases. The serological response is detected in more than 90% of recipients and occurs 5–7 days after a single injection. The response is strictly group-specific and confers no protection against group B organisms.

Varicella zoster virus

Varicella zoster virus (VZV) is a herpes virus which is the causal agent of varicella (chickenpox) and herpes zoster (shingles). Primary infection with VZV causes chickenpox and is predominantly a childhood disease. The virus persists in a latent state within the host and can subsequently reactivate years or decades later to cause shingles (zoster) especially in immunocompromised individuals.

Clinical features

Chickenpox is an acute generalized illness with sudden onset of mild fever and constitutional upset and a typical skin eruption that is maculopapular for a few hours, vesicular for 3–4 days, and leaves a granular scab in 4–7 days. The vesicles are monolocular and collapse on puncture. Lesions commonly occur in successive crops, often with several stages of maturity present at the same time; they tend to be more abundant on covered than on exposed parts of the body. In some cases, the lesions may be so few as to escape observation. Mild atypical and inapparent infections may occur. The illness can result in complications such as pneumonia, encephalitis, visceral dissemination, or haemorrhagic varicella. Most of the mortality associated with VZV occurs in these patients. It is important to note that morbidity and mortality is greater in adults and in children aged 15 years or older. Chickenpox is five times more likely to be fatal in pregnancy than in the non-pregnant adult.

Herpes zoster or shingles is a local manifestation of re-activation of latent varicella infection in the dorsal root ganglia. Vesicles with an erythematous base appear, sometimes in crops, in irregular fashion on the skin to areas supplied by sensory nerves of a single or associated group of dorsal root ganglia. In the immunosuppressed or those patients with malignancies, chickenpox-like lesions may appear outside the dermatome.

Immunosuppressed patients, e.g. with cancer (especially of lymphoid tissue), with or without steroid therapy, immunodeficient patients and those on immunosuppressive therapy may have an increased frequency and severity of zoster, both localized and disseminated. Neonates developing varicella between ages 5–10 days, and those whose mothers develop the disease 5 days prior to or within 2 days after delivery, are at increased risk of developing severe generalized chickenpox, with a fatality rate of up to 30%. Infection in early pregnancy may be associated with congenital malformations in up to 2% of cases. Infection of adults is generally more severe than infection of children.

Period of infectivity and transmission

The **incubation period** ranges from 2–3 weeks (usually 13–17 days). In chickenpox, the virus is shed from the nasopharynx 1–2 days *before* the rash appears and then from the skin lesions until the vesicles have dried to a scab, usually about 4–7 days; therefore the contagious period is from 2 days *before* to approximately 5 days *after* the onset of rash. The **mode of spread** is via the respiratory route and by direct contact with skin vesicles. During this time, the patient is considered highly infectious. In shingles, the virus is shed from the skin lesion vesicles and until they have dried to form a scab, the patient is considered infectious for approximately 1 week after the appearance of the vesiculopustular lesions. Crusted vesicles are no longer infectious. It must be noted, however, that contagiousness may be prolonged in individuals with suppressed immunity.

Infection control measures

VZV is spread from person-to-person by direct contact and by the respiratory route (droplet and airborne) from secretions of the respiratory tract or vesicle fluids both from cases of chickenpox and herpes zoster. It can also be transmitted indirectly through articles freshly soiled by discharges from vesicles and mucous membranes of infected people. The following measures should be considered in the control of VZV infection in the health care setting:

◆ All suspected or clinically confirmed cases of chickenpox must be nursed in a side room with airborne isolation precautions (see Chapter 7, Table 7.1). The room should preferably have negative pressure ventilation, if possible.

◆ In the case of zoster infection, the patient should be nursed in a side room with infection control precautions from the first appearance of the vesiculopustular lesions until scab formation.

◆ Patients with VZV infection and susceptible (non-immune) persons exposed within the previous 21 days should not be admitted to hospital unless absolutely necessary.

◆ In-patients who develop varicella and susceptible patients (non-immune) exposed in hospital should be discharged as soon as possible if clinical condition permits.

- Exposed susceptible persons (non-immune), when they are hospitalized, must be isolated in a side room with appropriate infection control measures from 10 days following their earliest varicella exposure until 21 days after their most recent exposure. This period may be extended in cases where varicella zoster immunoglobulin (VZIG) has been administered or in cases of immunosuppression.
- In pregnant women the disease is more serious with a higher risk of fulminating varicella pneumonia. Therefore all pregnant patients who are admitted should be isolated in a side room with full *en-suite* facilities using the infection control precautions.

Post-exposure prophylaxis

Passive immunization with VZIG is frequently prescribed for exposed individuals in whom varicella vaccine is contraindicated. VZIG prophylaxis is recommended in individuals with a significant contact with a case of varicella or zoster where the clinical condition increases the risk of severe complications of varicella. VZIG does *not* necessarily prevent infection even when given within 72 hours of exposure. However it may attenuate disease if given up to 10 days after exposure. Severe maternal varicella may still occur despite VZIG prophylaxis. There is some evidence that the likelihood of foetal infection during the first 20 weeks of gestation is reduced in women who develop chickenpox under cover of VZIG.

VZIG is given by IM injection as soon as possible and not later than 10 days after exposure. It must not be given IV. If a second exposure occurs after 3 weeks a further dose is required.

Active immunization with **varicella vaccine** is contraindicated in immunocompromised susceptible children, neonates whose mothers acquired varicella from 5 days before to 2 days after birth, adolescents, and adults, as well as premature infants and pregnant women. Varicella vaccine is also effective post-exposure and can prevent or modify illness in up to 90% of exposed individuals if given within 3 days, and in 67% of people if given within 5 days of exposure.

Management of contacts

Definition of contact

A *significant contact* is defined as being in the same room (e.g. house or classroom or 2–4 bed hospital bay) for a significant period of time (15 min or more) or any face-to-face contact for 5 min. When assessing the risk, it is important to bear in mind that in the UK, seropositivity for VZV is about 90% of adults over the age of 18 years. However, in many tropical/subtropical countries seropositivity rate is less than 60% of adults. This may be due to population density and climatic effects. After significant exposure, patients/staff who are at risk of developing severe complications of varicella should be urgently tested for varicella immunity so that appropriate treatment should be given to avoid/minimize complications.

Health care workers

Non-immune HCWs who are exposed to infection should be warned they may develop chickenpox and be re-allocated to minimize patient contact from days 8–21 post-contact. Pregnant staff who have no clear history of chickenpox must avoid contact with patients and colleagues with VZV infection. VZV vaccine should be offered to non-immune HCWs.

Pregnant women

Chickenpox is five times more likely to be fatal in pregnancy than in the non-pregnant adult.

If chickenpox occurs during the first 20 weeks of gestation, intrauterine fetal infection and occasionally fetal damage can occur. The fetal varicella syndrome is rare (<2% of affected pregnancies) and clues to its presence may be found at a 20-week ultrasound scan. The most dangerous time in pregnancy to acquire chickenpox is at term or immediately after term. This is because there is a high chance that the newborn infant may be exposed and may have little or no immunity. The newborn may then become seriously ill with VZV infection. If varicella occurs during pregnancy, the woman should be advised of the likelihood of fetal involvement, with reference to the stages of the pregnancy that the infection took place and the providers of her antenatal care should be informed. For these reasons, non-immune pregnant women and HCWs should not care for patients who are infectious, such as patients with chickenpox or shingles.

If a HCW has a history of clinical chickenpox, testing is not necessary since they will be immune. If the HCW is unsure whether or not they have had chickenpox and they are pregnant or contemplating pregnancy, then they may have their VZV antibody status checked. Varicella vaccine is recommended for non-immune HCWs, but is not recommended during pregnancy. Vaccinees should not become pregnant for 1 month after vaccination. Pregnant HCWs who are not immune should not care for patients with chickenpox or shingles (see Chapter 16, Table 16.2).

The **varicella vaccine** is a live attenuated vaccine and is good for controlling outbreaks in schools and health institutions. This vaccine can also be used to prevent or reduce the severity of varicella infection when administered within 3 days of exposure. Two doses of vaccine should be given at least 28 days apart. Non-immune pregnant women should be considered for varicella vaccine as soon as possible after delivery, although it is not licensed for use during breastfeeding.

If inadvertent exposure occurs, **VZIG** should be given to all non-immune pregnant women who have had significant contact with a case of chickenpox. It should be given as soon as possible and must be given within 10 days of exposure to the virus. If a pregnant woman develops chickenpox, VZIG is of no benefit. Oral acyclovir is recommended in a woman who is more than 20 weeks pregnant and if treatment can be started within 24 hours of the onset of the rash. Aciclovir is not licensed for use in pregnancy therefore informed consent should be obtained. No adverse fetal or neonatal effects have been reported, although there is a theoretical risk of teratogenesis if taken in the first trimester.

If the varicella infection occurs more than a week before delivery, in apparent or mild *in utero* infection typically occurs. If the infection occurs 7 days before to 7 days after delivery, these women run a high risk of severe disseminated infection in the neonate. VZIG is recommended for infants whose mothers develop chickenpox in the period 7 days before to 7 days after delivery. VZIG can be given without antibody testing of the infant.

Neonates

Babies born before 30 weeks of gestation or below 1 kg birth weight should receive VZIG if exposed to varicella, irrespective of the immune status of the mother. It is also given to VZV antibody-negative infants exposed to chickenpox or herpes zoster in the first 7 days of life. Prophylactic IV aciclovir should be considered for neonates whose mothers develop varicella 4 days before to 2 days after delivery as they are at the highest risk of fatal outcome despite VZIG prophylaxis. Mothers with varicella should be allowed to breastfeed. If nipple lesions are present, then milk can be expressed from the affected breast until the lesions are crusted. This expressed milk can be fed to the baby if s/he is covered by VZIG.

Other high-risk patients

The following patients are also classified as high-risk patients due to poor immunity. These patients should be advised to take reasonable steps to avoid close contact with chickenpox or herpes zoster and to seek urgent medical attention if exposed to chickenpox. Manifestations of fulminant illness include pneumonia, hepatitis, and disseminated intravascular coagulation; rash is not necessarily a prominent feature. These patients may require prophylactic cover with VZIG following contact with chickenpox or zoster (British Infection Society, 2008).

◆ Patients receiving immunosuppressive chemotherapy or radiotherapy for malignant disease. The risk continues up to 6 months after completion of treatment. Bone marrow transplant patients. The risk continues up to 1 year after completion of treatment.

◆ Patients taking high doses of systematic steroids (adult 40 mg/day for >1 week; 2 mg/kg/day for >1 week or 1 mg/kg for >1 month). The risk continues up to 3 months after treatment has stopped.

◆ Patients receiving immunomodulatory drugs such as azathioprine, cyclosporine, methotrexate, cyclophosphamide, etc.

◆ Patients with HIV infection particularly if the CD4 count is <200 cells/mm^3.

Viral haemorrhagic fevers

Viral haemorrhagic fevers (VHFs) are a group of viral diseases which are endemic mainly in West and Central Africa. VHFs can present a significant risk to all countries due to the ease of international travel. For the latest information, please visit the WHO website (http://www.who.int/csr/disease/). They have a significant mortality rate and there is no vaccine available. The most clinically important viruses are:

◆ Lassa fever virus: Nigeria, Sierra Leone, and Liberia.

- Marburg virus: Uganda, Kenya, Zimbabwe.
- Ebola virus: Zaire and Sudan.
- Crimean-Congo haemorrhagic fever virus: former Soviet Union and East and West Africa.

The diagnosis of VHF should be considered in a patient who has febrile illness and has returned from tropical Africa or a VHF endemic country within the last 3 weeks. All such persons should go through risk assessment (Table 11.4).

Clinical manifestations

VHFs usually present as a febrile illness with headache, myalgia, sore throat, cough, and vomiting. Some patients have a cough, chest pain, abdominal tenderness, and skin rash. In severe cases, patients may suffer extensive haemorrhage, accompanied by a purpuric rash and bleeding from almost any part of the body, including the intestine, eyes, gums, nose, mouth, lungs, and uterus. Encephalopathy and multiorgan failure are common in severe cases and the case mortality rate is high. History of adequate malarial prophylaxis must be taken. Malaria is a common confounding diagnosis and is suspected in patients who have failed to take adequate malarial prophylaxis. It is important to note that dengue haemorrhagic fever can be misdiagnosed as VHF.

If the GP has seen a patient at home and suspects a diagnosis of VHF in a patient suffering from acute atypical fevers, (especially with any accompanying superficial haemorrhages or in patients who have recently returned from endemic areas), he/she is advised not to move the patient from home and to seek specialist advice. In hospital stetting, the provisional diagnosis might first be made in a patient attending the A&E department or in a patient already in a general hospital ward.

Incubation period

The incubation period of the infection is usually 7–10 days (ranging from 3–17 days). For infection control purposes, if no infection has occurred in a period of up to 21 days from exposure, a contact is usually taken to be free from infection.

Mode of transmission

Patients are infectious while they are symptomatic and until the virus has been cleared from blood and body fluids. Lassa fever virus has been found in respiratory secretions of asymptomatic patients and in urine during the convalescent phase. Sexual transmission of Ebola virus and Lassa fever virus has been documented, and Ebola virus has been found in seminal fluid for up to 2 months after the onset of symptoms.

The main risk of transmission in the health care setting is from mucosal or parenteral exposure to contaminated blood or other body fluids. Lassa fever virus may also be transmitted by exposure to aerosols of contaminated body fluids, particularly nasopharyngeal secretions and urine. Virus may be isolated from the urine of a patient with Lassa fever for 3–9 weeks post-infection.

SPECIAL PATHOGENS | 237

Table 11.4 Risk categories and infection control precautions for patient with suspected/confirmed VHFs

Risk	Minimum	Moderate	High
Criteria	Not in a known endemic area or onset >21 days after leaving endemic area	In a known endemic area <21 days before onset (and no high-risk features) or not in a known endemic area, but in adjacent area within 21 days and have severe illness with organ failure and/or haemorrhage which could be due to VHF	In a known endemic area <21 days before onset and *either* stayed in house with case/suspected case or nursed case/suspected case or contact with fluids or body of case/suspected case or lab worker in contact with fluids or body of case/suspected case or were previously moderate risk, but have developed severe illness with organ failure and/or haemorrhage which could be due to VHF Have not been in a known endemic area < 21 days before onset, but have cared for or had contact with case/suspected case or handled fluids or body of case/suspected case
Specimen collection and processing	Standard procedures for transport; as for other blood-borne viruses Processing in minimum containment level 1 Specimens should be tracked and their handling audited	Special precautions for obtaining specimens (gown, gloves, eye and face protection) Rigid packaging for transport to laboratory Malaria film only Processing in minimum containment level 3	Special precautions for obtaining specimens (gown, gloves, eye, and face protection). Rigid packaging for transport to lab Arrangements may be in place for preparation and decontamination of a blood film in containment level 3 facility followed by staining and examination in lower level of containment elsewhere
Infection control precautions	If unwell, to standard isolation (single room, apron, gloves)	Isolation in room with controlled ventilation, if available	Isolation in room with negative pressure ventilation, if available Consider urgent transfer to the Regional Infectious Diseases unit

Adapted from UK Advisory Committee on Dangerous Pathogens. *Management and Control of Viral Haemorrhagic Fever.* London: The Stationary Office, 1997.

Diagnosis

A firm diagnosis is not always possible but both the clinical and the epidemiological evidence need to be considered for any patient presenting with undiagnosed fever within 3 weeks of return from an endemic area.

In the initial assessment of patients with suspected VHF, laboratory testing should be kept to an absolute minimum to minimize the risk associated with the collection and handling of laboratory specimens. Laboratory procedures must include a risk assessment at each stage, including risks associated with the chosen techniques, recommendations about training and surveillance measures, waste disposal, and decontamination.

All patients with suspected VHF and their specimens and bodily secretions should be handled at Physical Containment Level 4. All specimens must be handled with appropriate safeguards. The specimens should not be sent through the normal courier mechanisms (human or otherwise), to ensure that accidents do not occur as a consequence of mishandling or misplacement of specimen. The laboratory staff and infection prevention and control practitioner must be alerted immediately to ensure appropriate handling of specimens.

Notification

All suspected cases of VHF must be notified to the local officer (CCDC in the UK) or other designated authority as per national guidelines.

Infection control and precautions

The following action must be taken:

+ The patient must be isolated in a single room with en suite toilet facility. Strict infection control (standard, contact and droplets) precautions must be instituted immediately.

+ The patient must not be moved from the suspected ward or department. It is possible that the patient may require treatment in a high-security, designated infectious diseases unit.

+ The absolute minimum of staff should have contact with the patient, i.e. one doctor and one nurse. The doctor involved in making the initial diagnosis should seek advice from the consultant physician in infectious diseases. In such circumstances, no other hospital medical staff should be invited to assist in confirming suspicions to minimize the risk to HCWs.

+ Staff already involved with the case must not resume other professional duties and should remain, as far as possible, within the department, using a designated staff room.

+ Patients and their body fluids are highly infectious therefore appropriate protective clothing must be worn, e.g. scrub suit, gown, apron, two pairs of gloves, mask, head cover, eyewear, and rubber boots.

+ Disposable equipment should be used whenever possible. Other instruments should be heat disinfected in the SSD.

- The environment must be decontaminated using hypochlorite solution 1:100 dilution. Fumigation of the room is necessary after the patient has been discharged.

- All waste must be treated as clinical waste and must be disposed of by incineration. VHFs are classified as dangerous biological agents (containment 4 pathogens) and transport and handling of specimens also requires special precautions.

- If the diagnosis of VHF is confirmed, staff who have been in contact with the patient may require continuing isolation and surveillance. This should be carried out by the OHD. Assessment of any surveillance measures necessary for patients may be needed for other patients who may have been in contact with suspect case.

Prion disease

Prion disease was first described in humans in the 1920s by Creutzfeldt and Jakob. Prion diseases in human and animal cases presented with progressive neurological disorder. Human prion diseases include Kuru, sporadic, familial, iatrogenic, and variant Creutzfeldt –Jakob disease (CJD). Animal prion diseases includes bovine spongiform encephalopathy (BSE or 'mad cow disease'), sheep/goat scrapie, etc. The disease is caused by accumulation in the brain of an aberrant form of abnormal prion protein (PrP_{Sc}). The incubation period of sporadic cases of CJD is unknown, but iatrogenic cases appear to have an incubation period of 2–15 years or more, and variant CJD (vCJD) has an incubation period of up to 50 years. Treatment is mainly symptomatic only as there is no proven effective treatment available as yet.

The PrP_{Sc} protein is extraordinarily resistant to standard cleaning and inactivation processes. They are highly resistant to low pH, enzymatic digestion, ionizing radiation, and detergents. They are also resistant to physical, chemical, and heat sterilization and disinfection procedures employed in the health care setting.

Human prion diseases

Sporadic CJD is the most common form of all prion diseases (80%). The onsets of symptoms are sudden with rapidly progressive dementia with myoclonus. Mean age of onset is 60–65 years. Duration from first symptoms to death is usually about 4–6 months.

Inherited CJD is rare and accounts for 15% of cases and is caused by an autosomal dominant gene. Average age of onset is 30–50 years and duration of illness is 2–5 years.

Acquired prion diseases are acquired from exposure to infective high-risk tissues or blood and variant CJD is acquired from exposure to BSE contaminated material.

Iatrogenic CJD is acquired for contaminated growth hormone, blood and blood products, and from surgery using contaminated instrument and EEG needles.

Diagnosis

The blood test for diagnosis of patient with symptoms of vCJD and is available on request from the UK National Prion Clinic on an individual patient basis (http://www.nationalprionclinic.org). CJD can be diagnosed by performing lumber puncture for

14-3-3 protein. Other diagnostic criteria can also be used, e.g. electroencephalography, magnetic resonance imaging, and tonsil biopsy for vCJD; brain biopsy is the only definitive diagnostic tool.

Mode of transmission

It is important to emphasize that CJD is transmissible only under certain circumstances. Normal social and clinical contact and non-invasive procedures *do not* present a risk to HCWs, visitors, relatives, and the community. CJD has been transmitted accidentally in human sources including growth hormones, dura mater preparation, and transplantation of a corneal graft donated by an affected patient and through blood transfusion. Therefore, CJD patients should *not* donate blood, any organs, or tissues, including bone marrow, sperm, eggs, or breast milk.

Blood and body fluid samples from patients with, or 'at increased risk' of CJD/ vCJD, should be treated as potentially infectious for blood-borne viruses and appropriate precautions should be followed. For categorization of patients at increased risk, please visit http://www.dh.gov.uk/ab/ACDP/TSEguidance/.

High-risk tissue for CJD/vCJD includes brain, spinal cord, cranial nerves, specifically the entire optic nerve and the intracranial components of the other cranial nerves, cranial ganglia, posterior eye, optic nerve, and pituitary gland. *Medium-risk tissue* includes spinal ganglia and olfactory epithelium. Body secretions, body fluids including saliva, blood, and cerebrospinal fluid and excreta are all *low risk*.

Infection control precautions

CJD/vCJD is *not* spread from person-to person by close contact therefore application of standard infection control precautions is sufficient and isolation of patients is *not* necessary.

Currently, there is no epidemiological evidence to suggest that normal social or routine clinical contact with a CJD or vCJD patient presents a risk to HCWs, relatives, and others in the community.

Invasive medical procedures: blood, biopsy and lumbar puncture samples from patients should only be taken by trained personnel who are aware of the hazards involved. Disposable gloves and apron should be worn. *Single-use disposable instruments should be used when performing a lumbar puncture* for the collection of cerebrospinal fluid.

Pathology specimens sent to the laboratory should be put in an appropriate container and be marked with a 'Biohazard' label. PrP$_{Sc}$ protein survives formalin fixation, therefore all formalin-fixed specimens should be regarded as being infective. The specimen must be processed in a Category 3 Laboratory only.

Surgical procedures: it is essential that any surgical procedure should be carefully planned beforehand and appropriate personnel informed. Patients should be put last on the list and all non-disposable equipment should be covered. A minimum number of experienced staff should take part in the operation. The team should wear appropriate PPE (i.e. liquid-repellent theatre gown over a plastic apron, gloves, mask, and visor or goggles).One-way flow of instruments should be maintained.

Disposable instruments and equipment should be used wherever possible. At the end of the operation, all surfaces in the operating theatre should be should be thoroughly cleaned and disinfected according to local protocol. **Spillages** of *any* fluids should be cleared up as quickly as possible (see Chapter 6, Box 6.5) using 10,000 ppm of sodium hypochlorite solution to decontaminate the surface.

Instruments used in high- or medium-risk procedures on patients with, or 'at increased risk' of, CJD/vCJD can be quarantined and re-used exclusively on the same patient, subject to tracking of instruments throughout the decontamination cycle, and ensuring that *under no circumstances* should quarantined instrument sets be reprocessed for use on other patients unless the diagnosis of CJD or vCJD has been positively excluded (see Figure 11.4).

Waste disposal: high- and medium-risk tissues from patients with, or 'at increased risk' of, CJD or vCJD, should be incinerated. Low-risk tissues or body fluids should follow normal clinical waste disposal.

Occupational exposure: no known cases of human CJD have occurred through occupational accident or injury. However, it is essential to take all precautions to avoid needle and sharp injuries.

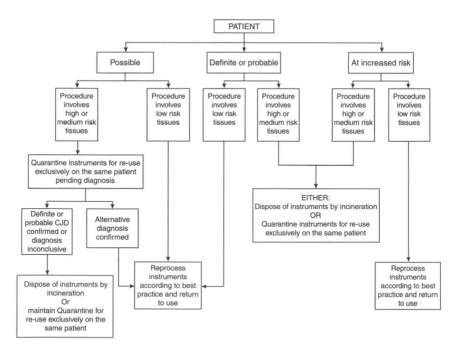

Fig. 11.4 Algorithm chart for precautions for reusable instruments for surgical procedures on patients with, or 'at increased risk' of, CJD, vCJD and other human prion diseases. With permission from Department of Health. *Transmissible Spongiform Encephalopathy Agents: Safe Working and the Prevention of Infection.* London: Department of Health, 2011.

Childbirth: in the event that a person with CJD becomes pregnant, no special precautions need to be taken during the pregnancy, except during invasive procedures. CJD is not known to be transmitted from mother to child during pregnancy or childbirth. Childbirth should therefore be managed using standard infection control procedures. The placenta and other associated fluids are designated as low risk and should be treated as clinical waste.

Postmortem: postmortems on patients with CJD should be done by a neuropathologist with access to a specialized mortuary. However, a general histopathologist who has been asked to perform a necropsy on a case of possible or probable CJD must follow suitable infection control precautions-based guidance which is available on the National Prion Clinic web site (http://www.nationalprionclinic.org).

Scabies and pediculosis

Scabies

Scabies is a contagious parasitic dermatosis caused by *Sarcoptes scabiei* var. *hominis*. It affects about 300 million individuals annually of all age groups and social classes. Mellanby's studies for the British Ministry of Health over 50 years ago demonstrated that clothing and linen are not a major source of scabies. In these studies, Mellanby had experimental subjects wear undergarments of persons with scabies and sleep in their unwashed sheets. The result was that fewer than two in 100 individuals exposed developed any sign of scabies.

Classically, scabies was seldom seen in individuals with good hygiene. Scabies tends to occur in clusters within family groups or other contexts in which intimate person-to-person contact occurs. It was most frequently seen in military combat groups, prisons, people living in poverty, and in orphanages. In addition scabies can occur sporadically in outbreaks in health care settings, including long-term care facilities, e.g. nursing and residential homes.

Clinical symptoms

The severe itching is caused by an allergic reaction to the presence of a small mite which burrows into the top layer of skin. Intense itching occurs especially at night or after a hot bath or shower. The allergic reaction does not appear immediately, but develops between 2–6 weeks to several months after infection due to delayed host immune response to the mite. However, symptoms may appear earlier (1–4 days) if the patient has had previous exposure.

Infectivity

Human beings are the only source of infection and any person infested with either mites or eggs is infectious. Spread of infection from person-to-person occurs through direct skin-to-skin contact, which is usually *prolonged and intimate* therefore casual contact is unlikely to spread the disease, unless the afflicted areas on the patient are heavily excoriated, exposing the mites so that they can be transmitted promptly.

'Norwegian' or 'crusty' scabies occurs in elderly or immunosuppressed patients, e.g. patients on immunosuppressive therapy, patients with AIDS, and patients with other malignancies. Immunocompromised patients may suffer hyper-infestation. This form of scabies is *highly contagious* because mites multiply rapidly and large numbers of the parasites are present in the exfoliating scales.

Transmission

In the health care setting, scabies is transmitted primarily through *intimate* direct contact with an infested person. Hand-holding or patient support for long periods is probably responsible for most health care-associated scabies. Transmission to HCWs has occurred during activities such as sponge-bathing patients or applying body lotions. Transmission via inanimate objects, such as clothing and bedding, is not common, and only occurs if contaminated immediately beforehand, as the mites do not survive very long out of contact with human skin. Transmission between patients may also be possible when patients are ambulatory. Infection control measures and management of institutional outbreak of scabies is summarized in Table 11.5.

Table 11.5 Summary of infection control measures and management of institutional outbreak of scabies

Actions	Measures for prevention and control
Recognition of index case promptly	Early recognition of a case is essential to prevent an outbreak. The onset of scabies in a staff member who has had scabies before can be an early warning sign of undetected scabies in a patient
	Send specimens to microbiology to confirm diagnosis
Keep records of all contacts	Once the case(s) is confirmed, keep records of all the patients, roommate(s), and skin scraping results
	Identify all the staff who have provided hands-on care to the patients/roommates before implementation of infection control measures
Active case finding by surveillance	Initiate active case findings which will include contact tracing of patients and family members that have been in contact with index case(s)
	Identify new or unsuccessfully treated cases of scabies
	Refer family members to their GP for treatment
Implement infection control precautions	Prolonged contact with the patient should be avoided. In addition, staff with scabies should avoid patient contact for 24 h after appropriate treatment is initiated
	For patient contact use non-sterile gloves, long-sleeved single use disposable gowns and shoe covers. Wash hands *before* and *after* contact with the patient and after contact with the environment. *Hands must be washed after removal of gloves*
	Strictly implement contact precautions (see Chapter 7, Table 7.1). It is important to note that 'Norwegian' or 'crusty' scabies are highly infectious and transmission can occur through inanimate objects and consideration should be given to extending the isolation period in the case of patients who are either heavily infested or patients who are immunocompromised

(Continued)

Table 11.5 (*continued*)

Actions	Measures for prevention and control
Prevent spread	Restrict rotation of staff and movement of institutionalized patients
	Reducing social contact with the confirmed cases by placing restrictions on visitors
	As a part of communication, provide a fact sheet giving information on the spread of scabies and how to prevent it to all relevant staff
Start early treatment	Simultaneously treat *all cases* and *all exposed individuals* to prevent re-exposure. To prevent continued transmission, prescribe topical and/or oral scabicide agents as recommended by a dermatologist or a physician
	Refer family members who have been in close physical contact with the patient to their general practitioner so that they can be treated if necessary
	Staff generally can return to work the day after treatment
	Healing criterion for individuals is resolution of clinical signs and itching within 2–4 weeks after treatment
Environmental disinfection	Routine cleaning and disinfection of the environment and vacuuming of the room should be done. Use of insecticide sprays and fumigants is not recommended
	Fomites should only be handled by laundry personnel using personal protective equipment
	Sarcoptes scabiei can survive at room temperature for several days in clothing therefore clothing and bedding used anytime during the previous 3 days before treatment should be machine-washed in hot water and dried thoroughly or ironed. It is important to note that the mites are killed within 10 minutes at a temperature of 50°C
	Clothing and other items that cannot be washed should be treated with insecticidal powder or stored in plastic bags for 10 days. It has been suggested that storing non-washable items in a freezer at −20°C for 72 h could be a useful disinfection procedure
Continued surveillance	Continued surveillance is imperative to eradicate scabies in institutions. An epidemic is considered as controlled if all the infested individuals are healed and if no new cases of scabies occur for 6–8 weeks after completion of treatment

Pediculosis

Lice (pediculosis)

There are many different species of lice but only three that are clinically important from the family pediculidae. They can be caught only by close contact, i.e. close enough for lice to walk onto another host. Lice can be found on the body, on bedding, chairs, floor, etc. They are dead, injured, or dying and not able to crawl onto another host. Nits are the eggs of lice, which are firmly attached to hair and are difficult to remove.

Infestations with lice may result in severe itching and excoriation of the scalp or body. Secondary bacterial infection may occur due to severe itching resulting in regional lymphadenitis (especially cervical).

Head louse (*Pediculus humanus* var. *capitis*): this species lives on the head and eyebrow hair. The female louse lays eggs at the base of the hairs where it is warmest. Transmission to another host occurs when two heads are in direct contact, allowing lice to crawl on to a new head. Lice prefer clean hair where they can move around easily. They are invariably acquired from family members or close friends who should be checked for infection. Head lice cannot be transmitted to others on clothing or linen and therefore no precautions are necessary. Patients with head lice need not be isolated, except in paediatric wards where close contact between children may transmit the lice. Outbreaks of head lice are common among children in schools and other institutions.

Pubic or crab louse (*Phthirus pubis*): they live on coarse body hair, usually the pubic area; they may also infect facial hair (including eye lashes), axillae, and body surfaces. They are transmitted by close physical contact, frequently but not always, by sexual contact. Children may acquire crab lice through close contact with their mother, e.g. axillary hair. Crab lice on clothing or bedding are not transmitted to other people and can be removed by washing clothes in a hot cycle (60° C or more).

Body louse (*Pediculus humanus* var. *corporis*): body lice are still prevalent among populations with poor personal hygiene, especially in cold climates where heavy clothing is worn and bathing is infrequent. They live in clothing, rather than hair and go to the body only to feed. Transmission occurs in overcrowded conditions by contact with infested clothing. They are easy to eradicate, as they will die if the clothing is not worn for 3 days.

Infection control measures

- Carefully remove all clothing of patients with body or pubic lice and seal in a bag. As lice dislike light, clothing should be handled in bright conditions. Single-use non-sterile disposable gloves and a plastic apron should be worn. In hospital, process linen as infected linen according to local policy.

- No special treatment of the environment is required as spread is by personal contact. Body lice are capable of surviving for a limited time in stored clothing, but head and pubic lice rapidly die when detached from their host.

- Patients with body lice do not require specific treatment but should be bathed. Infestation with head and crab lice should be referred to the medical practitioner for appropriate treatment.

- Clothing, bedding and fomites should be treated with a hot water cycle (60°C or more).

Fleas

Infestation is usually with dog, cat, or bird fleas, which will bite humans in the absence of the preferred host. The human flea is rare. Fleas are able to survive for some months in the environment without feeding. Elimination of the host or treatment of pets and the use of suitable insecticides on environment surfaces and soft furnishing are therefore essential. The following infection control procedures are recommended:

♦ Remove all clothing and bedding. All laundry should be treated as infected linen according to the local policy.

♦ Clothing not suitable for washing may be treated with low temperature steam. Seek advice from the SSD manager.

♦ The laundry bag must be removed immediately from the ward.

♦ Identify the flea, and if possible, treat or remove the host. If it is a cat flea, take steps to exclude feral cats from the site.

♦ Vacuum clean floors, carpets, upholstery, fabrics, etc.

♦ Contact your pest control officer to treat the environment, e.g. ducting, hard surfaces, and under fixtures, with a residual insecticide if necessary.

Key references and further reading

Clostridium difficile infection

APIC. *Guide to the Elimination of Clostridium difficile in healthcare settings*, 2008. Washington, DC: APIC, 2008.

Department of Health. *Clostridium difficile infection: How to deal with the problem*. London: DH Publication, 2009. Available at: http://www.dh.gov.uk/.

European Society of Clinical Microbiology and Infectious Diseases (ESCMID): treatment guidance document for *Clostridium difficile* infection (CDI). *Clinical Microbiology and Infection* 2009; **15**(12):1067–79.

Health Protection agency. *Regional Microbiology Network Care Bundle: A good practice guide to control Clostridium difficile, 2007*. London: HPA.

SHEA/IDSA Guidelines: clinical practice guidelines for *Clostridium difficile* infection in adults: 2010 Update by the Society for Healthcare Epidemiology of America (SHEA) and the Infectious Diseases Society of America (IDSA). *Infection Control Hospital Epidemiology* 2010; **31**(5):431–455.

SHEA/IDSA Practice Recommendation: Strategies to prevent transmission of *Clostridium difficile* infections in acute care hospitals. *Infection Control and Hospital Epidemiology* 2008; **29** (Supplement1):S81–S92.

Weber DJ, Rutala WA. The role of the environment in transmission of *Clostridium difficile* Infection in healthcare facilities. *Infection Control and Hospital Epidemiology* 2011, **32**(3):207–9.

Gastrointestinal infections

Boone SA, Gerba CP. Significance of fomites in the spread of respiratory and enteric viral disease. *Applied and environmental microbiology*, 2007; **73**(6):1687–96.

CDC. Updated norovirus outbreak management and disease prevention guidelines. *Morbidity and Mortality Reports* 2011; **60**(3):1–16.

Chadwick PR, Beards G, Brown D, *et al*. Management of hospital outbreaks of gastro-enteritis due to small round structured viruses. *Journal of Hospital Infection* 2000; **45**:1–10.

Department of Health. *Food Handlers: Fitness to Work*. London: Department of Health, 1995.

Department of Health. *Management of outbreaks of foodborne illness*. London: Department of Health, 1994.

Health Protection Agency. *Guidance on Infection Control in Schools and other Child Care Settings*. London: HPA, 2010.

PHLS Advisory Committee on Gastrointestinal Infections. Preventing person to person spread following gastrointestinal infection: guidance to public health physician and environmental offices. *Communicable Disease and Public Health* 2004; **7**(4):362–84.

Blood-borne viral infections

Department of Health. *Health clearance for tuberculosis, Hepatitis B, Hepatitis C and HIV: New healthcare workers*. London: Department of Health, 2007.

European Study Group: Occupational Post-Exposure Prophylaxis Study Group: Towards a standard HIV post-exposure prophylaxis for health care workers in Europe. *Euro surveillance* 2004; **9**:40–3.

Report of joint working party of the Hospital Infection Society and the Surgical Infection Study Group. Risks to surgeons and patients from HIV and Hepatitis: Guidelines on precautions and management of exposure to blood or body fluids. *British Medical Journal* 1992; **305**:1337–43.

SHEA. *Guideline for management of healthcare workers who are infected with Hepatitis B virus, Hepatitis C virus, and/or Human immunodeficiency virus*. Infection Control and Hospital Epidemiology 2010; **31**(3): 203–232.

WHO. *Preventing Mother-to-child transmission of hepatitis*. Manila (Western Pacific Region); World Health Organization, 2006.

Tuberculosis

CDC. Guidelines for preventing the transmission of *Mycobacterium tuberculosis* in health-care settings, 2005. *Mortality and Morbidity Review* 2005; **54**(RR-17):1–141.

Crofton J, Chaulet P, Maher D. *Guidelines for the management of drug-resistant tuberculosis*. Geneva: World Health Organization, 1997.

Department of Health. *Health clearance for tuberculosis, Hepatitis B, Hepatitis C and HIV: New health care workers*. London: Department of Health, 2007.

HPSC. *Guidelines on the Prevention and Control of Tuberculosis in Ireland 2010*. Dublin: Health Protection Surveillance Centre, 2010.

Jacobson AC. *Genius: Some Revaluations*. Port Washington, NY: Kennikat Press, 1970.

NICE. *Tuberculosis: Clinical diagnosis and management of tuberculosis, and measures for its prevention and control* (Clinical Guideline 117). London: National Institute of Clinical Excellence, 2011.

Phillips MS, Fordham von Reyn. Nosocomial infections due to non-tuberculous *Mycobacteria*. *Clinical Infectious Diseases* 2001; **33**:1363–74.

Sepkowitz KA. How contagious is tuberculosis? *Clinical Infectious Diseases* 1996; **23**:954–62.

WHO. *WHO policy on TB infection controls in health-care facilities, congregate settings and households*. Geneva: World Health Organization, 2009.

WHO. *Guidelines for prevention and control: Tuberculosis and air travel*. Geneva: World Health Organization 2007.

Respiratory viral illness

Heymann DL. *Control of communicable disease manual*, 19th edn. Washington DC: American Public Health Association, 2008.

Royal College of Physicians. *Preparations for Pandemic Influenza Guidance for hospital medical specialties on management during a pandemic influenza outbreak*. London: Royal College of Physicians, 2009.

WHO. *Pandemic Influenza Preparedness and Response.* Geneva: WHO, 2009.

WHO. *Hospital Infection control guidance for severe acute respiratory syndrome (SARS).* Geneva: WHO, 2003.

Legionnaires' disease

Department of Health. *Health Technical Memorandum (HTM 04–01) (Part A Design Installation and Testing and Part B Operational Management). The control of Legionella hygiene, 'Safe' hot water cold water and drinking water systems.* London: The Stationery Office, 2010.

European Working Group for Legionella Infection. *European guidelines for control and prevention of travel-associated Legionnaires' disease.* London: European Working Group for Legionella Infection, 2005.

Fallon RJ. How to prevent an outbreak of Legionnaires' disease. *Journal of Hospital Infection* 1994; **27**:247–56.

Health Protection Agency. *Guidance for the laboratory diagnosis of Legionella infections in the HPA. National Standard Method QSOP 30 Issue 3.* London: Health Protection Agency, 2005.

Lin YE, Stout JE, Yu VL. Controlling *Legionella* in hospital drinking water: an evidence-based review of disinfection methods. *Infection Control and Hospital Epidemiology* 2011; **32**(2):166–73.

Public Health Laboratory Services Atypical Pneumonia Working Group. Investigating a single case of Legionnaires' disease. *Communicable Disease and Public Health* 2002; **5**(2):157–62.

Sabria M, Yu VL. Hospital-acquired legionellosis: solutions for a preventable infection. *The Lancet Infectious Diseases* 2000; **2**:368–73.

Risa Risa KJ, Stout JE, Muder RR. Intermittent flushing of outlets improved control of Legionella colonization in a hospital hot water system treated by CU/Ag ionization. In: Program and abstracts of the 47th Interscience Conference on Antimicrobial Agents and Chemotherapy; September 12–16, 2007; Chicago, IL.

WHO. *Legionella* and the prevention of legionellosis. Geneva: WHO, 2007.

Meningococcal disease

Department of Health *Immunization against infectious diseases.* London: The Stationery Office, 2006. Please go to the UK Department of Health website (http://www.dh.gov.uk/) for updates and additions since 2006.

Health Protection Agency. *Guidance for public health management of meningococcal disease in the UK.* London: Health Protection Agency, 2011.

NICE. *Bacterial meningitis and meningococcal septicaemia. Management of bacterial meningitis and meningococcal septicaemia in children and young people younger than 16 years in primary and secondary care* (Clinical Guideline 102). London: National Institute of Clinical Excellence, 2010.

Varicella zoster virus

British Infection Society: Tunbridge AJ, Breuer J, Jeffery KJM. Chickenpox in adults: Clinical management. *Journal of Infection* 2008; **57**:95–102.

Department of Health. *Immunization against infectious diseases.* London: The Stationery Office, 2006. Visit http://www.dh.gov.uk/for regular updates and additions since 2006.

Royal College of Obstetricians and Gynaecologists. *Chickenpox in pregnancy* (Guideline No. 13). London: Royal College of Obstetricians and Gynaecologists, 2001.

Viral haemorrhagic fevers

Management of patients with suspected viral haemorrhagic fever. *Morbidity and Mortality Weekly Report* 1988; **37**(Suppl):1–16.

Notice to Readers Update: Management of patients with suspected viral haemorrhagic fever-United States. *Morbidity and Mortality Weekly Report* 1995; **44**(25):475–9.

UK Advisory Committee on Dangerous Pathogens. *Management and control of viral haemorrhagic fevers*. London: The Stationery Office, 1996.

WHO and CDC: *Infection control for viral haemorrhagic fevers the African health care setting*. Geneva: WHO, 1998.

Piron disease

Department of Health. *ACDP Transmissible Spongiform Encephalopathy Risk Management Subgroup recommendations*. London: Department of Health, 2011. Available at: http://www.dh.gov.uk/.

NICE. *Patient safety and reduction of risk of transmission of Creutzfeldt-Jakob disease (CJD) via interventional procedures* (Guideline 106). London: National Institute of Clinical Excellence, 2006.

Scabies and pediculosis

Bouvresse S, Chosidow O. Scabies in healthcare settings. *Current Opinion in Infectious* 2010; **23**:111–18.

Lettau LA. Nosocomial transmission and infection control aspects of parasitic and ectoparasitic disease. Part I. Introduction/Enteric Parasites. *Infection Control and Hospital Epidemiology* 1991; **12**:59–65.

Lettau LA. Nosocomial transmission and infection control aspects of parasitic and ectoparasitic diseases. Part II. Blood and Tissue Parasites. *Infection Control and Hospital Epidemiology* 1991; **12**:111–21.

Lettau LA. Nosocomial transmission and infection control aspects of parasitic and ectoparasitic disease. Part III. Ectoparasites/Summary and conclusions. *Infection Control and Hospital Epidemiology* 1991; **12**:179–85.

Chapter 12

Intravascular catheter-related infections

As it takes two to make a quarrel, so it takes two to make
a disease, the microbe and its host.

Charles V. Chapin (1856–1941)

In 1935, Dr Werner Forssmann inserted a catheter through a vein in his arm into the right auricle of his own heart confirming that it was possible to access the heart using this method without invasive surgery. Since then indwelling intravenous (IV) catheters are an integral part of patient care. They provide a route for administering fluids, blood products, nutrients, and IV medications. They are also used for monitoring haemodynamic function, for maintaining vascular access in an emergency, and to obtain blood specimens. Most IV catheters are short (<5 cm) and are inserted into smaller peripheral veins in the arms. Central venous catheters (CVCs) are much longer (>15 cm) and are placed into larger veins of the body. Some CVCs may be inserted via a peripheral vein site and the tip is advanced until it is situated within a central vein. These are referred to as peripherally-inserted central (venous) catheters (PICCs).

Many patients with IV catheters have serious underlying diseases, making them more susceptible to infection. Catheter-related bloodstream infection (CR-BSI) is one of the most important complications of venous access. The risk of infection associated with these IV catheters can be minimized by adherence to aseptic technique *during* and *after* catheter insertion. In addition, since the risk of infection increases with the duration of catheterization, IV catheters should be used only when absolutely necessary and *must be removed when no longer needed.*

Sources of infections

Intrinsic contamination

This is defined as contamination occurring during device or fluid production and before use. This contamination may be the result of faulty sterilization (of IV fluids, drugs, giving sets, and other devices) or damage during manufacture or storage. The microorganisms are usually Gram-negative bacteria growing in the infusate, such as *Klebsiella* spp., *Enterobacter* spp., or *Pseudomonas* spp.

Extrinsic contamination

The source of infection may be extrinsic (introduced during therapy) and can occur due to contamination of the IV catheter at the time of insertion, poor sterile precautions during drug admixture or administration of the intravenous fluid, or contamination of part of administration system or catheter by the hands of the operator. However, the most important reservoirs of microorganisms causing catheter-related infection are the insertion site and the device hub. The microorganisms are usually Gram-positive bacteria residing on the patient's skin, most often coagulase-negative staphylococci and *Staphylococcus aureus*. In addition, metastatic colonization of the device from a distant site of infection (GI and urinary tract, wound etc.) may occur. Points of access for microbial contamination in infusion therapy is outlined in Figure 12.1.

Education and training

The IV catheter should be *inserted by trained personnel* with documented *competence* and is part of a core skill component of medical training. Adequate supervision must

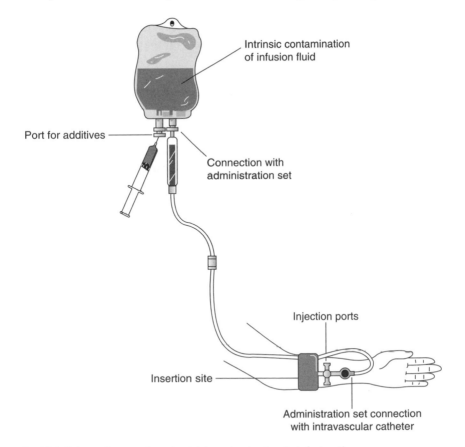

Fig. 12.1 Points of access for microbial contamination in infusion therapy.

be provided for trainees who perform IV catheter insertion. Policies and procedures regarding the insertion and maintenance of IV devices should be written and reviewed on a regular basis. These policies must be readily accessible to all staff. Procedure for insertion of peripheral venous catheter and CVC are outlined in Boxes 12.1 and 12.2.

Surveillance of catheter-related infection

It is essential that the surveillance of catheter-related infection should be conducted in high-risk patients/areas (e.g. ICU) and definitions developed by CDC (CDC/NHSN, 2008)

Box 12.1 Procedure for insertion of peripheral venous catheter

Ensure that the patient is in a comfortable position and aware of the nature of the procedure as this will reduce anxiety. Avoid shaving the skin sit—use hair clippers instead, but *only* if hair is present at the insertion site.

- Collect all necessary equipment.
- Operator should use an alcohol rub on physically clean hands or antiseptic detergent to disinfect hands or wash hands thoroughly for 60 seconds if antiseptic is not available.
- Dry hands thoroughly on a paper towel or clean linen towel, unless alcohol rub is used.
- Select an appropriate site, ideally avoiding bony prominences and joints.
- Disinfect IV insertion skin site with 2% alcoholic chlorhexidine, or 10% alcoholic povidone-iodine, or 70% isopropyl alcohol impregnated swab for *at least 30 seconds* prior to venepuncture. Allow the insertion site to dry before inserting the catheter.
- *Do not touch the venepuncture site* once the vein has been selected and the skin prepared. *Do not touch the shaft* of the catheter with the fingers during insertion.
- Select a catheter that will fit easily into the vein. The correct sized catheter reduces trauma and congestion of the vein.
- Insert the catheter as swiftly and as aseptically as possible using an aseptic non-touch technique. *Do not* attempt repeated insertions with the same catheter. Seek help from a senior colleague whenever difficulties arise. If the first insertion is not successful the procedure should be repeated with a new catheter.
- Look out for flashback of blood and then advance the catheter slowly.
- Apply sterile, clear, semipermeable dressing or gauze.
- Secure catheter to avoid movement.
- Label the site with the insertion date.
- Connect up the IV administration set.
- Ensure that all sharps are safely discarded into a sharps bin.
- Wash and dry hands.

Box 12.2 Procedure for insertion of central venous catheter

The insertion of a CVC is an aseptic procedure. The hands must be disinfected with an antiseptic/detergent hand wash preparation for 1 minute. Sterile gloves, gowns, and mask should be worn. Use large sterile drapes to cover the area.

- Collect all necessary equipment.
- Disinfect hands using an antiseptic/detergent for *1 minute* or use an alcohol hand rub on physically clean hands.
- Disinfect skin insertion site with 2% alcoholic chlorhexidine, or 10% alcoholic povidone-iodine with friction for *at least 2–3 minutes* prior to venepuncture.
- Allow the insertion site to *dry before inserting the catheter.*
- Surround the site with *large* sterile drapes.
- Insert the CVC as swiftly as possible, maintaining an aseptic non-touch technique throughout the procedure.
- Blood should be aspirated freely to ensure that the catheter is in a vascular space before injecting fluid. Check the position of CVP lines by x-ray.
- Leave the site clean and dry after insertion.
- Secure the catheter with sutures or clips and then apply an appropriate sterile, clear, semipermeable dressing.
- *Label the site* with insertion date. Record insertion date in the patient's medical notes.
- Connect up the IV administration set.
- Ensure that all sharps are safely discarded into a sharps bin.
- Wash and dry hands.

and the HELICS (ECDC, 2004) are available on their websites. It is important that the incidence of CR-BSI should be reported as incidence per 1000 catheter days. This data should be provided on a regular basis and in a timely manner to the units, clinical staff and heads of departments.

Catheter sites should be *monitored on a daily basis*, both visually and by palpation through an intact dressing, looking for catheter-related complications (i.e. tenderness, thrombosis, swelling, or signs of inflammation or infection). Semi-permeable adhesive dressings have the advantage of allowing inspection of the site without the removal of the dressing. If the patient develops tenderness at the insertion site, fever without an obvious source, or other manifestations suggesting local or bloodstream infection, the dressing should be removed to allow thorough examination of the site. In addition, it is also important that patients should be encouraged to report any changes in their catheter site or any new discomfort.

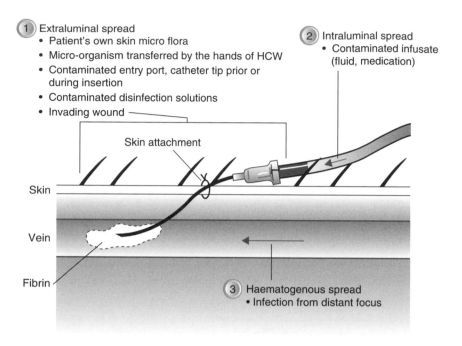

1 Extraluminal spread
  • Patient's own skin micro flora
  • Micro-organism transferred by the hands of HCW
  • Contaminated entry port, catheter tip prior or during insertion
  • Contaminated disinfection solutions
  • Invading wound

2 Intraluminal spread
  • Contaminated infusate (fluid, medication)

Skin attachment

Skin

Vein

Fibrin

3 Haematogenous spread
  • Infection from distant focus

Fig. 12.2 Sources of microbial contamination in patients with an IV catheter. Extraluminal sources are the most common source of introducing infection.

Pathogenesis

An IV catheter is a foreign body which produces a reaction in the host consisting of a film of fibrinous material (biofilm) on the inner and outer surfaces of the catheter (Figure 12.2). This biofilm may become colonized by microorganisms and will be protected from host defence mechanisms. Since infection usually follows colonization of the biofilm, this may cause local sepsis or septic thrombophlebitis or in some cases, the microorganisms in the biofilm may be released into the bloodstream causing systemic infection and CR-BSI. In addition, the *presence of biofilm makes treatment with antibiotics ineffective* and therefore once the IV catheter related infection is suspected or confirmed, removal of the IV line is necessary.

Prevention strategies

Current strategies to prevent IV catheter associated infections are based on the implementation of a 'care bundle' (see 'Care bundle approach', Chapter 1) developed by the IHI. In addition, the UK Department of Health has developed care bundles both for peripheral and CVC which are summarized in Tables 12.1 and 12.2.

Effective implementation of these interventions in the ICUs in Michigan, USA has virtually eliminated CR-BSI (Berenholtz et al., 2004). Pronovost and colleagues have demonstrated that this programme could be successful on a large scale and can be sustained on a long-term basis (Pronovost et al., 2006, 2010). The elements of prevention

Table 12.1 Care bundle to prevent infections associated with peripheral IV cannula

Insertion care bundle	Maintenance care bundle
◆ *Avoid* unnecessary cannulation	◆ Review need for catheter on a *daily basis*
◆ Insert IV catheter using *strict aseptic technique* and use sterile items	◆ Inspect cannula on a daily basis for signs of infection
◆ Disinfect skin with 2% chlorhexidine gluconate in 70% isopropyl alcohol and allow to it dry	◆ Use aseptic technique for daily care (e.g. hand hygiene before accessing the device and disinfect catheter hubs)
◆ Use a sterile, semipermeable, transparent dressing to allow observation of insertion site	◆ Replace cannula in a new site after 72–96 h or earlier if clinically indicated
◆ Record date of insertion in medical notes	◆ Replace cannula immediately after administration of blood/blood products and 72 h after other fluids

Adapted from *High Impact Intervention No 1. Peripheral intravenous cannula care bundle*. London: Department of Health, 2007.

programmes included: an educational programme, asking the clinical team to review daily about the continued need for a CVC, empowering the bedside nurse to stop a CVC insertion if guidelines were not followed correctly, having a CVC insertion cart/trolley to ensure all elements of insertion are kept in one common location, and a CVC checklist performed by the bedside nurse.

Consideration prior to insertion

Selection of catheter type: polyurethane and silicone catheters have a lower risk of complication than other types. When prolonged central venous access is required, catheters such as the Hickman type (which have a cuff and are tunnelled subcutaneously) should

Table 12.2 Care bundle to prevent central venous catheter infections

Insertion care bundle	Maintenance bundle
◆ Use single lumen unless indicated otherwise	◆ Review need for CVC on a *daily basis* and remove promptly if not required
◆ Use maximal sterile barrier precautions during insertion	
◆ Avoid femoral site; subclavian vein is the preferred site	◆ Inspect CVC site on a daily basis for signs of infection
◆ Disinfect skin with single use sterile solution of 2% chlorhexidine gluconate in 70% isopropyl alcohol and allow to dry	◆ Use aseptic technique for daily care (e.g. hand hygiene before accessing the device and use of sterile single use antiseptic solution to disinfect hub)
◆ Use semipermeable dressing (with sustained-release chlorhexidine gluconate-impregnated sponge)*	

* Sustained-release chlorhexidine gluconate-impregnated sponge can be used if CA-BSI is not decreasing despite all the preventative measures have been taken (see text).
Adapted with modification from the IHI *Care Bundle to Prevent Central Line Infections* (2007) and Department of Health *High Impact Intervention No 2. CVC care bundle* (2007).

be used because they are associated with a lower rate of sepsis than standard CVCs. Totally implantable access devices (e.g. Porta-A-Cath®) should be considered for patients who require long-term (>30 days) intermittent vascular access. *Single-lumen catheters should be used* unless multiple ports are essential. If total parenteral nutrition (TPN) is being administered, a dedicated single-lumen CVC or dedicated lumen on a multilumen CVC should be used.

Antimicrobial impregnated catheters: antimicrobial/antiseptic impregnated catheters have a lower rate of colonization than standard CVCs and as a result they can be left in place for longer periods. However, antimicrobial-impregnated catheters (e.g. chlorhexidine–silver sulfadiazine and minocycline–rifampin) should *not be used routinely*. The use of these CVC should be considered in the adult patients who require catheterization for longer than 5 days and despite full adherence to maximum infection control precautions (i.e. educating persons who insert and maintain catheters, use of maximal sterile barrier precautions, and use of >0.5% chlorhexidine preparation with alcohol for skin antisepsis during CVC insertion), there is still a high rate of catheter-related sepsis (CDC, 2011).

Selection of insertion site: select the insertion site and technique with the lowest risk of complications, both infectious and non-infectious. Do not routinely use the cut-down procedure as a method of inserting catheters. The catheter should *not be inserted* into an area of inflammation or infection.

Peripheral intravascular lines: in adults, use an upper limb site in preference to a lower extremity site for cathetr insertion. Replace a catheter inserted from lower to upper extremity site as soon as it is feasible. In paediatric patients, insert catheters into a scalp, hand, or foot site in preference to a leg, arm, or antecubital fossa site.

Central venous catheter: subclavian rather than jugular or femoral sites should be selected for catheter insertion unless medically contraindicated. The risk of infection is *highest in femoral sites* due to very high density of skin microflora. Since the jugular vein has proximity to the oropharynx, has higher local skin temperature, and the site can be difficult to maintain with an occlusive dressing, these factors may potentially contribute to increased risk of infection. It is essential that the person inserting the CVC in the subclavian should have appropriate expertise to avoid complication (pneumothorax, subclavian artery puncture, subclavian vein stenosis, thrombosis, air embolism, etc.). Potential reasons to use a site other than the subclavian vein include significant coagulopathy, obvious site infection, inaccessibility, or patients who are on haemodialysis and patients with advanced kidney disease.

The date and time of CVC insertion should be documented in the clinical notes. Once the CVC has been inserted, it *must be secured* with sutures or clips to prevent catheter movement, dislodgement and sepsis. Suture-less securement devices are preferred to reduce the risk of infection and also have the added benefit of reducing the risk of sharps injury to HCWs.

Aseptic technique: adherence to aseptic technique both during catheter insertion and maintenance is essential. If possible, IV catheter teams should be appointed consisting of trained staff to ensure stringent adherence to aseptic technique. Drug admixtures and the preparation of all parenteral nutrition fluids must be carried out using *strict aseptic* *technique* in the pharmacy, and if this facility is not available then a laminar-flow hood/cabinet should be used. Any access points (e.g. hubs, connectors, or injection ports), *must be disinfected* using 70% isopropyl alcohol before use.

Hand hygiene: hands *must* be disinfected prior to catheter insertion and subsequently during any catheter manipulation, e.g. before and after palpation of catheter sites, as well as before and after replacing of dressing. Remember that the use of gloves does not obviate the need for hand hygiene.

Use of gloves: clean rather than sterile gloves should be worn for the insertion of peripheral IV line provided that the access site is not touched *after* the application of skin antiseptics. Sterile gloves should be worn for the insertion of CVC catheters, e.g. arterial, central, and midline catheters. Wear either clean or sterile gloves when changing the dressing on IV catheters.

Skin antiseptic: skin must be disinfected using a single-use sterile applicator containing a solution of 2% chlorhexidine gluconate in 70% isopropyl alcohol and the site allowed to dry before catheter insertion and at the time of dressing changes. Chlorhexidine gluconate should not be used in patients aged less than 2 months old.

Alternately, an iodophor or an alcoholic povidone-iodine solution should be used for patients with a history of chlorhexidine sensitivity. The antiseptic preparation must be allowed to remain on the insertion site until it dries. If povidone-iodine is used then it should remain on the skin for *at least 2 minutes* or longer until it is dry. Do not use organic solvent (e.g. acetone or ether) on the skin before insertion or during maintenance of catheters.

IV injection ports: the use of multilumen catheters *should be avoided*, if possible. Before accessing the system, IV injection ports must be disinfected with a 70% isopropyl alcohol impregnated swab or an iodophor. They should always be kept clean and dry. Put a cap on all stopcocks when not in use.

Catheter site dressing regimens: sterile dressings should be used to cover the catheter site and should be replaced when the dressing becomes damp, loosened, or soiled, or when inspection of the site is necessary. For tunnelled or implanted catheters, the dressing should be replaced no more than once per week, until the insertion site is healed. Clean or sterile gloves must be worn when changing the dressing. Either gauze or sterile transparent semipermeable dressing should be used.

Semi-permeable adhesive: this dressing has the advantage of allowing inspection of the site without the removal of the dressing. The transparent dressing should be changed every 7 days, except in paediatric patients because in these patients, the risk of dislodging the catheter outweighs the benefit of changing the dressing.

Gauze dressing: if the site is bleeding or oozing, a gauze dressing is preferred. This dressing should be replaced every 2 days or earlier if damp, loosened, or soiled.

Antimicrobial impregnated sponge: use of sustained-release chlorhexidine gluconate-impregnated sponge (which releases a steady amount of chlorhexidine over several days and is covered by a transparent dressing) have been shown to substantially reduce CVC infections (Timsit et al., 2009). Its use should be considered after all other basic infection prevention measures (i.e. educating persons who insert and maintain catheters, use of maximal sterile barrier precautions, and use of >0.5% chlorhexidine preparation with alcohol for skin antisepsis during CVC insertion) have been adopted and implemented and CR-BSI remains high in patients older than 2 months of age.

In-line filters: in-line filters reduce the incidence of infusion-related phlebitis but there are no data to support their efficacy in preventing infections associated with IV therapy. Infusate-related sepsis can be minimized if most of the medication or infusate admixtures are carried out in the pharmacy under aseptic conditions. Furthermore, in-line filters may become blocked, especially with certain solutions (i.e. dextran, lipids, mannitol), thereby increasing the number of line manipulations. Thus, for the purpose of reducing catheter-related sepsis, the use of in-line filters is not recommended.

Antimicrobial prophylaxis: routine use of intranasal antibiotic ointment and/or use of systematic antibiotic prior to CVC insertion are *not* recommended to prevent CR-BSI. Topical antimicrobial ointments should *not* be used routinely prior to insertion or as part of routine catheter site care because of their potential to promote fungal infections and antimicrobial resistance.

Consideration after catheterization

Anticoagulant flush solutions: anticoagulant flush solutions are widely used to reduce the risk of catheter thrombosis. Since thrombi and fibrin deposits on catheters may serve as a nidus for microbial colonization of IV catheters, it is believed that the use of anticoagulants may have a role in the prevention of catheter-related sepsis. However, its use must be balanced against the risk of prolonged exposure to heparin. Although low-dose warfarin decreases the risk of thrombus formation in cancer patients, it has *not* been shown to reduce infectious complications and therefore routine use of anticoagulant therapy in general patient populations is *not* recommended (CDC, 2011).

Replacement of catheters: the peripheral venous catheters should be removed if the patient develops signs of phlebitis (i.e. warmth, tenderness, erythema, and palpable venous cord), infection, or a malfunctioning catheter. In adults, peripheral venous catheter sites should be changed every 96 hours (where possible) to minimize the risk of phlebitis. In paediatric patients, peripheral venous catheters should be left in place until IV therapy is completed, unless a complication occurs.

CVCs or arterial catheters should *not routinely be replaced* solely for the purpose of reducing the incidence of infection. Replacement is necessary if catheter-related sepsis is suspected. Any catheter inserted when adherence to proper asepsis is not ensured (e.g. those inserted in an emergency) should be re-sited at the earliest opportunity, preferably within 48 hours.

Guidewire exchange: replacement of central venous catheters over a guidewire when there is a clinical suspicion for catheter-related infection is *not* recommended. If continued IV access is required, remove the implicated catheter, and replace it with another catheter at a *different* insertion site. Although the practice should be avoided wherever possible, guidewire exchange may be required to replace a malfunctioning non-tunnelled catheter if there is *no evidence of infection* and the risk of inserting a new catheter into a new site is unacceptably high, e.g. due to obesity or coagulopathy. With the advent of ultrasound-guided insertion such circumstances are not common.

A new set of sterile gloves should be used prior to handling the new catheter when guidewire exchanges are performed.

Catheter related-bloodstream infections: if CR-BSI is suspected, two sets of blood cultures (one from peripheral vein and one from IV line) should be taken. Swabs should be taken from the site of catheter insertion, especially if there is local evidence of infection, e.g. presence of pus. If microbiological investigation is supportive of a diagnosis of catheter infection then the catheter should be removed and an alternative site chosen for re-insertion. Catheter-related infections should be treated with appropriate antibiotics, the choice of antibiotic depending on the culture and sensitivity of the microorganisms. If the catheter is removed, then the distal end of the catheter (~5 cm) should be cut under aseptic condition and sent in a sterile container to microbiology laboratory for culture. *Routine bacteriological sampling of catheter tips is not necessary.*

Use of antibiotic lock solutions: antibiotic locks are created by filling the lumen of the catheter with an antimicrobial solution and leaving the solution in place until the catheter hub is re-accessed. The aim is to prevent colonization of the intraluminal catheter surface which will lead to prevention of CR-BSI. Despite some promising results, lock solutions are *not currently recommended for routine* as their use has not been fully evaluated. However, antibiotic lock solutions can be used in patients with limited venous access, have a history of recurrent CR-BSI despite maximal adherence to aseptic technique and who are at high risk for severe sequelae from a CR-BSI, i.e. patients with recently implanted devices such as a prosthetic heart valve or aortic graft.

Needleless connection devices: needleless connectors were introduced in an effort to reduce the potential for IV access-related needle stick injuries to HCWs. Since their introduction in the last decade, there have been several reports of increased CR-BSI rates with the use of needleless access devices. Therefore it is essential that the clinical team *must be educated* and their practices monitored to ensure that the techniques they use for accessing/de-accessing are appropriate for the specific devices in accordance with the manufacturer's instructions. When needleless systems are used, a split septum device should be preferred over some mechanical valves due to increased risk of infection.

Parenteral solutions and administration sets

Before use, parenteral solutions must be checked for expiry dates and the integrity of the packaging. Parenteral fluid must be checked for macroscopic contamination and clarity of solution, e.g. visible turbidity, leaks, cracks, particulate matter. Any solutions that are not clear must not be used and if the manufacturer's expiry date has passed, the solutions should not be used but disposed of appropriately. Sterile packs and parenteral solutions must be stored in a clean area and condition to avoid damage (see Chapter 6, Box 6.1).

Use *single-dose vials* for parenteral additives or medications whenever possible. The access diaphragm of multidose vials should be cleaned with 70% alcohol before inserting a device into a vial. The diaphragm *must not be touched* after it has been disinfected. Multidose vials must be discarded if their sterility is compromised.

Administration sets, including secondary sets and add-on devices should be replaced no more frequently than at 96-hour interval unless catheter-related sepsis is suspected or documented or when the integrity of the product has been compromised.

IV tubing used to administer blood, blood products, or lipid emulsions should be replaced at the end of the infusion or within 24 hours of initiating the infusion. Lipid emulsion infusion should be completed within 24 hours and blood within 4 hours of hanging.

Key references and further reading

Berenholtz SM, Pronovost PJ, Lipsett PA, *et al.* Eliminating catheter-related bloodstream infections in the intensive care unit. *Critical Care Medicine* 2004; **32**:2014–20.

CDC/Healthcare Infection Control Practices Advisory Committee. *Guidelines for the Prevention of Intravascular Catheter-Related Infections, 2011.* Atlanta, GA: CDC, 2011.

CDC/NHSN surveillance definition of health care-associated infection and criteria for specific types of infections in the acute care setting. *American Journal of Infection Control* 2008; **36**:309–32.

Department of Health. epic2: Guidelines for preventing infections associated with the use of central venous access devices. *Journal of Hospital Infection* 2007; **65S**:S33–S49.

Department of Health. *High Impact Intervention No 1. Peripheral intravenous cannula care bundle and High Impact Intervention No 2. Central venous catheter care bundle.* London: Department of Health, 2007. Available at: http://hcai.dh.gov.uk/.

HELICS. *Surveillance of nosocomial infections in Intensive Care units.* Hospital in Europe for Link Infection Control through Surveillance: September, 2004. Available at: http://www.ecdc.europa.eu.

Institute for Healthcare Improvement. *Infection Prevention Bundle: Prevent Central Line Infections, 2007.* Available at: http://www.ihi.org.

Pronovost P, Needham D, Berenholtz S, *et al.* An intervention to decrease catheter-related bloodstream infections in the ICU. *New England Journal of Medicine* 2006; **355**:2725–32.

Pronovost P, Goeschel CA, Colantuoni E, *et al.* Sustaining reductions in catheter related bloodstream infections in Michigan intensive care units: observational study. *British Medical Journal* 2010; **340**:c309.

SHEA/IDSA Practice Recommendation: Strategies to Prevent Central Line-Associated Bloodstream Infections in Acute Care Hospitals. *Infection Control Hospital Epidemiology* 2008; **29**(Suppl 1):S22–S30.

Timsit J-F, Schwebel C, Bouadma L, *et al.* Chlorhexidine-impregnated sponges and less frequent dressing changes for prevention of catheter-related infections in critically ill adults: a randomized controlled trial. *Journal of American Medical Association* 2009; **301**(12):1231–41.

Chapter 13

Catheter-associated urinary tract infections

A few days ago, two surgeons came to give me a cystic examination.
. . . both of them washed their instruments and their hands. Gosselin washed his after, but your pupil, Guyon, before this small operation.

Claude Bernard (From a conversation between Bernard and Louis Pasteur)

It has been estimated that about 10% of hospitalized patients require urinary catheterization. Urinary tract infections (UTIs) following catheterization are the most common infections, accounting for up to 40% of all health care associated infections.

After catheterization, the risk of acquiring bacteriuria increases with time with an average daily risk of 3–10% per day. The overall incidence of bacteriuria in patients with an indwelling urinary catheter in place for 2–10 days is 26%, and nearly 100% in 4 weeks. It has been estimated that up to 4% of bacteriuric patients will ultimately develop clinically significant bacteraemia with a case fatality of 13–30%. Therefore a urinary catheter should be inserted only when it is indicated (see Box 13.1). Daily review should be carried out regarding the patient's clinical need for continuing urinary catheterization and it should be removed *as soon as possible*, preferably within 5 days. Alternatives to indwelling catheters are intermittent catheterization with an associated infection risk ranging from 0.5–8%; this should be considered in certain groups of patients.

Risk factors

- Increased duration of catheterization (i.e. >6 days).
- Female.
- Older age.
- Diabetes mellitus.
- Malnutrition.
- Azotaemia (creatinine >2.0 mg/dL).

Box 13.1 Appropriate and inappropriate indications for the use of indwelling urinary catheters

Examples of appropriate uses of indwelling catheters

- Patient has acute urinary retention or bladder outlet obstruction.
- Need for accurate measurements of urinary output in critically ill patients.
- Perioperative use for selected surgical procedures.
- Patients undergoing urological surgery or other surgery on contiguous structures of the genitourinary tract.
- Anticipated prolonged duration of surgery—catheters inserted for this reason should be removed in post-anaesthesia care unit.
- Patients anticipated to receive large-volume infusions or diuretics during surgery.
- Need for intraoperative monitoring of urinary output.
- To assist in healing of open sacral or perineal wounds in incontinent patients.
- Patient requires prolonged immobilization, e.g. potentially unstable thoracic or lumbar spine, multiple traumatic injuries such as pelvic fractures.
- To improve comfort for end of life care if needed.

Examples of *inappropriate* uses of indwelling catheters

- As a substitute for nursing care of the patient or resident with incontinence.
- As a means of obtaining urine for culture or other diagnostic tests when the patient can voluntarily void.
- For prolonged postoperative duration without appropriate indications, e.g. structural repair of urethra or contiguous structures, prolonged effect of epidural anaesthesia, etc.

Source: HICPAC/CDC. *Guidelines for prevention of catheter-associated urinary tract infections 2009*. Atlanta, GA: CDC, 2009.

- Failure to adhere to aseptic technique both during insertion and maintenance.
- Failure to use closed urinary system.

Pathogenesis

Under normal circumstances the urethral flora, which tends to migrate into the bladder, is constantly flushed out during urination. When a urinary catheter is inserted, this flushing mechanism is circumvented and perineal and urethral flora migrate into the bladder mucosa leading to bladder colonization and subsequent infection if the catheter is left in place for prolonged periods. An additional factor in initiating the infection is that there is bacterial reflux from contaminated urine in the drainage bag (Figure 13.1); this can be prevented by using a closed drainage system and strict adherence to aseptic technique both during insertion and maintenance.

Two distinct types of bacteria are encountered in the urinary tract of a catheterized patient: free-floating planktonic bacteria (which usually do not cause infection), and those which form a biofilm on the catheter surface. Once the microorganisms are attached to the catheter surface by producing exopolymer substances they can grow, multiply and disseminate. Biofilms have considerable survival advantages over plank-tonic bacteria as they are resistant to both phagocytosis and antimicrobial agents. Biofilms that develop on long-term indwelling urinary catheters make treatment diffi-cult when the catheter remains in place. Antibiotics are unable to penetrate the biofilm to eradicate microorganisms, and normal immune defences are ineffective within the biofilm. Therefore treatment of catheter-associated urinary tract infections (CA-UTIs) with an antibiotic in the presence of a catheter is usually *not* effective and can lead to development of multi-resistant microorganisms.

Microbiology

A UTI is usually endogenous, caused by microorganisms from the patient's own bowel. In community-acquired infection, the commonest microorganisms are 'coliforms' e.g. *Escherichia coli*, *Proteus* spp., and *Klebsiella* spp., which are usually susceptible to most antibiotics and are relatively easy to treat. In a community where indiscriminate antimicrobial use is common, multi-resistant Gram-negative bacteria are also preva-lent in the human bowel outside the hospital.

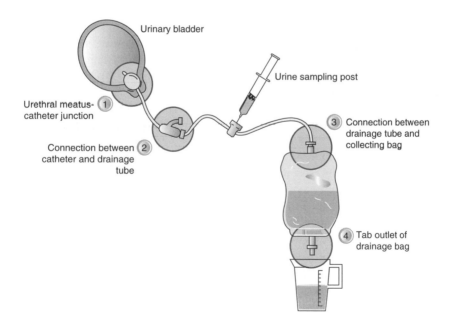

Fig. 13.1 The four main sites through which bacteria may reach the bladder of a patient with an indwelling urethral catheter. The recommended measures for prevention are listed in Table 13.2.

E. coli is the commonest cause of UTI; however, these infections are increasingly caused by more resistant Gram-negative species, such as *Klebsiella* spp. and *Pseudomonas* spp. Similarly, ampicillin-sensitive *Enterococcus faecalis* is gradually being replaced by the resistant *Enterococcus faecium*. CA-UTIs are more resistant to antibiotics because hospitalized patients become colonized with resistant organisms, a process encouraged by increasing length of hospital stay and exposure to antibiotics. In addition, resistant organisms may be transferred from other patients, most commonly via contaminated staff hands, a break in the closed system, and from contaminated environment and items/equipments.

Diagnosis

The diagnosis of UTIs in patients with long-term indwelling urinary catheters can be difficult as the signs and symptoms may not be present with a catheter *in situ*. Neither urinalysis nor urine cultures are reliable as cultures from these catheters specimen are universally positive. In addition, UTIs in patients with spinal cord lesions may be particularly difficult to diagnose because of the inability of the patient to sense localizing symptoms. Clinical symptoms, e.g. fever and rigors, are the most consistent symptom of CA-UTI. However, given the high prevalence of bacteriuria in patients with an indwelling catheter, this definition lacks specificity.

The diagnosis of UTIs in hospitals depends on laboratory support. Where this is good and a careful, midstream specimen is collected, finding $\geq 10^5$ bacterial colony forming units (CFU)/mL in a patient *without* an indwelling catheter is diagnostic of a UTI. Bacterial concentrations $>10^2$ CFU/mL suggest infection provided the specimen is obtained *aseptically* by needle aspiration *from the proximal drainage tubing port* (see Figure 13.1) and *not from the urine bag* in a patient with an indwelling catheter. Use of urine dipstick to diagnosis UTI on a catheterized patient is *not* reliable it is often positive due to heavy mixed growth.

Although UTIs in non-catheterized patients are usually caused by a single microorganism, in catheterized patients infections are frequently polymicrobial, provided the specimen is collected as described above.

The presence of multiple microorganisms does not necessarily indicate contamination. Urine must be processed promptly as, even with good technique, urine samples may contain small numbers of contaminants. These microbes can multiply at room temperature (especially in hot climates) and give falsely high colony counts. If delay is expected, the specimen should be transported in an ice box and refrigerated on arrival. Boric acid (1% W/V or 1 g/10 mL of urine) is added to the urine as preservative but it is inhibitory to certain microorganisms and it is difficult to achieve exact 1% W/V concentration, therefore its use should be avoided.

Prevention strategies

Current strategies to prevent CA-UTIs are based on the implementation of a 'care bundle' (see 'Care bundle approach', Chapter 1). The catheter care bundle for the prevention of CA-UTIs was developed by the USA Institute of Health Improvement

Table 13.1 Care bundle to prevent catheter-associated urinary tract infections

Insertion care bundle	Maintenance bundle
Avoid unnecessary catheterization	Use aseptic technique for daily catheter care (e.g. hand hygiene, sterile items/equipment)
Use sterile items/equipment	
Insert catheter using strict aseptic non-touch technique	Don't break the closed drainage system. If urine specimen required, take specimen aseptically via the sampling port (see Fig. 13.1)
Use closed drainage system	
Chose catheters of appropriate size	Keep the drainage bag above the floor but below bladder level to prevent reflux/contamination
Consider use of antimicrobial impregnated catheters in 'high-risk' patients requiring short-term catheterization (2–10 days)	Review the need for the catheter on a daily basis. Remove catheter promptly when no longer necessary

Adapted with modification from the IHI *Infection Prevention Bundle: Preventing Catheter-Associated Urinary Tract Infections*, 2009 and *High Impact Intervention No 6. Urinary Catheter Care Bundle*. London: Department of Health, 2007.

and the UK Department of Health are summarized in Table 13.1 with further strategies to prevent CA-UTIs outlined in Table 13.2.

Consideration prior to catheterization

Staff training: catheterization is an aseptic procedure and should be carried out using aseptic technique. Ensure that health care personnel are trained and competent to carry out insertion and daily maintenance of urethral catheterization. Policies and procedures regarding the insertion, maintenance, and changing regimens of indwelling urinary devices should be written, reviewed, and updated on a regular basis. These policies should be readily accessible. Regular education as well as an orientation programme should be implemented to include instruction on the importance and principles of catheterization and the care of the patient with indwelling urinary devices.

Asepsis: urethral catheterization should be considered as a minor surgical procedure. Therefore the catheter must be inserted using an aseptic technique and sterile equipment (see Box 13.2). Before the procedure, efficient and effective cleaning of the area and surfaces involved should be undertaken. Aseptic technique should be maintained throughout the procedure. Only a closed urinary drainage system should be used. It has been estimated that the risk of infection can be reduced from 97% when an open system is used to 8–15% when a sterile, continuously closed system is employed.

Catheter material: choice of catheter material will depend on clinical experience, patient preference, and the anticipated duration of catheterization. Latex catheters are the least expensive, but irritation and allergic reaction may occur. Silicone catheters are comfortable and may be a better choice for long-term catheterization. Silicone catheters obstruct less often than latex, Teflon, or silicone-coated latex in patients prone to encrustation.

Antimicrobial coated catheters: several studies support the use of latex-coated, silver alloy coated urinary catheters as adjunct for the prevention of CA-UTI.

Table 13.2 Summary of strategies to prevent catheter-associated urinary tract infections (see Figure 13.1)

Entry points for bacteria	Preventative measures
1. External urethral meatus and urethra	
Bacteria carried into bladder during insertion of catheter	◆ Pass catheter when bladder is full for wash-out effect
	◆ Before catheterization prepare urinary meatus with an antiseptic (e.g. 0.2% chlorhexidine aqueous solution or povidone iodine)
	◆ Inject single-use sterile lubricant gel or use 2% lignocaine anaesthetic gel into urethra and hold there for 3 min before inserting catheter
	◆ Use sterile catheter
	◆ Use non-touch technique for insertion
Ascending colonization/ infection up urethra around outside of catheter	◆ Keep peri-urethral area clean and dry; bladder washes and ointments are of *no* value
	◆ Secure catheter to prevent movement in urethra
	◆ After faecal incontinence, clean area and change catheter
2. Junction between catheter and drainage tube	
	◆ Do not disconnect catheter unless absolutely necessary
	◆ Always use aseptic technique for irrigation
	◆ For urine specimen collection, disinfect sampling port by applying alcoholic impregnated wipe and allow it to dry completely, then aspirate urine with a sterile needle and syringe
3. Junction between drainage tube and collection bag	
Disconnection	◆ Drainage tube should be welded to inlet of bag during manufacture
Reflux from bag into catheter	◆ Drip chamber or non-return valve at inlet to bag
	◆ Keep bag below level of bladder. If it is necessary to raise collection bag above bladder level for a short period, drainage tube must be clamped temporarily
	◆ Empty bag every 8 h or earlier, if full
	◆ Do not hold bag upside down when emptying
4. Tap at bottom of collection bag	
Emptying of bag	◆ Collection bag must never touch floor
	◆ Always wash or disinfect hands with an alcoholic hand rub before and after opening tap
	◆ Use a separate disinfected jug to collect urine from each bag
	◆ Don't instil disinfectant/antiseptic into urinary bag after emptying

Box 13.2 Procedure for urinary catheterization

Prior to insertion, the procedure must be explained to the patients to allay any fear and anxiety they may have.

Urethral catheterization is considered as a minor surgical procedure therefore the catheter must be inserted using an aseptic technique and sterile equipment. Aseptic non-touch technique should be maintained throughout the procedure.

Before the procedure, check the expiry dates, integrity of containers/packages and the correct amount of sterile water required to be inserted if the device has a balloon.

- All equipment used must be sterile.
- Lay out the sterile field on top of the trolley, making sure all items required are open and accessible.
- Hands must be washed thoroughly with an antiseptic hand wash preparation.
- Sterile gloves must be worn for the procedure and an aseptic non-touch technique should be used.
- The peri-urethral area should be cleaned using sterile water or saline. In a male, retract the foreskin and cleanse the glans. In a female, separate the labia and cleanse the vulva using a front-to-back technique.
- Instil 2% lignocaine (± 0.25% chlorhexidine gluconate) to the urethra to minimize pain. This can be stored in the fridge to improve effectiveness. Allow 3–5 min for it to take anaesthetic effect before catheterization.
- Insert the catheter and advance it by holding the inner sterile sleeve, avoiding contact with the non-sterile surface. The aseptic non-touch technique should be used, in which the operator has no contact with the sterile shaft of the catheter.
- Inflate the balloon by instilling the manufacturer's recommended amount of sterile water. If the site is to be dressed (e.g. suprapubic) the dressings surrounding the device must be sterile.
- Connect the catheter to a sterile, closed urinary drainage system.
- Hang the drainage bag below the level of the bladder to stop reflux or apply the leg bag with the support. The bag must be supported in the drainage stand to allow free flow of urine and to prevent the bag from touching the floor.
- Secure the catheter to the patient's thigh or abdomen to prevent movement and urethral meatal ulceration.
- Hands must be washed after gloves are removed.

Silver alloy catheters significantly reduce the incidence of asymptomatic bacteriuria in patients who are on short-term catheterization (2–10 days). There is no evidence that they decrease symptomatic infections and therefore they should not be used routinely. However, their use should be considered in reducing bacteriuria in catheterized patients, especially in those patients at highest risk of either bacteriuria or complications associated with bacteriuria.

Catheter size: catheter size/gauge relates to the circumference of the catheter. Larger diameter catheters block the urethral gland and put pressure on the urethral mucosa, which may result in ischaemic necrosis. They are also resistant to bending and are more likely to cause pressure necrosis, especially in males. In general, the smallest diameter catheter (with a 10-mL balloon) that allows free flow of urine is the most desirable. The smallest size/gauge catheter is also less likely to be associated with leakage. Urological patients may require larger diameter catheters and these must be used on the advice of the urologist.

Use of prophylactic antimicrobial agents: the administration of systemic antibiotics at the time of catheter insertion may provide early benefit to prevent CA-UTIs but it also exposes the patient to a risk of antibiotic associated toxicity and subsequent development of infections with resistant bacterial strains. Therefore the routine use of prophylaxis in this setting is *not* recommended. Long-term antibiotic prophylaxis is ineffective and predisposes to infection with resistant microorganisms and fungi and is *not* recommended.

Consideration after catheterization

Maintenance of catheter: after insertion, regular inspection of the catheter and drainage system must be attended to and documented at least daily. The date and time of catheter changes should be documented either in nursing or medical notes.

Meatal care: meatal cleansing should be performed at intervals appropriate for keeping the meatus free of encrustations and contamination. Meatal cleansing with antiseptic solutions is *not* necessary. Applying antimicrobial ointment to the urethral meatus has *not* reliably been shown to reduce the incidence of UTIs. Daily routine bathing or showering is all that is needed to maintain meatal hygiene. If faecal incontinence occurs, the perineum must be cleaned and the catheter changed *without delay*.

Drainage bag: reflux of urine is associated with infection. Therefore it is important that the sterile drainage bags should be positioned in a way that prevents back-flow of urine. The urinary drainage bags should be put on a holder attached to the bed frame or a stand to prevent contact with the floor. The bag and tubing must at all times be *below* the level of the bladder so that flow can be continuously maintained by gravity. Where dependent drainage cannot be maintained, e.g. during moving and handling, clamp the urinary drainage bag tube and remove the clamp as soon as dependent drainage can be resumed. Routine use of antiseptics (e.g. chlorhexidine and hydrogen peroxide) in the drainage bag is *not* recommended, as they do not reduce the incidence of bacteriuria.

Emptying the drainage bag: the drainage bag should be emptied regularly (i.e. 8-hourly or earlier if it fills rapidly) via the drainage tap at the bottom of the bag to maintain urine flow and to prevent reflux. The spout from the tap must be completely emptied to minimize a build-up of microorganisms in the stagnant urine. Extreme care must be taken when emptying the drainage bag to prevent cross-infection. Hands must be disinfected and non-sterile, single-use gloves should be worn before emptying each bag. Alcohol impregnated swabs may be used to decontaminate the outlet (inside and outside) *before* and *after* emptying the bag. When the bag is empty, the tap should be closed securely and wiped with a tissue. If the bag does not have a tap, replace it when full using an aseptic technique. Do not reconnect a used bag. Wash and dry hands thoroughly after touching the drainage bag.

When emptying the drainage bag, *use a separate container for each patient* and avoid contact between the urinary drainage tap and the container. Each bag should be *emptied separately* as required. For the purposes of measuring urinary output, an integral measuring device is necessary. The urine receptacle should be heat disinfected and stored dry after each use. Single-use disposable receptacles may be used. After emptying the receptacle, non-sterile, single-use gloves should be discarded in a clinical waste bag and hands washed and dried thoroughly.

Bladder irrigation: routine bladder irrigation or washout with antiseptics (e.g. chlorhexidine) or antimicrobial agents does not prevent CA-UTIs and should *not* be used. The introduction of such agents causes erosion of the bladder mucosa and promotes the emergence of resistant microorganisms. In addition, they may also cause damage to the catheter. If the catheter becomes obstructed and can be kept open only by frequent irrigation, the catheter should be changed, as it is likely that the catheter itself is contributing to obstruction. However, continuous or intermittent bladder irrigation may be indicated during urological surgery or to manage catheter obstruction and should *only* be undertaken on the advice of an urologist. Condom use for 24-hour periods should also be avoided and other methods, such as napkins or absorbent pads, used at night.

Specimen collection: closed drainage bag should *not* be disconnected to obtain a sample as this causes interruption to the closed system and may pose a risk of infection to the patient. If a sample of urine is required for bacteriological examination, it should be obtained from a sampling port using an aseptic technique. *Do not* obtain a sample for bacteriological culture from the drainage bag. The sampling port must first be disinfected by wiping with a 70% isopropyl alcohol impregnated swab. The sample may then be aspirated using a sterile small bore needle and syringe and transferred into a sterile container. Bacteriological testing of urine is indicated if the patient has possible or probably CA-UTI and otherwise routine culture of urine is *not* recommended.

Removal of catheter: the optimal time limit for replacing catheters depends upon individual circumstances and the type of catheter used. However, urinary catheters should not be changed as long as they are functioning well. A catheter that requires frequent irrigation for recurrent obstruction should be changed and replaced. The routine administration of prophylactic antibiotic at the time of catheter removal is not recommended. Culturing of urine sampled after catheter removal is indicated only for patients where there is a high degree of suspicion or symptoms suggestive of infection.

Management of patients with bacteriuria and infections

Asymptomatic bacteriuria

The treatment of asymptomatic bacteriuria (i.e. significant bacteriuria in the *absence* of clinical symptoms) in patients who require continued catheterization is *not* indicated. Antibiotics are only indicated if there is evidence of clinical infection. The treatment of CA-UTI in patients with long-term catheters may be difficult without removing or changing of the catheter because bacteria are embedded in the biofilm (or encrustation) on the surface of the catheter and may be protected from the action of antibiotics. In addition, the use of an antibiotic in the presence of the catheter often results in infection with a more resistant strain of bacteria. After the catheter is removed, in most patients the bacteriuria spontaneously resolves. If treatment is indicated, it is only for those cases in which the bacteriuria has persisted after catheter removal and in which there are no underlying anatomical or physiological barriers to eradication of the bacteriuria.

Routine administration of prophylactic antibiotic at the time of catheter removal is *not* recommended. Culturing of urine sampled after catheter removal is indicated only for patients where there is a high degree of suspicion or symptoms suggestive of infection.

Symptomatic patients

Febrile episodes are found in less than 10% of catheterized patients living in a long-term facility. Therefore, it is extremely important to rule out other sources of fever. In case of symptomatic CA-UTI, it is essential to treat with appropriate antibiotic and remove and replace with new a catheter if the indwelling catheter has been in place for more than 7 days. There are no adequate clinical studies to guide the length of therapy for CA-UTI and therefore the duration of treatment depends on the severity of clinical symptoms.

Management of candiduria

While it is clear that symptomatic candiduria requires treatment, it is controversial whether asymptomatic candiduria requires treatment. Frequently, *candiduria resolves without treatment if the catheter is removed*. In the case of candiduria associated with urinary symptoms or if candiduria is secondary to systemic infection, parenteral therapy with an antifungal is indicated. However, the presence of *Candida* in a urine sample may reflect local infection elsewhere, e.g. vaginal thrush in a female and balinitis in a male.

Diabetes predisposes to the development of candiduria as glycosuria enhances urinary growth of *Candida* spp. In addition, diabetes also impairs host defences, particularly phagocytosis, and the development of a neurogenic bladder allows for urinary stasis and increases the likelihood of the urinary tract infections.

Key references and further reading

APIC. *Guide to the Elimination of Catheter-Associated Urinary Tract Infections (CAUTIs); Developing and applying facility-based prevention interventions in acute and long-term care settings, 2008* (APIC Elimination Guide Series). Washington DC: APIC Headquarters, 2008.

Department of Health. *High Impact Intervention No 6. Urinary Catheter Care Bundle.* London, Department of Health, 2007. Available at: http://hcai.dh.gov.uk/.

Department of Health. epic2: Guidelines for preventing infections associated with the use of short-term urethral catheters *Journal of Hospital Infection* 2007; **65**(Suppl 1):S28–S33.

HICPAC/CDC. *Guidelines for prevention of Catheter-associated Urinary Tract infections 2009.* Atlanta, GA: CDC, 2009. Available at: http://www.cdc.gov/.

Hooton TM, Bradley SF, Cardenas DD, *et al.* IDSA Guidelines. Diagnosis, prevention, and treatment of catheter-associated urinary tract infection in adults: 2009. International Clinical Practice Guidelines from the Infectious Diseases Society of America. *Clinical Infectious Diseases* 2010; **50**:625–63.

Institute of Health Improvement. *Infection Prevention Bundle: Preventing Catheter-Associated Urinary Tract Infections,* 2009. Available at: http://www.ihi.org/ihi.

Lo E, Nicolle L, Classen D, *et al.* Strategies to prevent catheter-associated urinary tract infections in acute care hospitals. *Infection Control and Hospital Epidemiology* 2008; **29**(Supplement 1): S41–S50.

Tenke T, Kovacs B, Bjerklund Johanse TE, *et al.* European and Asian guidelines on management and prevention of catheter-associated urinary tract infections. *International Journal of Antimicrobial Agents* 2008; **31S**:S68–S78.

Chapter 14

Prevention of ventilator-associated pneumonias

> When a man lacks mental balance in pneumonia he is
> said to be delirious. When he lacks mental balance
> without pneumonia, he is pronounced insane by
> all smart doctors.
>
> *Martin H. Fisher*

Health care-associated pneumonia in hospitalized patients has a mortality rate of up to 40%. Although pneumonia may occur in patients throughout the hospital stay, the patients at greatest risk are those who are intubated to enable them to be managed on mechanical ventilatory support; other risk factors are summarized in Box 14.1.

Definition and microbiology

Hospital-acquired pneumonia

Hospital-acquired pneumonia (HAP) is defined as pneumonia developing 48 hours after admission to hospital and is classified as early or late onset. **Early-onset pneumonia** occurs within the first 72 hours after hospital admission and is often caused by microorganisms acquired from the community. They are usually caused by antibiotic susceptible bacteria, e.g. *Streptococcus pneumoniae, Staphylococcus aureus*, and *Haemophilus influenzae*. **Late-onset pneumonia** occurs after 4–5 days and is often caused by more resistant bacteria acquired within hospital, e.g. *Staph. aureus* (both meticillin-resistant and meticillin-sensitive) and Gram-negative bacilli including *Klebsiella pneumoniae, Escherichia coli, Serratia marcescens, Citrobacter* spp., *Enterobacter* spp., *Pseudomonas aeruginosa*, and *Acinetobacter* spp.

In addition, HAP can also be caused by *Legionella* spp., usually acquired from hospital air conditioning systems or from contaminated water supplies. *Aspergillus fumigatus* is acquired particularly in immunocompromised patients and is associated with building work. Other organisms responsible for pneumonia include viruses (e.g. influenza), yeasts, and *Mycobacterium tuberculosis* and atypical mycobacteria.

Box 14.1 Risk factors for hospital-acquired and ventilator-associated pneumonia

Patient-related factors

Chronic lung/
cardiopulmonary diseases
Extreme age (elderly or
preterm neonate)
Obesity or malnutrition
Chronic disease or impaired
immunity
Heavy smokers

Medical interventions

Prolonged hospitalization
Mechanical ventilation
Presence of foreign body, e.g. endotracheal and/
or nasogastric tubes
Aspiration of gastric content due to depressed
consciousness (coma, cerebrovascular accidents,
use of sedative or hypnotic drugs)
Achlorhydria, H_2 antagonist, proton-pump
inhibitor, or antacid therapy
Difficulty breathing due to major trauma,
abdominal/thoracic surgery, neuromuscular
disease
General anaesthesia
Immunosuppressive or cytotoxic drugs
Severe illness, e.g. septic shock

Ventilator-associated pneumonia

There is no consensus or well-established definition of ventilator-associated pneumonia (VAP). The diagnosis should be considered in a patient who develops a new or progressive pulmonary infiltrate with fever, leucocytosis, and purulent tracheobronchial secretions 48 hours after endotracheal intubation and/or mechanical ventilation (although some case definitions require no minimum time period for intubation, simply the requirement to be intubated and ventilated at the time of symptoms, or in the preceding 48 hours). These criteria should be combined with direct bronchoscopic assessment, if possible.

The risk of developing VAP is estimated at 3% per day for the first 5 days of mechanical ventilation, 2% per day for days 6 to 10, and 1% per day for every day beyond 10 days of mechanical ventilation. Compared to non-ventilated patients, the risk of pneumonia increases at least 7–10-fold in patients following surgery or in patients in the intensive care unit (ICU) requiring mechanical ventilation. In addition to high morbidity and mortality, VAP is associated with greater time spent on the ventilator, and longer ICU and hospital stays.

Although case definitions for VAP have been developed by the CDC (CDC/NHSN, 2008) and HELICS in Europe (ECDC, 2004), in practice the diagnosis of VAP can be difficult and significant interobserver variability has been noted. Factors such as the surveillance strategy, diagnostic techniques, and laboratory procedures likely account for some of the differences in VAP rates between different health care facilities.

Pathogenesis

The pathogenesis of VAP usually requires two important processes to take place: 1) bacterial colonization of the aerodigestive tract, and 2) aspiration of contaminated secretions into the lower airway. Severely ill/stressed patients in the ICU are at increased risk of colonization with microorganisms, especially with Gram-negative bacilli due to the increased binding of these bacilli to the buccal cells, mediated by a loss of cell surface fibronectin. The presence of invasive medical devices is an important contributor because it causes mechanical and chemical injury to the ciliated epithelium of the respiratory tract leading to loss of the first-line defence mechanism. The injury promotes colonization and aspiration of bacteria from the oropharynx or stomach into the tracheobronchial tree. In addition, the presence of a foreign body (e.g., endotracheal tube) is associated with biofilm formation and facilitates bacterial colonization of the tracheobronchial tree. The problem is further compounded by the fact that most of the ICU patients also have a nasogastric tube which predisposes to gastric reflux and increases the potential for aspiration (see Figure 14.1).

Prevention strategies

Strategies for prevention of VAP are usually focused on reducing the bioburden of bacterial colonization in the aerodigestive tract with the aim of decreasing the incidence of aspiration and/or pneumonias. This includes: 1) avoidance/early removal of endotracheal and nasogastric tubes as soon as clinically feasible, 2) avoidance of unnecessary re-intubation to prevent respiratory trauma, and 3) maintenance of adequate volume and safe pressures in the endotracheal tube cuff to prevent aspiration.

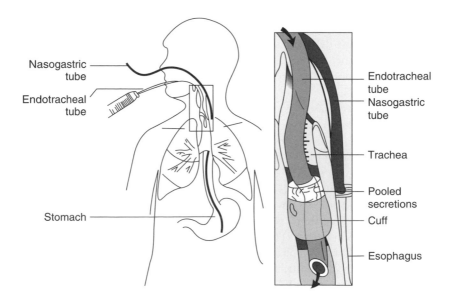

Fig. 14.1 An endotracheal tube.

Table 14.1 Care bundle to prevent ventilator associated pneumonia

Regular observations	Ongoing care
Elevation of the head of the bed to 30–45°	Adherence to hand hygiene and aseptic technique
Daily assessment of sedation with readiness to extubate	
Gastric ulcer prophylaxis	Oral hygiene
Management of ventilator tubing	Subglottic suctioning of respiratory secretions
Appropriate humidification of inspired gas	
Deep vein thrombosis prophylaxis	

Adapted from the UK Department of Health *High Impact Intervention No 5. Care bundle for ventilated patients* (2007) and IHI *Infection Prevention Care bundle for VAP* (2007).

It should be noted that over-inflation of these cuffs leads to tracheal mucosal trauma and this may increase the risk of infection.

Current strategies to prevent VAP are based on the implementation of a 'care bundle' (see 'Care bundle approach', Chapter 1) developed by the IHI and the UK Department of Health and are summarized in Table 14.1.

General measures for prevention

Education and training: an infection control training programme should be introduced to promote good infection control practices (adherence to aseptic technique for all sterile/clean procedures, hand hygiene, wearing of gloves for contact with the respiratory secretions, adequate decontamination of environmental surfaces, items and equipments, etc.). Clutter around the patients should be minimized and staff responsible for cleaning, disinfection, and maintenance of respiratory equipment must be trained.

Surveillance: surveillance of VAP should be introduced in the ICU and data should be collected both on outcome and adherence to the process surveillance. This must be fed back to the clinical team on a regular basis and rates and compliance with the elements of the bundle (if implemented by the unit) should be displayed prominently in the unit to improve clinical practice. ICUs that have introduced *practical education and training* to staff combined with regular and timely feedback of surveillance data have seen a substantial reduction in VAP.

Staffing level: inadequate staffing has been associated with failure to adhere to the infection control practices and protocols and has resulted in increased nosocomial infections in ICU patients. This issue must be addressed to ensure that the clinical team follow protocols to minimize the risk of *all* health care-associated infections including VAP.

Antibiotic prescribing: widespread use of broad-spectrum antibiotics is common in ICUs, is not always appropriate, and should be avoided where possible. This objective can be achieved by developing an antibiotic guideline based on local resistance patterns. Compliance with antibiotic prescribing should be monitored and data should be fed back to the clinicians. This process works best when the infection control and clinical ICU teams work together in the development and monitoring processes, with the clear goal of improving patient care. If broad-spectrum antibiotics are used as empiric therapy, they should be changed to narrow-spectrum agents as appropriate once the bacteriology results are available. Adequate doses of antibiotics must be given and the duration should be kept to a minimum, i.e. 1 week for most cases of HAP. This can be achieved by daily review of antibiotic need, preferably by senior ward medical staff during regular ward rounds with the clinical microbiologist. The routine use of aerosolized antibiotics for the prevention and treatment of VAP has not been proven to have any value but can be considered as an adjunctive treatment for VAP caused by multidrug-resistant pathogens that are not responsive to standard therapy.

Surgical patients: preoperatively, patients should be encouraged to stop smoking and any existing infection should be treated. Postoperatively, coughing exercises and breathing techniques should be taught. Early mobilization is essential and postoperative pain should be controlled with judicious use of analgesics. It is essential that patients should be kept in a semi-recumbent position during enteral feeding.

Specific measures for prevention

Specific measures for prevention of VAP are summarized below. Table 14.2 summarizes the infection prevention measures necessary for devices and procedures used in a ventilated patient.

Table 14.2 Major interventions used in prevention of ventilator associated pneumonias

Procedure/device	Intervention to decrease risk
Suctioning	◆ Use single-use disposable gloves and wash hands before and after the procedure ◆ Use sterile suction catheter and sterile fluid to flush catheter ◆ Change suction tubing between patients ◆ Use closed suction system, if possible
Suction bottle	◆ Use single-use disposable, if possible ◆ Non-disposable bottles should be washed with detergent and allowed to dry or heat disinfect in washing machine or send to sterile supply department
Ventilator breathing circuits	◆ Replace mechanical ventilators, if soiled or malfunctioning ◆ Periodically drain breathing tube condensation traps, taking care not to spill it down the patient's trachea; wash hands after the procedure ◆ Use HME ventilator circuits, if possible (see text)
Nebulizers	◆ Fill with sterile water only ◆ Change nebulizers between patients by using sterilization or a high-level disinfection or use single-use nebulizers, if possible
Humidifiers	◆ Fill with sterile water which must be changed every 24 h or sooner, if necessary ◆ Clean and sterilize humidifiers between patients. Single-use disposable humidifiers are available but they are expensive
Ventilators	◆ After every patient, clean and disinfect ventilators ◆ Sterilize/disinfect (high-level) re-usable components as per the manufacturer's instructions

Semi-recumbent position: patients who are confined to bed have an increased frequency of pulmonary and non-pulmonary complications. Significant reductions in VAP have been achieved amongst patients if the semi-recumbent position is maintained during the first 24 hours of mechanical ventilation. Provided there are no contraindications (e.g. spinal injury), the patient should be maintained with elevation of the head of the bed to a 30–45° angle to reduce reflux and aspiration of gastric and oesophageal material containing organisms. If this is not possible, then the head of the bed should be raised to the highest level possible and the position maintained during transfer of patients to ICU. Patients should be encouraged to take deep breaths and cough, and also be turned regularly to facilitate postural drainage.

Sedative interruption: the development of VAP has been associated with the duration of mechanical ventilation, i.e. the more days a patient is ventilated the greater their risk. Efforts to minimize the duration of mechanical ventilation are enhanced by daily sedative interruptions and daily assessment of the patient's readiness to extubate. Not all patients are suitable for these assessments, and the clinical team will determine this on the ICU ward rounds. Concerns have been expressed that those patients who are not deeply sedated may have an increased potential for self-extubation and for increased pain and anxiety associated with lightening sedation. A balance needs to be struck based on individual patient assessment.

Stress ulcer prophylaxis: patients receiving mechanical ventilation are at high risk for upper gastrointestinal (GI) haemorrhage from stress ulcers. In a healthy person, bacterial colonization of the stomach with potentially pathogenic organisms is prevented by acidic pH and normal peristalsis movement. Administration of pH-lowering drugs (e.g. H_2-receptor antagonists, proton-pump inhibitors, and antacids) to prevent stress ulcers may increase the colonization density of the aerodigestive tract; this is further compounded by the loss of normal peristalsis movement, and together the risk of VAP is increased.

The administration of sucralfate is associated with a reduced risk of VAP when compared with the use of other agents such as histamine antagonists that raise gastric alkalinity in ventilated patients. However, use of sucralfate therapy has been associated with an increased risk of clinically important GI bleeding when compared with ranitidine. In addition, sucralfate may interact with enteral feeds and medications. Therefore, whenever clinically appropriate, stress ulcer prophylaxis should be avoided in order to help preserve gastric function. Its use should be considered in patients felt to be at moderate/high risk for stress ulceration, e.g. patients with head trauma, burns, prolonged mechanical ventilation, acute kidney injury, steroid use, and coagulopathy.

Oral care: poor oral hygiene contributes significantly to the incidence of VAP in intubated patients. Regular oral care using antiseptic solution (6-hourly use of oral antiseptics, e.g. chlorhexidine gel or liquid) has been recommended for patients who are receiving mechanical ventilation. However, its role in reduction of VAP needs further investigation. If chlorhexidine mouth care is used, it is important that the teeth should be cleaned prior to use to reduce staining. Chlorhexidine may be inactivated by tooth paste if applied within 30 minutes to 2 hours. A suitable regimen might be chlorhexidine gel applied four times a day, with tooth brushing twice daily. It is also important to ensure that patients are not allergic to chlorhexidine.

Selective decontamination therapy: the concept of selective decontamination was introduced in the 1980s and involved routine administration of prophylactic non-absorbable antibiotics orally along with a short course of IV antibiotics. This has been used in the Netherlands but rarely in ICUs outside that country, due to concerns of emergence of antibiotic resistance.

Endotracheal intubation: avoid use of endotracheal intubation, if possible. Non-invasive positive pressure should be used in appropriate patients as it allows for the provision of respiratory support without the need for intubation and so helps reduce VAP (although these patients often require a nasogastric tube to reduce the risk of gastric distension from air). Since re-intubation of patients is also associated with an increased risk of developing VAP by facilitating aspiration, it should be avoided if possible. The use of silver-coated endotracheal tube can reduce the occurrence of VAP during the first 10 days of mechanical ventilation and should be considered in high risk patients.

Subglottic suctioning: despite the endotracheal (ET) tube cuff, upper respiratory tract secretions contaminated with microorganisms that pool above the cuff are frequently aspirated into the lower tracheobronchial tree (Figure 14.1). In order to prevent the leakage and aspiration of colonized subglottic secretions into the lower airway, pressure of the ET tube cuff should be maintained *at least* 20 cmH$_2$O (>25 and <30 cmH$_2$O). It has been shown that subglottic suctioning is effective in reducing the incidence of VAP by nearly half and should be especially used for patients expected to remain ventilated for more than 3 days. However, data demonstrating any consistent improvement in patient outcomes with this intervention are lacking at present, and the special ET tubes required are costly. Prediction of which patients will require more prolonged ventilation is difficult and exchange of tubes in order to insert these special ones risks aspiration at that time.

Suction catheters: there are two types of suction catheter systems available (open and closed) and both systems have similar rates of VAP. However, use of closed suctioning system has several advantages: 1) helps maintain positive pressure in the ventilator circuit, 2) prevents exogenous contamination of the ET tube, 3) helps prevent aerosolization and reduce environmental contamination, and 4) reduces exposure of microorganisms to HCWs during suctioning. Closed suctioning systems only need to be changed when malfunctioning or visibly soiled. As part of preventative measures, the number of disconnections of suction equipment should be minimized as much as possible.

Ventilator tubing: increased manipulation and changing of ventilator circuits may increase the incidence of VAP. Therefore, ventilator circuits should only be changed when the circuit is damaged, visibly soiled, or mechanically malfunctioning. When significant condensate accumulates within a ventilator circuit, it should be removed to avoid aspiration and VAP. In order to avoid this problem, heat and moisture exchanger ventilator circuits should be used as they reduce manipulation and help minimize the development of condensate within ventilator circuits.

Nasogastric tube: a nasogastric tube for enteral feeding may erode the mucosal surface or block the sinus ducts and has been associated with nosocomial sinusitis. In addition, it can also contribute to regurgitation of gastric contents leading to aspiration which may increase the risk of VAP. Although patients ventilated through an ET tube are unable to eat and therefore require enteral feeding via a naso- or orogastric tube, the use of fine-bore tubes rather than the larger 'Salem sump' variety may minimize nasal trauma and reflux. The preferential use of the oral route to enteral tubes has been advocated to reduce sinusitis risk.

Humidifier and nebulizer: in a humidifier, gas bubbles passes through water, enabling them to pick up water vapour but not the actual droplets of water. Therefore the air is saturated with fine water vapour with a particle size of less than 1 micron. Whereas as in a nebulizer, gas passes rapidly through a tube which is immersed in a solution containing medication thus creating a mist of droplets of 1–40 microns. Since these tiny droplets will reach alveoli, it is essential that only *sterile* water is used. Refer to Table 14.2 for maintenance of these devices.

Humidification with heat and moisture exchangers: heat and moisture exchangers (HME) recycle exhaled heat and moisture from the patients and eliminate the need for a humidifier by reducing the development of condensate within ventilator circuits. These devices consist of a filter or small sponge in a plastic casing that is inserted into the ventilator circuit between the swivel adapter and Y-junction. However, the use of HME filters has not been shown to consistently reduce the occurrence of VAP compared with water humidification methods. The use of HME filters should be considered as a cost-effective method of providing a short-term (24-hour) period of humidification to patients receiving ventilation.

It is important to note that HME filters add dead space to the circuit, may increase circuit resistance, and may not provide sufficient humidity for critically ill patients as some of the patients often require higher humidity than these filters can provide. These filters should *not* be used in patients with haemoptysis, copious or tenacious secretions, and patients at risk of airway obstruction or difficulty discontinuing mechanical ventilation because of increased airway resistance. Before its use, each type of patient must be carefully evaluated by ICU physicians.

Key references and further reading

APIC. *Guide to the Elimination of Ventilator-associated Pneumonia.* 2009. Washington, DC: APIC, 2008.

American Thoracic Society & Infectious Diseases Society of America. Guidelines for the management of adults with hospital-acquired, ventilator-associated, and healthcare-associated pneumonia. *American Journal of Respiratory and Critical Care Medicine* 2005; **171**:388–416.

Department of Health. *High Impact Intervention No 5. Care bundle for ventilated patients (or tracheostomy where appropriate).* London: Department of Health, 2007. Available at: http://hcai.dh.gov.uk/.

HELICS. *Surveillance of nosocomial infections in Intensive Care units.* Hospital in Europe for Link Infection Control through Surveillance: September, 2004. Available at: http://www.ecdc. europa.eu.

Horan TC, Andrus M, Dudeck MA, *et al.* CDC/NHSN surveillance definition of health care-associated infection and criteria for specific types of infections in the acute care setting. *American Journal of Infection Control* 2008; **36**:309–32.

Institute of Health Improvement. *Infection Prevention Bundle: Prevent Ventilator-Associated Pneumonia*, 2007. Available at: http://www.ihi.org/ihi.

Masterton RG, Galloway A, French G, *et al.* Guidelines for the management of hospital-acquired pneumonia in the UK: Report of the Working Party on Hospital-Acquired Pneumonia of the British Society for Antimicrobial Chemotherapy. *Journal of Antimicrobial Chemotherapy* 2008; **62**:5–34.

SHEA/IDSA. Practice recommendation: Strategies to prevent ventilator-associated pneumonia in acute care hospitals. *Infection Control and Hospital Epidemiology* 2008; **29**(Supp.1):S31–S40.

Chapter 15

Surgical site infections

Every operation in surgery is an experiment in
bacteriology and the success of the experiment,
in respect of the patient, depended not only on
the skill, but also on the care exercised by the
surgeon in the ritual of the operation.

Sir Berkely Moynihan

Sir James Simpson, who was Professor of Obstetrics in Edinburgh in 1861, wrote:
'The man laid on the operating table of one of our surgical hospitals is exposed to
more chances of death than the English soldier on the fields of Waterloo'. Since then,
great advances have been made to make surgical procedures safer, but despite all the
advances in operative techniques and a better understanding of the pathogenesis,
surgical site infections (SSIs) continue to be a major source of morbidity and mortality
worldwide. It has been estimated that each patient with SSI stays approximately
7–10 additional days in the hospital and has 2–11 times higher risk of death, compared
with operative patients without a SSI.

Microbiology

Over the last decades there has been little change in the incidence and distribution of
microorganisms isolated from SSIs with the exception that these pathogens show
increasing resistance to antibiotics. The microorganisms isolated from SSIs differ
primarily depending on the type of surgical procedure, e.g. in clean surgical procedures,
Staphylococcus aureus from the exogenous environment (or the patient's skin flora) is the
usual cause of infection while surgical procedures in clean-contaminated, contaminated, and dirty procedures are usually polymicrobial and consist both of aerobic and
anaerobic Gram-negative and Gram-positive endogenous flora.

Risk factors

In 1964, Altemeir and Culbertson were among the first investigators to conceptualize
the pathogenic relationship and the key factors involved in SSIs. In their model, they
indicated that the risk of SSI is directly proportional to the microbial contamination of

the operative wound and to virulence of the microorganism and inversely proportional to the integrity and resistance of the host defences:

$$\text{Risk of SSI} = \frac{\text{Dose of bacterial contamination} \times \text{Virulence of microorganism}}{\text{Resistance of patient defence}}$$

It has been shown the risk of SSI is markedly increased if a surgical site is contaminated with greater than 10^5 microorganisms per gram of tissue. However, in the presence of a foreign body the dose of contaminating microorganisms required may be much lower, i.e. only 100 staphylococci are required per gram of tissue to produce infection if silk suture is present in the wound.

Besides patient- and procedure-related factors (see Table 15.1), some of the most critical factors in the prevention of SSIs, although difficult to quantify, are the sound judgement and proper technique of the surgeon and surgical team.

In 1992, the CDC attempted to redefine SSIs and this system has provided a greater discrimination for the patients at risk of developing wound infection which includes:

1. *Type of operating procedure:* an operation classified as either clean, contaminated or dirty/infected (see Table 15.2). Operative procedure classified as either contaminated or dirty by the traditional wound classification system = Score 1.

2. *Host susceptibility:* the aim of ASA (American Society of Anesthesiologists) score is to measure the intrinsic host susceptibility which is readily available at the time of surgery (see Table 15.3). ASA preoperative assessment score of 3, 4, or 5 = Score 1.

3. *Duration of surgery:* duration of surgery is a marker of the complexity of the operative procedure as well as the skill of the operating team. Infection risk increases with the increased duration of surgery above the 75th percentile for that proce-

Table 15.1 Risk factors associated with surgical site infections

Host-related	Procedure-related
Age	Type of procedure
Obesity	Preoperative hair removal
Disease severity	Duration of surgery
ASA (American Society of Anesthesiologists) severity score	Antibiotic prophylaxis
Nasal carriage of *Staph. aureus*	Tissue trauma
Remote infection	Foreign material
Duration of preoperative hospitalization	Blood transfusion
Malnutrition and low serum albumin	Emergency surgery
Diabetes mellitus	Drains
Malignancy	
Immunosuppressive therapy	

Table 15.2 Wound classification based on estimation of bacterial density, contamination and risk of subsequent infections

Class	Surgical procedure	Definition	Expected infection rate (%)
I	Clean	Non-traumatic, uninfected operative wounds in which no inflammation is encountered; there is no break in technique; and the respiratory, alimentary, or genitourinary tracts or the oropharyngeal cavities are not entered. In addition, clean wounds are primarily closed and, if necessary, drained with closed drainage. Operative incisional wounds that follow non-penetrating (blunt) trauma should be included in this category if they meet the criteria	1–3
II	Clean-contaminated	Operation in which the respiratory, alimentary, or genitourinary tracts are entered under controlled conditions and without unusual contamination Specifically, operations involving the biliary tract, appendix, vagina, and oropharynx are included in this category, provided no evidence of infection or major break in technique is encountered	8–10
III	Contaminated	Operation associated with: ♦ Open, fresh trauma wounds ♦ Major breaks in a sterile technique or gross spillage from the gastrointestinal tract ♦ Acute, non-purulent inflammation.	15–20
IV	Dirty and infected	Operation involving old trauma wounds with retained devitalized tissue, foreign bodies, or faecal contamination, and those with existing infection. This definition suggests that the organisms causing postoperative infection were present in the operative field before the operation	25–40

Adapted with permission from Mangram AJ, Horan TC, Pearson ML, *et al*. Guideline for prevention of surgical site infection, 1999. *Infection Control Hospital Epidemiology* 1999; **4**:250–80.

dure because bacterial contamination increases over time and the operative tissues are damaged by drying and other surgical manipulations (use of retractor, diathermy, etc.). Operative procedure lasting longer than time T = Score 1.

To calculate the total score, sum the scores for the factors present; the total score ranges from 0 to 3.

It is important to note that although the NNIS (National Nosocomial Infections Surveillance) risk index is a useful tool it may not predict SSI accurately because procedures and patient-related factors are too diverse. In addition, the tool has rarely been validated in populations outside the NNIS participating hospital nor has it been compared with other risk factors outlined in Table 15.1.

Table 15.3 Physical status classification score according to the American Society of Anesthesiologists (ASA)

ASA Score	Patient's preoperative physical status
1	Normally healthy patient
2	Patient with mild systemic disease
3	Patient with severe systemic disease that is not incapacitation
4	Patient with an incapacitating systemic disease that is a constant threat to life
5	Moribund patient who is not expected to survive for 24 h with or without operation

Definitions

SSIs are considered to be hospital acquired if the infection occurs within 30 days of the operative procedure or within 1 year if a device/foreign material is implanted. Theatre-acquired infections are usually deep-seated and often occur within 3 days of the operation or before the first dressing. However, some infections, particularly after prosthetic/implant surgery may not be recognized for weeks or months.

Surveillance

Surveillance of SSIs is a useful tool to demonstrate the magnitude of the problem. For surveillance of SSIs, it is important that internationally agreed definitions should be followed and this must be agreed with the surgical team. The definitions developed by the NHSN/CDC (with and without modifications) are the most widely used (see Box 15.1 and Figure 15.1). Before feedback to the surgical team, it is essential the data *must be validated* and *risk adjusted*.

Limitations for SSI surveillance

In recent years, the surveillance of SSIs has been complicated by changes in surgical practice (e.g. increased use of laparoscopic procedures), procedures carried out in day surgical units, and the short duration of postoperative stay. As a result of these changes most SSIs occur when the patient is discharged into the community. It has been estimated that up to 70% of SSIs are missed if the data collection relies *only* on the hospital surveillance. To address this issue, some hospitals have developed their own postdischarge surveillance. However, this method of data collection has been shown to have poor sensitivity and specificity due to lack of standardization.

Another major pitfall of surveillance is that most personnel who are responsible for detection, diagnosing, and data collection of SSIs are not adequately trained. In equivocal cases the surgeon's judgement ultimately determines whether an SSI is present or not and this can result in bias both of under- and over-reporting of infections as in doubtful cases the infection can be in the eye of the beholder!

Box 15.1 CDC criteria for defining surgical site infections

Superficial incisional SSI

Infection occurs within 30 days after the operative procedure, and involves only skin or subcutaneous tissue of the incision, and patient has at least one of the following:

- Purulent drainage from the superficial incision.
- Organisms isolated from an aseptically obtained culture of fluid or tissue from the superficial incision.
- At least one of the following signs or symptoms of infection: pain or tenderness; localized swelling, redness, or heat; and superficial incision is deliberately opened by surgeon and is culture-positive or not cultured. A culture-negative finding does not meet this criterion.
- Diagnosis of superficial incisional SSI by the surgeon or attending physician.

Deep incisional SSI

Infection occurs within 30 days after the operation if no implant is left in place or within 1 year if implant is in place and the infection appears to be related to the operative procedure *and* involves deep soft tissues (e.g. fascial and muscle layers) of the incision *and* patient has at least one of the following:

- Purulent drainage from the deep incision but not from the organ/space component of the surgical site.
- A deep incision spontaneously dehisces or is deliberately opened by a surgeon and is culture-positive or not cultured when the patient has at least one of the following signs or symptoms: fever (>38°C), localized pain, or tenderness. A culture-negative finding does not meet this criterion.
- An abscess or other evidence of infection involving the deep incision is found on direct examination, during reoperation, or by histopathological or radiological examination.
- Diagnosis of a deep incisional SSI by a surgeon or attending physician.

Organ/space SSI

Infection occurs within 30 days after the operation if no implant is left in place or within 1 year if implant is in place and the infection appears to be related to the operative procedure *and* infection involves any part of the body (excluding the skin incision, fascia, or muscle layers) that is opened or manipulated during the operative procedure *and* patient has at least one of the following:

- Purulent drainage from a drain that is placed through a stab wound into the organ/space.
- Organisms isolated from an aseptically obtained culture of fluid or tissue in the organ/space.

Box 15.1 CDC criteria for defining surgical site infections (*continued*)

- ◆ An abscess or other evidence of infection involving the organ/space that is found on direct examination, during reoperation, or by histopathological or radiological examination.
- ◆ Diagnosis of an organ/space SSI by a surgeon or attending physician.

With permission from Horan TC, Andrus M, Dudeck MA. CDC/NHSN surveillance definition of health care-associated infection and criteria for specific types of infections in the acute care setting. *American Journal of Infection Control* 2008; **36**:309–32.

Surgical asepsis and the operating theatre

The principle of surgical asepsis is to prevent SSIs and must be used for *all* operating room procedures. This is achieved by:

- ◆ Use of sterile instruments, sutures, dressing, and other materials.
- ◆ Wearing of sterile gowns and gloves by the operating team.
- ◆ Disinfection of surgical site and hands of the operating team using antiseptics.
- ◆ Performing surgery in an adequately ventilated operating theatre (see 'Operating theatres', Chapter 19) to reduce the microbial bioload of the microorganisms generated by the theatre personnel.

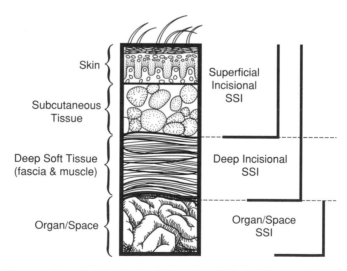

Fig. 15.1 Cross-section of abdominal wall depicting CDC classification of surgical site infection. With permission from Horan TC, Gaynes RP, Martone WJ, *et al*. CDC definitions of nosocomial surgical site infections, 1992: a modification of CDC definitions of surgical wound infections. *Infection Control Hospital Epidemiology* 1992; **13**:606–8.

It is essential that all members of the operating team who are 'sterile' must only touch sterile articles; persons who are 'unsterile' must only touch unsterile articles. All sterile packs must be opened using a non-touch technique that will prevent contamination of sterile instruments.

Responsibility of health care workers

The surgeon in charge of the patient, the anaesthetist, and the scrub nurse should be responsible for ensuring that all members of the operating team know the operating room procedures and infection control precautions that are to be taken, including any additional precautions that may be required.

Routine screening of theatre personnel is *not* necessary, unless an outbreak clearly links personnel to infected cases. Staff with dermatitis or skin wounds should be excluded from the operating team and carriers/dispersers of *Staph. aureus* (including MRSA), *Streptococcus pyogenes* (β haemolytic group A streptococci) or with septic lesions should not work in the theatre until the condition resolves. All HCWs who perform exposure-prone procedures should be immunized against hepatitis B and be tested for immunity by the Occupational Health Department (OHD). Those who are, or have reason to believe that they may have been exposed to HIV, hepatitis B or C virus in whatever circumstances, must seek medical advice from the OHD regarding their suitability to perform exposure-prone invasive procedures (See Chapter 16, p. 314).

Operating room attire

Theatre gowns: the operating team should wear impermeable, cuffed-wrist, sterile gowns. Gowns contaminated with blood or body substances should be removed as soon as possible and bagged for laundering, or discarded as clinical waste if disposable. Alternatively, plastic aprons should be worn under gowns and should be of sufficient length to overlap with footwear. Operating suite/operating room clothing should *not* be worn outside the operating room environment.

Surgical face masks: all members of the *scrub team should wear a fluid-repellent mask* to protect the HCW from blood splatter and aerosolized blood and/or body fluids which may be generated during surgical procedures. A new mask must be worn for each operation. Masks should be tied securely to fit comfortably and cover the nose and mouth. When removing the mask it should be handled by the strings only and discarded after use. Staff not assisting at surgery do not need to wear a facemask.

Gloves: remember that wearing of sterile gloves *does not* render surgical hand preparation unnecessary. Wearing of sterile gloves during surgery serves two purposes: it prevents transfer of microorganisms from HCWs to patients during surgery and also provides protection against the risk of transmission of blood-borne pathogens from patients to the surgical team. Only single-use sterile gloves should be used. They must not be washed or disinfected and reused.

Glove puncture is common during surgical procedure and puncture range varies from 5–82% and more than 80% of cases go unnoticed by the surgeon. It has been estimated that puncture rate depends on the duration and type of surgical procedures, e.g. after 2 hours of surgery, 35% of all gloves demonstrate puncture. If the gloves are punctured, it allows transfer of microorganisms from surgeons' hands and a recent trial demonstrated that punctured gloves double the risk of SSIs (Misteli et al., 2009.) Double gloving significantly reduces the risk of puncture during surgery but does not completely eliminate the risk of puncture.

Eye protection: masks and protective eyewear or face shields should be worn during procedures which are likely to generate droplets/aerosols of blood and/or body fluids to prevent exposure of the mucous membranes of the mouth, nose, and eyes.

Hair/beard cover: hair and scalp constitute special problems in terms of generating and liberating microorganisms. The hair acts as an 'air filter' and collects bacteria from the hospital surrounding and is released from the hair and scalp in the dry state. Therefore it is essential that all members of staff entering the theatre must wear their hair in a neat style. Long hair should be tied in such a way that when the head is bent forward, hair does not fall forward. Hair must be completely covered by a close-fitting cap made of synthetic material. Beards should be fully covered by a mask and a hood of the balaclava type, which is tied securely at the neck.

Footwear: footwear should be enclosed and capable of protecting HCWs from accidentally dropped sharps and other contaminated items. Open footwear must never be worn in the operating room. If there is a risk of spillage of blood or other high-risk body fluids, surgical waterproof boots should be worn. Plastic shoe covers should *not* be used for the purpose of protecting footwear.

Safe handling and disposal of sharps

All HCWs working in the operating room must be responsible for the safe handling and disposal of sharp instruments that they have used. Following procedures is recommended to minimize sharps injuries:

♦ Sharp instruments *should not be passed by hand*. A specified puncture-resistant sharps tray must be used for the transfer of all sharp instruments.

♦ Only one sharp must be in the tray at one time. If two surgeons are operating simultaneously, each surgeon needs his/her own sharps tray.

♦ Before any surgical or operative procedure, the surgeon and scrub nurse should decide on the routine for passage of sharp instruments during the procedure. This may entail the designation of a 'neutral zone'.

♦ Hand-held straight needles should *not* be used if an alternative is possible.

♦ Needles *must never* be picked up with the fingers, nor the fingers used to expose and increase access for the passage of a suture in deep tissues. When suturing, forceps or a needle holder should be used to pick up the needle and draw it through the tissue.

♦ Where practical, suture needles should be cut off before knots are tied; the sharp point of the needle should be grasped in the jaws of the needle holder before being cut off.

♦ Sharps *must be disposed of safely* according to the local policy.

♦ All sharps injuries must be managed as according to the local sharps injury/inoculation post-exposure management policy.

Environmental issues

Environmental cleaning: the operating room *must be cleaned between cases.* All surfaces (operating table, instrument table, equipment used, etc.) should be cleaned using warm water and detergent preparation; disinfectant can be used if indicated. The floor must be mopped with a detergent preparation at the end of each session and scrubbed daily at the end of the list. The floor of the operating theatre should be cleaned at the end of each session and scrubbed daily. Routine use of disinfectant is not required apart from their use in removal and disinfection of blood and other high-risk body fluids. Spillages on the floor should be disinfected and removed as soon as possible. Walls and ceilings are rarely heavily contaminated and for general housekeeping purposes they should be cleaned twice a year. Lint-free cloth is recommended for operating theatre cleaning. *Routine microbiological sampling* of the operating room or environment is *not* recommended as inanimate objects and surfaces are seldom the cause of surgical wound infection (see p. 357 on guidance on microbiological sampling). Settle plates used to evaluate air-borne contaminants are *not* useful.

Clinical waste: clinical waste (excluding sharps) should be placed into an appropriate leak-resistant bag, sealed, and removed from the operating room. Other waste should be disposed of in accordance with the hospital waste disposal policy. Linen should be handled in accordance with the hospital policy.

Tacky mats and plastic shoe covers: using tacky mats at the entrance of an operating theatre does little to minimize the overall degree of contamination of floors and should *not* be used. Use of plastic or fabric shoe covers can be replaced by ordinary shoes dedicated exclusively to the operating theatre as no difference exists in floor contamination whether personnel wear shoe covers or not and this practice has *no impact* on the rate of SSIs.

Surgical scrub

The objective of using surgical scrub is to ensure the removal/killing of both transient flora and a substantial reduction and suppression of the resident skin flora (see p. 135); this is achieved by using an antimicrobial preparation. Depending on the antiseptic preparation, a 3-minute scrub could be as effective as a 5-minute scrub. A European guideline recommends that the total application for surgical scrub time must not be shorter than 2 minutes and a minimum of *two applications* are necessary (Labadie et al., 2002). From evidence, it appears that the first surgical scrub of the day should be for 3–5 minutes with subsequent washes for 3 minutes between consecutive operations; alternatively, application of alcohol hand rub products to clean hands for 3 minutes can be used (WHO, 2009). See Fig. 15.2.

Preparation prior to scrub procedure

- Keep nails short and pay attention to them when washing your hands as most microorganisms on hands come from beneath the fingernails.
- Do not wear artificial nails or nail polish and all jewellery (rings, watches, bracelets) must be removed before entering the operating theatre.
- The hands and forearms should be free of open lesions and breaks in the skin.

Box 15.2 Scrubbing procedures using an antiseptic agent

- ◆ Start timer. Adjust water to a warm temperature and thoroughly wet hands and forearms above the elbows in order to remove dirt and transient flora.
- ◆ Clean under each fingernail and around the nail bed with a nail cleaner prior to performing the first surgical scrub of the day.
- ◆ Holding hands up above the level of the elbow, apply antiseptic agent to the hands and forearms up to the elbow.
- ◆ Use circular motion, begin at the fingertips of one hand and lather and wash between the fingers each side of each finger, between the fingers, and the back and front of the hand for 2 minutes.
- ◆ Proceed to scrub the arms, keeping the hand higher than the arm at all times. This helps to avoid recontamination of the hands by water from the elbows and prevents water from contaminating the hands.
- ◆ Wash each side of the arm from wrist to the elbow for 1 minute. Repeat the process on the other hand and arm, keeping hands above elbows at all times.
- ◆ If the hand touches anything at any time, the scrub must be lengthened by 1 minute for the area that has been contaminated. Rinse hands and arms by passing them through the water in one direction only, from fingertips to elbow.
- ◆ Do not move the arm back and forth through the water. Proceed to the operating theatre holding hands above elbows. At all times during the scrub procedure, care should be taken not to splash water onto surgical attire.
- ◆ Hands and arms should be dried using sterile towels starting with the fingertips and keeping the hands above the elbow. Use a *separate towel* for each hand.
- ◆ Keep hands above the level of the waist and do not touch any non-sterile object.
- ◆ Put on sterile gown (see 'Donning sterile gown following scrub procedure') and surgical gloves using aseptic technique (see Figure 15.3).

- ◆ Hands and arms should be washed with a non-medicated soap before entering the operating theatre area or if hands are visibly soiled.

Use of nailbrushes: any agent or method of skin decontamination that causes skin abrasions (e.g. use of a brush on skin) *must be avoided*. The first wash of the day should include a thorough clean under the fingernails and subungual areas with a nail file. Nailbrushes should *not* be used as they may damage the skin and encourage shedding of squamous epithelial cells from the skin. If their use is considered essential, then the nailbrushes *must be single use sterile*; if reusable nailbrushes are used (autoclavable nailbrushes are available) then they *must* be sent to the SSD for sterilization.

Water quality and wash-hand sink: use of warm (*not hot*) water is recommended as it makes antiseptics and soap work more effectively. Very hot water must be avoided as it removes protective fatty acids from the skin resulting in skin damage. It is important to note that surgical scrub requires *clean water to rinse the hands* after application of hand antiseptic agents. *Pseudomonas* spp. are frequently isolated from taps/faucets in hospitals and taps are common sources of *P. aeruginosa* and other Gram-negative bacteria and have been linked to infections in multiple health care settings. To minimize this problem, it is important to remove tap aerators from sinks designated for surgical scrub; installation of automated sensor-operated taps will help minimize this risk. In countries lacking continuous supply of drinking water and improper tap mainte-nance, recontamination may be a real risk even after correct surgical hand scrub is performed. In addition, it is important to note that single surgical scrub many con-sume up to approximately 20 litres of warm water. In countries with limited resources, particularly when the availability, quantity, or quality of water is doubtful, the use of alcohol-based hand rub should be the preferred method.

Surgical hand antisepsis: rapid multiplication of skin bacteria occurs under surgical gloves if hands are washed using a non-antimicrobial agent. During surgery, the resident microflora slowly multiply under the gloves and if the gloves are punctured, the microbes can gain access to the wound, and in the presence of a foreign body or necrotic tissue, it can cause SSIs even when the microbial count is only 100 cfu. Therefore, the antimicrobial agent used for surgical hand preparation must eliminate the transient flora and significantly reduce the resident flora at the beginning of an operation and maintain the microbial release from the hands below baseline until the end of the procedure in case of an unnoticed puncture of the surgical glove releasing bacteria from the hands to the open wound.

The most active antiseptic agents (in order of decreasing activity) are chlorhexidine gluconate, iodophors, and triclosan. Triclosan-containing products are mainly bacterio-static and are inactive against *P. aeruginosa* and are no longer used. The most commonly used products for surgical hand antisepsis are chlorhexidine or povidone-iodine-con-taining detergents because they have lower levels of toxicity, faster mode of action, or broader spectrum of activity. Application of chlorhexidine or povidone-iodine results in similar initial reductions of bacterial counts (70–80%). Rapid re-growth occurs after application of povidone-iodine, but not after use of chlorhexidine due to its residual effects. Despite both *in vitro* and *in vivo* studies demonstrating that povidone-iodine is *less efficacious*, induces more allergic reactions, and does not show similar residual effects than chlorhexidine, povidone-iodine remains one of the widely-used products for surgical hand antisepsis.

Alcohol-based hand rubs: several alcohol-based hand rubs have been licensed for use as preoperative surgical hand preparations. The antimicrobial efficacy of alcohol based formulations is superior to all other currently available products. Numerous studies have demonstrated that formulations containing 60–95% alcohol alone, or 50–95% when combined with small amounts of a QAC, hexachlorophene or chlo-rhexidine gluconate, reduce bacterial counts on the skin immediately post-scrub more effectively than other agents. In addition, skin irritation and dermatitis are more fre-quently observed after surgical hand scrub using chlorhexidine than an alcohol-based hand rinse. In countries with limited resources, particularly when the availability, quantity, or quality of water is doubtful, the use of alcohol-based hand rub should be the preferred method.

It is essential that before applying alcohol hand rub, the hands of the surgical team should be cleaned upon entering the operating theatre by washing the hands with a non-medicated soap to eliminate any risk of colonization of bacterial spores. Before applying alcohol hand rub, it is essential that hands *must be completely dry*. When applying alcohol hand rub, it is essential that the hands *should be wet* from the alcohol-based rub during the *whole procedure*, which requires approximately 15 mL (depending on the size of the hands) and requires a total of 3 minutes. Use of alcohol hand rub for surgical hand disinfection has several advantages which include rapid action, time saving, less side effects, and no risk of recontamination by rinsing hands with water.

> The handrubbing technique for surgical hand preparation must be performed on perfectly clean, dry hands.
> On arrival in the operating theatre and after having donned theatre clothing (cap/hat/bonnet and mask), hands must be washed with soap and water.
> After the operation when removing gloves, hands must be rubbed with an alcohol-based formulation or washed with soap and water if any residual talc or biological fluids are present (e.g. the glove is punctured).

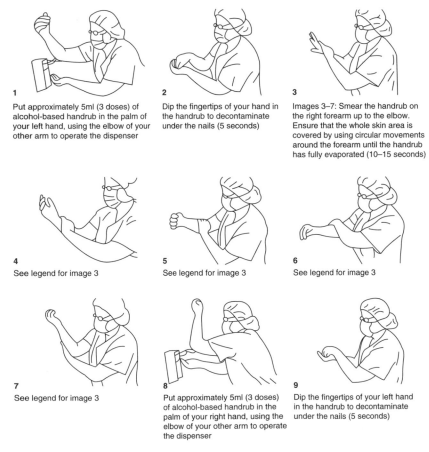

1
Put approximately 5ml (3 doses) of alcohol-based handrub in the palm of your left hand, using the elbow of your other arm to operate the dispenser

2
Dip the fingertips of your hand in the handrub to decontaminate under the nails (5 seconds)

3
Images 3–7: Smear the handrub on the right forearm up to the elbow. Ensure that the whole skin area is covered by using circular movements around the forearm until the handrub has fully evaporated (10–15 seconds)

4
See legend for image 3

5
See legend for image 3

6
See legend for image 3

7
See legend for image 3

8
Put approximately 5ml (3 doses) of alcohol-based handrub in the palm of your right hand, using the elbow of your other arm to operate the dispenser

9
Dip the fingertips of your left hand in the handrub to decontaminate under the nails (5 seconds)

Fig. 15.2 Surgical hand preparation technique with an alcohol-based hand rub formulation. With permission from WHO. *WHO Guidelines on Hand Hygiene in Health Care: First Global Patient Safety Challenge. Clean Care is Safer Care.* Geneva: World Health Organization, 2009.

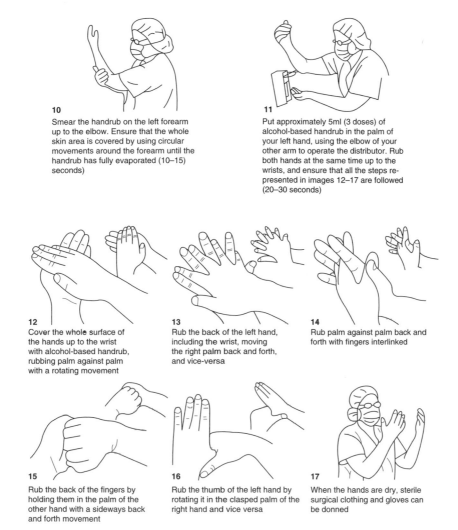

10
Smear the handrub on the left forearm up to the elbow. Ensure that the whole skin area is covered by using circular movements around the forearm until the handrub has fully evaporated (10–15) seconds)

11
Put approximately 5ml (3 doses) of alcohol-based handrub in the palm of your left hand, using the elbow of your other arm to operate the distributor. Rub both hands at the same time up to the wrists, and ensure that all the steps represented in images 12–17 are followed (20–30 seconds)

12
Cover the whole surface of the hands up to the wrist with alcohol-based handrub, rubbing palm against palm with a rotating movement

13
Rub the back of the left hand, including the wrist, moving the right palm back and forth, and vice-versa

14
Rub palm against palm back and forth with fingers interlinked

15
Rub the back of the fingers by holding them in the palm of the other hand with a sideways back and forth movement

16
Rub the thumb of the left hand by rotating it in the clasped palm of the right hand and vice versa

17
When the hands are dry, sterile surgical clothing and gloves can be donned

Fig. 15.2 (*continued*).

The manufacturer of the product must provide recommendations as to how long the product must be applied. Alcohol-based hand rub should *not be used* unless they pass the test EN 12791 or an equivalent standard and many currently available products for hygienic hand rub do not meet the European standard EN 1500.

Donning sterile gown following scrub procedure

◆ All packs contain folded gowns with inner side towards scrub nurse.

◆ Remove folded gown from pack, step back from bench.

◆ Holding gown at shoulder level with both hands, allow to unfold (inner side of gown will be towards you).

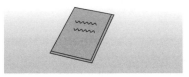

1. Prepare a large, clean, dry area for opening the package of gloves. Perform hand disinfection. Ask someone (e.g., circulating nurse) to open the package of gloves.

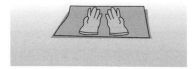

2. Open the inner glove wrapper, exposing the cuffed gloves with the palms up.

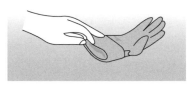

3. Pick up the first glove by the cuff, touching only the inside portion of the cuff (the inside is the side that will be touching your skin when the gloves is on).

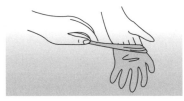

4. While holding the cuff in one hand, slip your other hand into the glove. (Pointing the fingers of the glove toward the floor will keep the fingers open). Be careful not to touch, anything, and hold the gloves above your waist level.

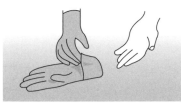

5. Pick up the second glove by sliding the fingers of the gloved hand under the cuff of the second glove. Be careful not to contaminate the gloved hand with the ungloved hand.

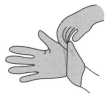

6. Put the second glove on the ungloved and by maintaining a steady pull through the cuff. Adjust the glove fingers and cuffs until the gloves fit comfortably.

Fig. 15.3 Method of donning sterile gloves.

◆ Place hands/arms into sleeves to upper area of knitted cuff; keep hands within cuff (for gloving procedure).

◆ Circulating nursing auxiliary will 'tie' gown at the back.

Measures to prevent surgical site infections

General measures

Infected patient: since the infective status of the patient is not always known, it is therefore essential that personnel working in the operating room (OR) must ensure that standard infection control precautions are implemented for every patient. The surgeon-in-charge of the patient, the anaesthetist and the nurse-in-charge of the OR should be responsible for ensuring that all members of the operating team know the infection control precautions. If the patient's colonization status is known (e.g. MRSA) or if the patient already has an infection, then additional precautions may include the use of experienced surgeons and operating teams to minimize the likelihood of accidents and complications, and the additional use of PPE. Surgery lists should be scheduled on the basis of clinical urgency and scheduling infected ('dirty') cases at the end of the day is recommended, if possible. Adequate time must be allowed to ensure that there is sufficient time for cleaning and safe disposal of clinical/pathological waste between cases. Once the OR is clean and all the surfaces are dry, the OR should be used for the next patient without delay.

Theatre staff: staff with bacterial skin infections or eczema may cause dispersal of *Staph. aureus* or *Strep. pyogenes*. Staffs with a boil or septic lesion of the skin are colonized with *Staph. aureus* and should not be allowed in the theatre until the lesion is treated and healed. Staff who are or have reason to believe that they may have been exposed to blood-borne hepatitis (B and C) or HIV infections *must declare* this and discuss it in complete confidence with the occupational health department or senior manager, either at the initial screening or when s/he first becomes aware of their infection. In general, such staff may require a work assessment and must avoid exposure-prone procedures (see p. 314).

Theatre discipline: the number of staff in the OR must be kept to the essential minimum as excessive presence and movement of staff contributes to an increased dispersal of airborne bacterial particles. Personnel who wish to view the operation can be accommodated in surgical viewing suites, where available.

The ventilation in the operating theatre is designed to optimize the quality of air and to reduce infection arising from bacteria shed by theatre staff. Therefore, unnecessary entry of personnel *must* be restricted to an absolute minimum to avoid contamination of wounds and sterile surgical instruments during surgery. In addition, the door to the OR should be *closed* at all times to maintain positive pressure and to avoid mixing of the corridor 'dirty' air with the OR 'clean' air. Theatre discipline *must* be strictly reinforced especially if the operating theatre does not meet the recommended designs and ventilation standards.

Theatre wear: outside clothing must be changed for clean, laundered OR attire/scrub suit which is worn in the operating suite. OR clothing should *not* be worn outside the operating theatre except in an emergency. In such circumstances, it must be changed for a clean scrub suit on return. OR gowns should be made of waterproof fabric with an ability to breathe, and should be comfortable to wear.

Specific measures

Current strategies to prevent SSIs are based on the implementation of a 'care bundle' (see 'Care bundle approach', Chapter 1) developed by the IHI and is summarized in Box 15.3 with further details on the prevention of SSIs recommended by NICE are available from NICE web site: http://www.nice.org.uk/.

Box 15.3 Surgical site infections care bundle

1 Appropriate use of antibiotics.

2 Appropriate hair removal.

3 Postoperative glucose control (major cardiac surgery patients).

4 Postoperative normothermia (colorectal surgery patients).

From the Institute of Health Improvement. *Bundle Prevent Surgical Site Infections*, 2007.

Preoperative patient care

Preoperative hospitalization: preoperative stay in hospital should be kept to a minimum. If this is necessary for medical reasons, keep the patient in a clean environment to protect them from colonization with bacteria from other infected/colonized patients.

Preoperatively, a detailed medical history should be taken to identify patients with infectious and other diseases (diabetes mellitus, heart disease, COPD, etc.) and where possible, these should be treated before elective surgery. Preoperative testing of a patient for infectious agents should be on the basis of clinical indication and medical practitioners should exercise their professional judgement in ordering any clinically relevant test, with the patient's consent. Preoperative screening for MRSA for certain types of high-risk procedures should follow local guidelines and be done before elective admission.

Patient's risk factors: patients with pre-existing skin lesions or infection in another site, and treatment with steroids and immunosuppressive drugs, are more prone to get SSIs due to impaired host defence mechanisms. These should be corrected or treated before an elective operation is planned. Cessation of tobacco use 30 days before surgery is also recommended as smoking not only increases the risk of postoperative chest infection but is also responsible for delayed healing of the surgical wound.

Preoperative shaving: hair should not be removed at the operative site unless the presence of hair will interfere with the operation. Preoperative shaving should be avoided because shaving can cause small nicks and breaks leaving the skin bruised and traumatized which increases the risk of colonization and infection. If hair is to be removed from the operative site, only the area needing to be incised should be shaved. This should preferably be done using depilatory cream the day before the operation. It is important to note that depilatory cream should be used with caution as it can cause serious skin irritation and rashes which may lead to wound infection. Alternately, hair can be removed with clippers in the anaesthetic room immediately before the operative procedure. If clippers are used, then the clipper head must be sterile. Razors and shaving brushes *must not* be used. Patients coming for elective surgery should be advised not to shave the area before admission.

Preoperative showers: preoperative showers or baths the night before an operative procedure using antimicrobial agents have been suggested as a means of reducing SSI in certain categories of patients, but the evidence is conflicting. However, such showers do reduce the skin carriage of potential pathogens even if this is not always translated in to reduced infection rates. Several studies observed lower infection rates when the patient showered preoperatively with antiseptic agents while other studies have failed to show a reduction in the wound infection rate. Although a Cochrane review (2007) has shown no clear evidence that this practice definitively decreases SSI risk, both NICE and CDC guidelines do recommend that patients should shower or bathe with an antiseptic agent prior to surgery. However, if this is done and it is important that, to gain the maximum antiseptic effect of chlorhexidine, it must be allowed to dry completely and not be washed off.

Antibiotic prophylaxis: the use of antibiotic prophylaxis before surgery has evolved greatly in the last 20 years. Improvements in the timing of initial administration, the appropriate choice of antibiotic agents, and shorter duration of administration have defined more clearly the value of this technique in reducing postoperative SSIs. For various reasons, misuse of prophylactic antibiotics is quite common and the surgeons must be reminded that prolonged courses of prophylactic antibiotics will not compensate for best practice in patient preparation, surgical technique, or postoperative care.

It is generally recommended that in most cases, a single dose should be administered IV between 30–60 minutes (2 hours for vancomycin and ciprofloxacin) before incision or earlier for operations in which a tourniquet is used (see Table 15.4). Repeat doses of IV cefuroxime or cefazolin should be given in the case of massive haemorrhage ($\geq$2 litres of blood is lost in an adult) or when the duration of the operation exceeds 3 hours. For Caesarean sections, IV antibiotics should be given immediately after the cord is clamped. The time of administration and doses must be recorded in the patient's anaesthetic notes. Use of third-generation cephalosporins for surgical prophylaxis is not recommended because they are costly and promote emergence of bacteria resistance.

Intraoperative patient care

Surgical technique: the skill of the surgeon has a central role in minimizing SSIs which includes expeditious surgery and the gentle handling of tissue. In addition, reduction of blood loss or haematoma formation, debridement and elimination of devitalized tissue with removal of all purulent material by irrigation/suction, and removal of all foreign materials from the wound are essential to minimize SSI in all patients.

Skin disinfection: since a break in the skin's barrier allows the ingress of microorganisms into the deeper layers, it is essential that the operating site is well cleaned and disinfected with an antiseptic before incision. The antiseptic skin preparation should be applied *with friction* in concentric circles moving away from the proposed incision site to the periphery and well beyond the operation site to accommodate an extension to the incision or new incisions or drain site to be made.

Various antiseptics are used to disinfect skin e.g. chlorhexidine (0.5–2%) or (7.5–10% povidone iodine) with or without alcohol (70% ethanol or isopropyl alcohol). In evaluation of antiseptic agents, three major criteria are important: immediacy,

Table 15.4 Antibiotic prophylaxis for surgical procedures

Surgical procedures	Antibiotics
Cardiac surgery	Cefuroxime 1.5 g 8 hourly (max. 48 h for cardiac procedures)
Neurosurgery	Cefuroxime 1.5 g (single dose)
Head and neck	Cefuroxime 1.5 g and metronidazole 500 mg 8 h (single dose) if operation involving the mucous, and up to three doses if membranes and deep tissue are involved
Biliary tract surgery	Cefuroxime 1.5 g (single dose)
Endoscopic retrograde cholangiopancreatography (ERCP)	Cefuroxime 1.5 g (single dose)
Gastroduodenal	Cefuroxime 1.5 g (single dose)
Appendectomy (simple)	Cefuroxime 1.5 g or gentamicin 2–3 mg/kg body weight and metronidazole 500 mg (single dose)
Colorectal surgery	Cefuroxime 1.5 g or gentamicin 2–3 mg/kg body weight and metronidazole 500 mg (single dose)
Orthopaedic surgery (Insertion of prosthetic joints, open operation)	Cefuroxime 1.5 g (single dose). Substitute clindamycin 900 mg if history of penicillin or cephalosporin allergy
Lower limb amputation	Benzylpenicillin 2 mega units IV 6-hourly; metronidazole or clindamycin for patient allergic to penicillin
	All antibiotics should be given for 24 h duration
Peripheral vascular surgery	Cefuroxime 1.5 g 8 hourly (three doses)
Urological surgery	IV antibiotic cover depends on sensitivity testing of screening urine. In an emergency situation, give gentamicin 2–3 mg/kg body weight (single dose)
Hysterectomy	Cefuroxime 1.5 g and metronidazole 500 mg or co-amoxiclav 1.2 g alone (single dose)
Caesarean section	Cefuroxime 1.5 g or co-amoxiclav 1.2 g IV after umbilical cord is clamped (single dose)
	Helpful hints

◆ All antibiotics should be administered IV between 30–60 min before incision (usually give at the time of induction of anesthesia); 2 h are allowed for the administration of IV vancomycin and IV fluoroquinolones Vancomycin should not routinely be used for antimicrobial prophylaxis and should be reserved for prophylaxis on patients with MRSA

◆ Repeat dose of antibiotics should be given for the operations when the duration of operation exceeds 3 h or in the case of massive haemorrhage (>2 L of blood is lost in an adult). Do not give prophylactic antibiotics for more than 24 h; discontinue within 48 h for cardiac procedures

◆ Prophylactic antibiotic dosage for adults: cefuroxime 1.5 g IV (750 mg if body weight, 50 kg); clindamycin 900 mg IV; metronidazole 500 mg IV and co-amoxiclav 1.2 g IV

persistence, and cumulative action. Data on prevention of IV bloodstream infections has repeatedly shown 2% chlorhexidine gluconate with 70% isopropyl alcohol to be more effective than povidone-iodine or alcohol and recent study has shown that use of chlorhexidine-alcohol is superior to povidone-iodine as preoperative antiseptics for prevention of SSI (Darouiche et al., 2010).

However, it should be noted that alcohol preparations may ignite if used in the presence of diathermy and must therefore never be allowed to dry by evaporation. Check the drapes to ensure that they are not saturated with alcohol or that the alcohol has not formed a pool underneath the patient before operating.

Draping: to restrict the transfer of microorganisms to the wound and to protect the sterility of instruments, equipment and the gloved hands of personnel, a sterile field must be established by placing sterile drapes around the wound. The use of plastic incisional adhesive drapes is not associated with a reduction in infection rate.

Wound drains: it is generally accepted that wound drains provide access for bacterial entry via colonization of the wound. A closed system of wound drainage is therefore required to minimize this risk; open wound drains are not considered appropriate.

Perioperative normothermia: maintenance of perioperative normothermia (temperature >36.0°C) for patients undergoing colorectal surgery has been recommended to reduce SSIs but this issue remains unresolved as more reliable data are needed.

Postoperative patient care

Postoperative stay: postoperative stay should be minimized and patient discharge is advised as soon as possible. If the patient needs to remain in hospital for medical reasons, the patient should be cared for in a clean environment to protect them from colonization with bacteria from infected/colonized patients.

Control blood glucose: for patients undergoing cardiac surgery, it is important that blood glucose level should be controlled during the immediate postoperative period and should be maintained at less than 200 mg/dL. It is recommended that blood glucose level should be measured at 6:00 am on postoperative day 1 and postoperative day 2, with the procedure day being postoperative day 0. Initiating close blood glucose control in the intraoperative period has *not* been shown to reduce the risk of SSI; in fact, trials have shown that initiating close glucose control during cardiac surgery may actually lead to higher rates of adverse outcomes, including stroke and death.

Wound dressing: staff should be trained in the appropriate method of dressing the wound. Frequency of dressing should be kept to a minimum and dressings should not be opened for 48 hours after the operation unless infection is suspected. The longer a wound is open, and the longer it is drained, the greater the risk of contamination. Postoperative infections acquired in theatre are usually deep-seated and often occur within 3 days of the operation or before the first dressing.

Key references and further reading

Altemeier WA, Culbertson WR. Surgical infection. In: Moyer CA, Rhoads JE, Allen JG, *et al.* (eds) *Surgery, Principles and Practice,* 3rd edn, pp. 51–77. Philadelphia, PA: JB Lippincott, 1965.

APIC. *Guide for the prevention of Mediastinitis Surgical Site Infections following Cardiac Surgery*. Washington, DC: APIC, 2008.

CDC. Guideline for prevention of surgical site infection, 1999. *Infection Control Hospital Epidemiology* 1999; **20**:247–80.

Classen DC, Evans RS, Pestotnik SL, *et al*. The timing of prophylactic administration of antibiotics and the risk of surgical-wound infection. *New England Journal of Medicine* 1992; **326**:281–6.

Darouiche RO, Wall MJ Jr, Itani KM, *et al*. Chlorhexidine-alcohol versus povidone-iodine for surgical-site antisepsis. *New England Journal of Medicine* 2010; **362**(1):18–26.

Gaynes RP, Culver DH, Horan TC, *et al*. Surgical site infection (SSI) rates in the United States, 1992–1998: the NNIS basic risk index. *Clinical Infectious Diseases* 2001; **33**(Suppl 2): S69–S77.

Institute of Health Improvement. *Bundle Prevent Surgical Site Infections*, 2007. Available at: http://www.ihi.org/ihi.

Horan TC, Andrus M, Dudeck MA. CDC/NHSN surveillance definition of health care-associated infection and criteria for specific types of infections in the acute care setting. *American Journal of Infection Control* 2008; **36**:309–32.

Hospital Infection Society. Behaviours and rituals in the operating theatre. *Journal of Hospital Infection* 2002; **51**:241–55.

Mangram AJ, Horan TC, Pearson ML, *et al*. Guideline for prevention of surgical site infection, 1999. *Infection Control Hospital Epidemiology* 1999; **4**:250–80.

Labadie JC, Kampf G, Lejeune B, *et al*. European Guidelines. Recommendations for surgical hand disinfection–requirements, implementation and need for research. A proposal by representatives of the SFHH, DGHM and DGKH for a European discussion. *Journal of Hospital Infection* 2002; **51**:312–15.

Misteli H, Weber WP, Reck S, *et al*. Surgical glove perforation and the risk of surgical site infection. *Archives of Surgery*, 2009; **144**:553–8.

NICE guidelines: *Surgical site infection prevention and treatment of surgical site infection*. London: the Royal College of Obstetricians and Gynaecologists Press, 2008.

SHEA/IDSA practice recommendation: Strategies to prevent surgical site infections in acute care hospitals. *Infection Control Hospital Epidemiology* 2008; **29**(Suppl 1):S51–S6.

Webster J, Osborne S. Preoperative bathing or showering with skin antiseptics to prevent surgical site infection. *Cochrane Database Systematic Review* 2007; **2**:CD004985.

WHO. *WHO Guidelines on Hand Hygiene in Health Care: First Global Patient Safety Challenge. Clean Care is Safer Care*. Geneva: World Health Organization, 2009.

Chapter 16

Staff health

Men at some time are masters of their fates:
The fault, dear Brutus, is not in our stars.
But in ourselves, that we are underlings.

Julius Caesar, Act I, Scene 2, Shakespeare

Protection of HCWs should be an integral part of the health and safety programme of all health care facilities. Health care facilities have a legal obligation to ensure that all their employees are appropriately trained and proficient in the procedures necessary for working safely. In addition, it is the responsibility of every employee to be aware of their own role in IPC and incorporate good practices into their daily activity to ensure that they do not jeopardize the health and safety of themselves or any other person.

Health care facilities should have an *adequately resourced* Occupational Health Department (OHD); one of their roles and responsibilities is to ensure that all steps are taken to ensure that the risk of infection to HCWs are minimized. In addition, they also have responsibility to ensure that if transmissible infection in a HCW is identified, they should be excluded from the work place or from direct patient contact until they are no longer infectious. They should liaise with a member of the IPC team for advice, if necessary.

Role of occupational health departments

- Primary health screening of all staff by questionnaire and/or medical examination.
- Keeping accurate and up-to-date records of all members of staff.
- Immunization of all existing staff at the required time interval.
- Training of all grades of staff in personal hygiene and prevention and management of sharps injuries.
- Examination of staff returning to work after absence due to diarrhoea or other infectious conditions to ensure that the infection has cleared and to give advice to the chronic carrier.
- Determining staff contacts of the infectious disease (e.g. tuberculosis, blood-borne viruses) and checking immunity and follow-up if necessary. Arranging tests and possibly treatment for staff with infectious diseases.

- Keeping records of all inoculation injuries, arranging post-exposure prophylaxis following inoculation injuries, and counselling of staff if necessary.
- Survey potential infective and toxic hazards (e.g. chemical disinfectant) to staff in health care facilities.

Pre-employment assessment

HCWs should be assessed before employment with the aim of preventing disease in the individual but a second, and no less important function is to prevent transmission of infectious agents to patients (see Box 16.1). It is important that the employee must be given assurance of the complete confidentiality of any health questioning and their occupational health record.

It is important that all newly employed staff in the health care setting attend the OHD. The screening process includes assessment by a health questionnaire completed by the employee, covering questions related to general health, history of infectious diseases, and immunization status. It is also important to ascertain immune status if the HCW has either had or been vaccinated against tuberculosis, rubella, measles, mumps, chickenpox, and hepatitis B virus. In addition, the presence of skin disorders such as eczema, and a history of an underlying immunosuppressive disorder might require a reassessment of the staff member's work practices.

Box 16.1 Responsibilities of doctors who have been exposed to a serious communicable disease

If you have any reason to believe that you have been exposed to a serious communicable disease, you *must seek* and follow professional advice without delay on whether you should undergo testing and if so, which tests are appropriate. Further guidance on your responsibilities if your health may put patients at risk is included in the booklet *Good Medical Practice.*

If you acquire a serious communicable disease, you must promptly seek and follow advice from a suitably qualified colleague, such as a Consultant in Occupational Health, Infectious Diseases or Public Health on:

- Whether, and in what ways, you should modify your professional practice.
- Whether you should inform your current employer, your previous employers, or any prospective employer, about your condition. You *must not rely on your own assessment* of the risks you pose to patients.
- If you acquire a serious communicable disease, you must promptly seek and follow advice. If you have a serious communicable disease and continue in professional practice you must have appropriate medical supervision. If you apply for a new post, you must complete any health questionnaire honestly and fully.

Source: *Serious Communicable Diseases.* London: General Medical Council UK, 1997.

Routine screening for staphylococcal, streptococcal, and *Salmonella* carriers is not recommended. Screening may be instituted if an outbreak occurs and if HCWs are felt to be either at risk or potentially associated with spread of the infection; this should be done in consultation with IPC team. Agencies which provide temporary staff for the hospital should be informed of the staff screening policy and, wherever possible, *only those agencies* with an effective screening programme should be used to employ staff.

Health status of health care workers

There are certain medical conditions of HCWs that increase their predisposition to infection if they come into contact with certain infectious patients, e.g. immune status, certain skin conditions, and pregnancy. There are many areas within health care establishments where HCWs with these conditions can safely work and there are few tasks that such HCWs are unable to perform safely. Health care establishments have a responsibility to manage and supervise such HCWs in ways that both acknowledge their right to work, and safeguard the welfare of both patients and HCWs. This responsibility includes the need to identify such HCWs and inform them of the problems they are likely to encounter in particular circumstances. It is important that the OHD should liaise closely with the IPC team.

Staff should not work if they have acute or chronic diarrhoeal disease or febrile respiratory illness. Catering staff need to be carefully questioned about gastrointestinal infection, history of enteric fever, skin conditions (e.g. allergic eczema, psoriasis and exfoliative dermatitis), recurrent sepsis and tuberculosis (see 'Protection against tuberculosis'). Staff with either shedding and/or weeping skin conditions or damaged skin may readily be colonized by microorganisms present in the health care environment. These HCWs may not be harmed by the acquisition of such microorganisms but may disseminate them widely and placement of such HCWs in wards containing patients with MRSA is not recommended. These employees should be identified by personal history screening and advised of the problems posed by their condition.

Staff who are or have reason to believe that they may have been exposed to bloodborne hepatitis (B and C) or HIV infection *must declare* this and discuss it in complete confidence with the OHD, either at the initial screening or when he or she first becomes aware of their infection (see Box 16.1). In general, such staff may require a work assessment and must avoid exposure-prone procedures (see 'Exposure-prone procedures').

Measures to protect health care workers

Immunization

All HCWs should be immunized against vaccine-preventable diseases. It is important that all HCWs should be up-to-date with their routine immunizations, e.g. tetanus, diphtheria, polio, and *measles, mumps, and rubella* (MMR). This is important in the context of the ability of staff to transmit infections to vulnerable groups but also for their *own* benefit. In addition, *BCG vaccine* is recommended for all staff who are working in immunocompromised patients (e.g. transplant and oncology unit) and those who are in regular contact with 'high-risk' patients, e.g. patients in chest medicine, thoracic surgery units, infectious disease/HIV wards, laboratory staff working in microbiology, pathology, and postmortem room staff are at potential risk of contracting tuberculosis. *Hepatitis B vaccination* is recommended for HCWs who are at risk of injury from blood-contaminated sharp instruments, or of being deliberately injured or bitten by patients, e.g. in the psychiatry unit. Antibody levels for hepatitis B should be checked 1–4 months after the completion of a primary course of hepatitis B vaccine. *Varicella vaccine* is recommended for susceptible HCWs who have regular patient contact but are not necessarily involved in direct patient care. Those with a definite history of chickenpox or herpes zoster can be considered protected. HCWs with a negative or uncertain history of chickenpox or herpes zoster should be serologically tested and vaccine only offered to those without varicella zoster antibody (see Chapter 11, 'Varicella Zoster Virus'). *Influenza immunization* should be offered on an annual basis to all clinical staff who are directly involved in patient care as its helps prevent influenza in staff and may also reduce the transmission of influenza to vulnerable groups of patients from an infected HCW. HCWs, who regularly handle faecal specimens are likely to be exposed to *polio* viruses, and should be offered a booster with a polio-containing vaccine every 10 years. HCWs in clinical infectious disease units should be tested and, if necessary, given a booster dose of a *diphtheria-containing vaccine*. An antibody test should be performed at least 3 months after immunization to confirm protective immunity and the individual given a booster dose at 10-year intervals thereafter. If a history of full diphtheria immunization is not available, the primary course should be completed and an antibody test should be performed at least 3 months later to confirm protective immunity. Boosters should be given 5 years later and subsequently at 10-year intervals.

Education and training

All HCWs must be given adequate education and practical training on all issues relating to IPC as part of their induction/orientation programme. This must be reinforced through a regular continuing education programme. They should be trained in the handling of blood and body fluids, chemical disinfectants, and should be aware of local policies and procedures on IPC which also includes safe disposal of sharps, clinical waste, safe handling of linen, etc. Health care facilities must provide a safe work environment, resources, and material (e.g. facilities and products for hand hygiene and personal protective equipment) should be available so that they can perform their tasks effectively. Regular audits should be carried out to ensure compliance with IPC policies and procedures. The manager of the health care facility must keep record of training in IPC for all staff.

Reporting

HCWs must report any accidents or illness to their line manager and, if appropriate, to the OHD. In addition, the incident report process includes notes on remedial and follow-up action taken before the process is considered complete. Table 16.1 summarizes the characteristics of common infectious diseases, mode of transmission, communicability, and recommended work restrictions for an infected HCWs.

Table 16.1 Characteristics of infectious diseases as related to transmission in health care environment

Disease	Mode of transmission (IP: incubation period)	Communicability (Duration of shedding)	Work restrictions
Conjunctivitis	Physical contact of contaminated hand at mucosal surfaces.	Low	◆ Restrict from patient contact until discharge ceases
Chickenpox	Respiratory droplet, contact and airborne. IP: 10–21 days (average 14 days)	High (−2 to +7 days or until scabbed)	◆ Exclude from duty until all lesions dry and crust
Post-exposure susceptible HCW			◆ Exclude from duty from 8–10 days after first exposure (as chickenpox is infectious 2 days prior to onset of rash) through to 21st day; 28th day if VZIG given after last exposure. They should be instructed to take twice daily temperatures and to remain at home if they are febrile, as this could be the first sign of a prodromal varicella illness
Cytomegalovirus infection	Physical contact with virus at mucosal surfaces	Low (weeks)	◆ No restriction. Apply standard infection control precautions esp. hand hygiene
Diarrhoeal diseases	Faecal-oral and fomites	Medium to high depending on the microorganisms	◆ Restrict from patient contact until symptoms resolve ◆ For food handlers, refer to local guidelines regarding need for negative stool culture before return to work
Diphtheria	Respiratory route IP: 2–5 days (range 2–7 days)	High	◆ Exclude from duty until antimicrobial therapy completed and two cultures obtained ≥24 h apart are negative

(continued)

Table 16.1 (*continued*) Characteristics of infectious diseases as related to transmission in health care environment

Disease	Mode of transmission (IP: incubation period)	Communicability (Duration of shedding)	Work restrictions
Enteroviral infections	Faecal–oral and fomites	Low to medium (1–8 weeks)	◆ Restrict from care of infants, neonates, or immunocompromised patients and their environments until symptoms resolve
Hepatitis A	Faecal–oral IP: 28–30 days (range 15 to 50 days)	Medium (2 weeks before onset of symptoms; virus can be excreted up to 6 months)	◆ Restrict from work until 7 days after onset of jaundice ◆ Most cases are non-infectious after the first week of jaundice
Hepatitis E	Faecal–oral IP: 15–64 days (range 3–6 weeks)	Medium (about 2 weeks after the onset of jaundice)	◆ No known but restriction from work until 14 days after onset of jaundice is advisable ◆ Women in the 3rd trimester of pregnancy are susceptible to fulminant disease
Hepatitis B & C	Blood-borne IP: HBV 75 days (range 45–180 days) IP: HCV 20 days to 13 weeks (range: 2 weeks to 6 months)	Medium	◆ No restriction provided standard precautions are followed ◆ HCWs who are involved in exposure-prone procedures must seek advice from OHD
Herpes simplex (Genital)	Physical contact of contaminated hand at mucosal surfaces	Medium Until lesions active. (1–8 weeks)	◆ No restriction provided standard precautions are followed
(Herpetic whitlow on hands)		High if breakdown in hand and personal hygiene (1–8 weeks)	◆ Restrict from patient contact and contact with patient's environment until the lesion is dry and crusted over. Evaluate for need to restrict from care of high-risk patients

HIV infection	Blood-borne IP: usually 2 weeks–3 months from exposure	Low	◆ No restriction provided standard precautions are followed ◆ For exposure-prone invasive procedures seek advice from OHD
Influenza	Respiratory, droplet, airborne, and contact IP: 2–3 days	High (–1 to 7 days)	◆ Exclude from duty until they are asymptomatic ◆ Encourage to take seasonal flu vaccination
Measles	Respiratory droplet IP: 7–18 days	Very high (–2 to + 5 days)	◆ Exclude from duty until 7 days after the rash appears
Post-exposure susceptible HCW			◆ Exclude from duty from 5th day after first exposure through to 21st day after last exposure and/or 4 days after rash appears
Mumps Active	Respiratory droplet IP: 14–19 days	High in certain cohorts (–6 to + 4 days)	◆ Exclude from duty until 9th day after onset of parotitis
Post-exposure susceptible HCW			◆ Exclude from duty 26th day after last exposure or until 9 days after onset of parotitis
Norovirus	Faecal-oral and fomites IP: 1–3 days	Very high Up to 2 weeks	◆ Allow back to work 72 h after symptoms are resolved
Parainfluenza	Respiratory IP: 1–7 days	Very high (7–21 days)	◆ Exclude from duty until they are asymptomatic
Parvovirus ('Fifth' or 'slapped cheek' disease)	Respiratory droplet IP: 13–18 days	Low to medium (–6 to + 3 days before symptoms)	◆ Refer to p. 317 for more details ◆ Attack rates is about 50% amongst susceptible household members

(continued)

Table 16.1 (*continued*) Characteristics of infectious diseases as related to transmission in health care environment

Disease	Mode of transmission (IP: incubation period)	Communicability (Duration of shedding)	Work restrictions
Pediculosis	Contact	Low	◆ Restrict from patient contact until treated and observed to be free of adult and immature lice
Pertussis	IP: 7–10 days (range 6–20 days)	Low to medium	◆ Exclude from duty from beginning of catarrhal stage through 3rd week after onset of paroxysms or until 5 days after start of effective antibiotic therapy
Post-exposure susceptible HCW			◆ Exclude from duty from beginning of catarrhal stage through 3rd week after the onset of paroxysms or until 5 days after start of effective antibiotic therapy
Scabies	IP: 2–6 weeks	Low to medium	◆ Restrict from patient contact until cleared by medical evaluation
Staph. aureus infection	Contact	Variable	◆ Seek advice from OHD on restriction of duties
Active skin lesions			◆ Restrict from patient contact and contact with patient's environment
			◆ They must not handle food
Carrier state			◆ No restriction, unless HCW is epidemiologically linked to transmission of infection (see Chapter 10)
Streptococcal infection, group A (*Strep. pyogenes*)	Contact	Medium/high	◆ Restrict from patient contact, contact with patient's environment, and food handling until 24 h after antibiotic therapy
Rubella Active	Respiratory droplet IP: 15–20 days	Low Highest before or at the onset rash (–7 to + 2 days)	◆ Exclude from duty until 5 days after rash appears

			Post-exposure susceptible HCW
Tuberculosis	Respiratory, airborne IP: 4–12 weeks (variable)	Low to medium	◆ Exclude from duty from 7th day after first exposure through 21st day after last exposure ◆ Exclude from duty until proven non-infectious (see 'Protection against tuberculosis')
Varicella zoster Localized in healthy person	Respiratory droplet, contact, and airborne	High	◆ Until all lesions dry and crust. Lesion must be covered

IP, incubation period; high, 50% or more; medium, 10–50%; low, <10%.

Management of sharps injuries

The primary aim of good infection control practice is to prevent sharps injuries occurring. However, when they do occur, it is essential to ensure that the injuries are managed appropriately and in a timely fashion, to minimize the risk of harm to HCWs or others directly or indirectly affected by sharps injuries. It is important that all HCWs should adopt a safe system of work when using or disposing of sharp objects (see Chapter 18, pp. 330–332). When undertaking any task or activity which has the potential to result in exposure to body fluids or tissues, HCWs should use standard infection control precautions, including the use of PPE.

Definitions

Sharp objects include injection needles, glass ampoules, syringes, phials, disposable scalpels and scalpel blades, other surgical instruments, bone and teeth fragments. Projectile objects and debris arising from dentistry or surgery are also included.

Sharps injury may be defined as an incident where the skin is punctured by an instrument or object that is *contaminated* with human blood, high-risk body fluids (see below), or tissue. For practical purposes, staff who have had contamination of the eyes, mouth, skin, cuts or abrasions, or by splashes or spills will be managed in line with the sharps management policy.

High-risk body fluids and tissues include blood and body fluids contaminated with blood, amniotic fluid, vaginal secretions, semen, human breast milk, cerebrospinal fluid, peritoneal fluid, pleural fluid, pericardial fluid, synovial fluid, saliva (in association with dentistry) and unfixed tissues and organs. *Low-risk materials* include urine, vomit, saliva (with the exception of dentistry) and faeces, unless they are visibly stained with blood or originated from patients with suspected/confirmed infection.

Reporting a sharps injury

Following appropriate first aid, injured individuals must be referred to the OHD or A&E Department as per local protocol *without delay* by the line manager (see Box 16.2). All accidents *must* be reported using the standard accident/incident reporting procedures and appropriate documentation completed. You *must not rely on your own assessment* of the risks. The clinical team is responsible for ensuring that appropriate risk assessments of the patient, where known, are undertaken to determine the risk of transmission of blood-borne viruses in all sharps injuries and the appropriate risk assessment form completed.

Post-exposure prophylaxis

Summary of post-exposure prophylaxis (PEP) is outlined in Box 16.3 and Table 16.2. If PEP is being considered, the injured person must be counselled using the PEP advice sheet. Following this counselling and advice, the injured worker may, in the absence of any contraindication decide to start PEP. For HIV exposure, If PEP is indicated, it should be initiated as soon as possible (preferably within 1 h of the injury) provided that there is no contraindication; a decision can always be made later not to

Box 16.2 Summary of management of occupational exposure to HIV, hepatitis B and C virus

Assessment	Action
First aid	Allow wound to bleed and then rinsed under running water and washed with soap. *Don't* scrub or suck the wound. Exposed mucous membranes including conjunctivae should be irrigated copiously with water or saline, after removing contact lenses, if present
Determine risk associated with exposure by assessing concentrated the virus	Type of fluid, e.g. blood, visibly bloody fluid, other potentially infectious fluid or tissue. Assess concentration of the virus by: ◆ Type of exposure, i.e. percutaneous injury was superficial or deep. ◆ If there was contamination of broken skin or a mucous membrane. ◆ Was it massive or small and how long was blood/body fluid in contact with the skin or mucous membrane? ◆ If a sharps injury, was the instrument hollow bore or solid? If a hollow bore instrument, what gauge was it? ◆ If the injury was caused by a needle, had it been used to inject drugs or to withdraw blood? ◆ If the injury was caused by a needle, was it attached to a syringe containing blood? ◆ If a sharp was misused, were other items associated with drug abuse present?
Evaluate source patient	Assess the risk of infection using available information. Following informed consent, test known source patient for HBsAg, anti-HCV, and HIV antibody; consider using rapid testing. For unknown sources, assess risk of exposure to HBV, HCV, or HIV infection. Do not test discarded needles or syringes for virus contamination
Evaluate the exposed HCW	Assess immune status for HBV infection, i.e. by history of hepatitis B vaccination and antibody response to vaccine. Give PEP for exposures posing risk of infection or transmission (see Table 16.2)

Box 16.3 Post-exposure prophylaxis

Virus	Post-exposure prophylaxis
Hepatitis B virus	PEP with HBIG and/or hepatitis B vaccine series after evaluation of the HBsAg status of the source and the vaccine-response of the exposed person (see Table 16.2)
	Perform follow-up anti-HBs testing in persons who receive hepatitis B vaccine
	Test for anti-HBs 1–4 months after last dose of vaccine
	Anti-HBs response to vaccine cannot be ascertained if HBIG was received in the previous 1 month
Hepatitis C virus	PEP not recommended
	Perform baseline and follow-up testing for anti-HCV 4–6 months after exposure
	Perform HCV RNA at 4–6 weeks if earlier diagnosis of HCV infection desired or if source known to be HCV positive
	Confirm repeatedly reactive anti-HCV EIAs with supplemental tests.
Human immunodeficiency virus	If appropriate, initiate PEP as soon as possible, preferably within 1 h of exposure
	Offer pregnancy testing to all women of childbearing age not known to be pregnant
	Seek expert consultation if viral resistance is suspected
	Administer PEP for 4 weeks if tolerated
	Perform follow-up testing and provide counselling
	Advise exposed persons to seek medical evaluation for any acute illness occurring during follow-up
	Perform HIV-antibody testing for at least 6 months post-exposure (e.g. at baseline, 6 weeks, 3 months, and 6 months)
	Perform HIV antibody testing if illness compatible with an acute retroviral syndrome occurs
	Advise exposed persons to use precautions to prevent secondary transmission during the follow-up period
	Evaluate exposed persons taking PEP within 72 h after exposure and monitor for drug toxicity for at least 2 weeks

Anti-HBs, antibody against hepatitis B surface antigen; anti-HCV= antibody against hepatitis C virus; ALT= alanine aminotransferase; EIAs= enzyme immunoassays; HBIG, hepatitis B immunoglobulin; PEP, post-exposure prophylaxis.

Table 16.2 Hepatitis B virus prophylaxis for reported exposure incidents

HBV status of person exposed	Significant exposure		Non-significant exposure		
	HbsAg-positive source	Unknown source	HbsAg-negative source	Continued risk	No further risk
≤1 dose HB vaccine pre-exposure	Give one dose of HBIG Give accelerated course of HB vaccine at 0, 1, and 2 months; give booster dose at 12 months if there is continuing risk of exposure	Give accelerated course of HB vaccine at 0, 1, and 2 months; give booster dose at 12 months if there is continuing risk of exposure	Initiate course of HB vaccine	Initiate course of HB vaccine	No need to give HBV prophylaxis
≥2 doses HB vaccine pre-exposure (anti-HBs not known)	Give one dose of HB vaccine followed by 2nd dose 1 month later	Give one dose of HB vaccine	Finish course of HB vaccine	Finish course of HB vaccine	No need to give HBV prophylaxis
Known responder to HBV vaccine (anti-HBs ≥10 micro unit/mL)	Consider booster dose of HB vaccine	Consider booster dose of HB vaccine	Consider booster dose of HB vaccine	Consider booster dose of HB vaccine	No need to give HBV prophylaxis
Known non-responder to HB vaccine (anti-HBs <10 micro unit/mL) 2–4 months post-vaccination	Give one dose of HBIG Consider booster dose of HB vaccine A 2nd dose of HBIG should be given at 1 month	Give one dose of HBIG Consider booster dose of HB vaccine A 2nd dose of HBIG should be given at 1 month	No need to give HBIG Consider booster dose of HB vaccine	No need to give HBIG Consider booster dose of HB vaccine	No need to give HBV prophylaxis

HB, hepatitis B; HBIG, hepatitis B immunoglobulin; HBV: hepatitis B virus.
Adapted from PHLS Hepatitis Subcommittee. *Communicable Disease Review* 1992; **2**:R97–R101.

continue a full course. In this case blood *must* be taken for baseline investigations, which include liver function tests, serum amylase, urea and electrolytes, full blood picture, and differential white cell count. A starter pack for PEP for HIV must be available in the A&E department. *All testing must be done with the fully informed consent* of the worker and only following counselling.

Exposure-prone procedures

All breaches of the skin or epithelia by sharp instruments are, by definition, invasive. However, most clinical procedures, including many which are invasive, do not provide an opportunity for the blood of the HCW to come into contact with the patient's open tissues. The UK Department of Health defines *exposure-prone procedures* as those invasive procedures where there is a risk that injury to the worker may result in the exposure of the patient's open tissues to the blood of the worker. These include procedures where the worker's gloved hands may be in contact with sharp instruments, needle tips, or sharp tissues (e.g. spicules of bone or teeth) inside a patient's open body cavity, wound, or confined anatomical space where the hands or fingertips may not be completely visible at all times. Procedures where the hands and fingertips of the worker are visible and outside the patient's body at all times, and internal examinations or procedures that do not involve possible injury to the worker's gloved hands from sharp instruments and/or tissues, are not considered to be exposure-prone, provided routine infection control procedures are adhered to at all times.

Examples of procedures that are *not* exposure-prone include:

+ Taking blood (venepuncture).
+ Setting up and maintaining IV lines or central lines (provided any skin-tunnelling procedure used for the latter is performed in a non-exposure-prone manner, i.e. without the operator's fingers being at any time concealed in the patient's tissues in the presence of a sharp instrument).
+ Minor surface suturing.
+ Routine vaginal or rectal examination.
+ Simple endoscope procedures.

When there is any doubt about whether a procedure is exposure-prone or not, expert advice should be obtained.

Protection against tuberculosis

All staff in regular contact with patients, and especially those working in chest medicine, thoracic surgery units, infectious disease wards, laboratory staff working in microbiology, pathology, and postmortem room staff are at potential risk of contracting tuberculosis. Therefore it is essential that all prospective employee (including agency staff and locums) should undergo pre-employment health screening which should include screening for tuberculosis. Health care facilities that have contracts with agencies should specify that the agency only supply staff that meets this requirement. Enquiries about symptoms suggestive of tuberculosis should form part of the pre-employment health questionnaire and which should be checked by the OHD. The results of tuber-culin skin testing and BCG vaccination should be obtained when feasible. Staff with symptoms compatible with tuberculosis should seek advice either from the OHD or from their own medical practitioner.

It is essential that all new employees to the health care facilities who will be working with patients or clinical specimens should *not start work* until they have completed a tuberculosis screen or health check. If they have been assessed previously by other OHD, then they must provide documentary evidence of such screening. Assessment of personal or family history of tuberculosis and inquiry into symptom and signs, possibly by questionnaire and documentary evidence of tuberculin skin testing (or interferon-gamma testing) and/or BCG scar must be checked by the OHD, *not* relying on the applicant's personal assessment. Refer to NICE web site: http://www.nice.org.uk/ for the most up-to-date guidance.

Following *exposure of staff* to a patient with open pulmonary (positive sputum smear for AAFB) tuberculosis, a list of staff at risk should be drawn by the line manager. This list should *only include staff that have had direct contact*. The list should be sent to the OHD who will assess the circumstances of the exposure incident and review the HCWs and take appropriate action. For details please refer to the NICE guideline on tuberculosis (NICE, 2011).

Pregnant health care workers

Certain infections can be a problem during pregnancy, some of which may, poten-tially, be acquired at the workplace, for example, cytomegalovirus (CMV), hepatitis viruses, HIV, rubella, parvovirus B19, and varicella-zoster virus. In general, adherence to standard precautions and maintaining high standards of general hygiene in the workplace will provide the HCWs with the necessary protection against infection.

It is the responsibility of the pregnant HCW to advise their medical practitioner and employer of their pregnancy. The employer should advise pregnant HCWs of the special risks associated with pregnancy and give them an opportunity to avoid patients with specific infections. All women of childbearing age should be counselled regarding their immune status and, if necessary, should be offered immunization before they become pregnant. All information about immune status and pregnancy of HCWs must remain confidential.

The following information relates to infections that are both significant in preg-nancy and have some possibility of being acquired through patient care. It is not meant to be a comprehensive account of all infections having relevance to pregnant women.

Rubella

Confirming rubella immunity is part of routine antenatal screening. However, serious congenital abnormalities most commonly follow rubella infection occurring in the first trimester. For this reason, rubella antibody status should be checked at employ-ment in all HCWs, particularly women of childbearing age. If rubella antibody is absent or below protective levels, then the HCW should be offered vaccination on beginning employment. Rubella vaccination should be avoided in early pregnancy, and conception should be avoided for 2 months following vaccination, although no case of congenital rubella syndrome has been reported following inadvertent vaccination shortly before or during pregnancy. Where necessary, those vaccinated can be tested for seroconversion 2 months after vaccination, and be re-vaccinated if necessary.

Post-exposure prophylaxis with normal immunoglobulin will *not* prevent infection in non-immune contacts and is therefore of little value in the protection of pregnant women exposed to rubella. However, it may prolong the incubation period, which in turn may marginally reduce the risk to the fetus. It may also reduce the likelihood of clinical symptoms in the mother. Normal immunoglobulin should only be used if termination of pregnancy due to confirmed rubella infection is unacceptable. In such cases, it should be given soon after exposure. Serological follow-up of recipients is essential, and should continue for up to 8 weeks.

Hepatitis B virus

All non-immune HCWs should be offered HBV vaccination as soon as possible at the start of employment and should be tested for antibodies to HBsAg 3 months after the third dose of vaccine. Those who do not respond should be offered a fourth dose or a further three doses depending upon the antibody level. Table 16.2 summarizes the schedule for hepatitis B virus immunization. While the safety of the HBV vaccine for the developing fetus has not yet been confirmed by a large-scale trial, HBV infection in a pregnant woman may result in severe disease for the newborn (see Chapter 11, 'Protection of the newborn'). Pregnancy should therefore not be considered a contraindication to the administration of HBIG or HBV vaccination.

Cytomegalovirus

After primary infection, young children excrete cytomegalovirus (CMV) in urine and saliva in larger amounts and for longer periods than adults. There is a high incidence of asymptomatic excretion of CMV among infants and toddlers. For this reason, isolation of children known to be excreting CMV is not recommended. To avoid CMV infection, washing hands after all patient contact and after contact with urine and saliva is essential. Avoidance of direct contact with saliva (e.g. kissing toddlers on the mouth) is also important. While CMV may commonly be encountered in urine and saliva, surprisingly there is little evidence that this virus has been acquired by female HCWs and, in particular, has then resulted in fetal infection. Generally, CMV infection in HCWs, even those working in high-risk areas such as neonatal units, transplant units, and caring for HIV positive patients, is not significantly more common than that in the general community.

However, pregnant HCWs should be informed of the risks of CMV infection and provided with an opportunity to determine their susceptibility by performing antibody testing. They should be counselled about how to minimize contact with known CMV-infected patients by applying standard infection control precautions, including the use of gloves and regular hand washing. Pregnant HCWs, or those contemplating pregnancy, should be counselled regarding mode of transmission of CMV and safe work practices. Routine antenatal screening is not recommended even in HCWs in high-risk areas, but can be offered on an individual basis. The implications of screening test results should be clearly explained.

Evidence of past CMV infection is a good indicator that symptomatic infection or congenital defects in the infant are unlikely to occur. However, it does not totally exclude the possibility of congenital infection, because reactivation of a past infection can occur during pregnancy. Conversely, if a HCW is antibody negative, avoidance of high-risk work areas will not eliminate the risk of primary CMV infection during pregnancy, especially if the HCW has close contact with children or other sources outside work. CMV seronegative women who care for children over the age of 2 years have a lower risk of infection. Redeploying seronegative pregnant employees to care for older children may further minimize the risk of working in high-risk areas. CMV immunoglobulin is available for the prevention and treatment of CMV infection in certain individuals at high risk of infection. However, its value is unclear.

Parvovirus B19 infection

Parvovirus B19 (fifth disease) is the cause of a common childhood illness and presents with erythema infectiosum which is characterized by fever and a rash with erythematous cheeks—hence it is commonly called 'slapped cheek 'disease. Hospital outbreaks of Parvovirus B19, involving infection of patients and HCWs, including pregnant HCWs, have been reported. If the parvovirus B19 infection is confirmed in a HCW, then the implications need to be considered for patients at risk (e.g. immunocompromised and patients with haemoglobinopathies) who were in contact with the infected HCW during the 7 days before onset of the rash. Contact is classified as persons in the same room (e.g. in a 2–4-bed hospital bay, a house, or in a classroom) for a significant period of time (≥15 minutes), or face-to-face contact with a laboratory-confirmed case of parvovirus B19 infection during the period of maximum infectivity i.e. from 7 days before the appearance of a rash or symptom.

About 60% of pregnant women will be immune to parvovirus B19 because of previous infection and can be reassured that they are at no risk. Transmissibility of the virus depends on the nature of the contact and, due to low transmissibility of the virus to adults, it has been estimated that 40% of women who are susceptible will not necessarily become infected. It is important to emphasize that the risks of a pregnant woman becoming infected are greater outside the health care setting than within it, particularly if she has children or works with children.

≤**20 weeks of pregnancy:** it has been estimated that up to 10% of pregnancies in which infection occurs during the first 20 weeks may suffer from fetal loss and cause aplastic anaemia that later becomes manifest as hydrops fetalis. There is no evidence of B19-associated teratogenicity, or of developmental abnormalities appearing later in childhood. These women have their susceptibility determined by testing booking sera for antibodies to parvovirus B19. Pregnant HCWs should therefore avoid contact with patients who are infected with human parvovirus B19.

≥**20 weeks of pregnancy:** women who were in contact with the infected individuals outside the infectious period (13–18 days) or when they were more than 20 weeks

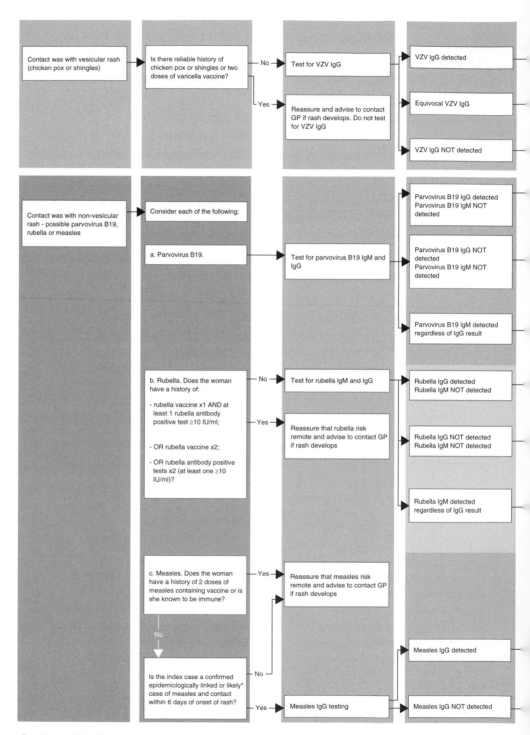

Fig. 16.1 Algorithm showing the follow-up of women exposed to rash in pregnancy. *Establish the likelihood of measles in the index case. With permission from HPA. *Guidance on viral rash in pregnancy*, London: Health Protection Agency, 2007.

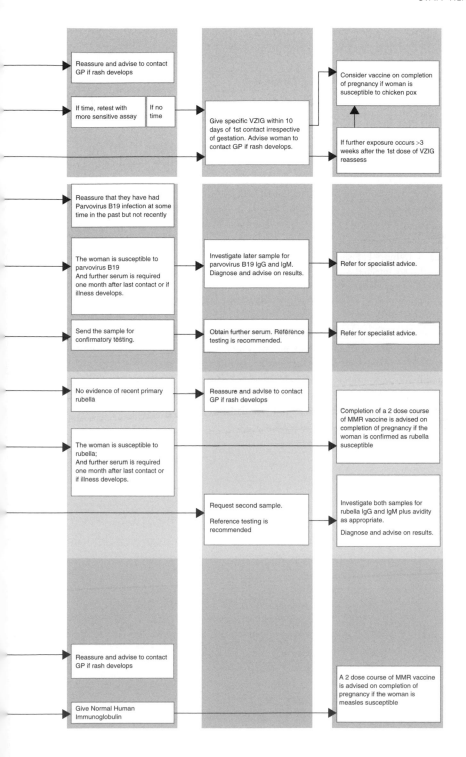

Reassure and advise to contact GP if rash develops

If time, retest with more sensitive assay | If no time

Give specific VZIG within 10 days of 1st contact irrespective of gestation. Advise woman to contact GP if rash develops.

Consider vaccine on completion of pregnancy if woman is susceptible to chicken pox

If further exposure occurs >3 weeks after the 1st dose of VZIG reassess

Reassure that they have had Parvovirus B19 infection at some time in the past but not recently

The woman is susceptible to parvovirus B19
And further serum is required one month after last contact or if illness develops.

Investigate later sample for parvovirus B19 IgG and IgM. Diagnose and advise on results.

Refer for specialist advice.

Send the sample for confirmatory testing.

Obtain further serum. Reference testing is recommended.

Refer for specialist advice.

No evidence of recent primary rubella

Reassure and advise to contact GP if rash develops

Completion of a 2 dose course of MMR vaccine is advised on completion of pregnancy if the woman is confirmed as rubella susceptible

The woman is susceptible to rubella;
And further serum is required one month after last contact or if illness develops.

Request second sample.

Reference testing is recommended

Investigate both samples for rubella IgG and IgM plus avidity as appropriate.

Diagnose and advise on results.

Reassure and advise to contact GP if rash develops

Give Normal Human Immunoglobulin

A 2 dose course of MMR vaccine is advised on completion of pregnancy if the woman is measles susceptible

pregnant can be reassured. Extremely rarely, infections after 20 weeks of gestation can be associated with transient anaemia in the mother or the newborn without sequelae.

Key references and further reading

Crowcroft NS, Roth CE, Cohen BJ, *et al.* Guidance for control of parvovirus B19 infection in health care settings and the community. *Journal of Public Health Medicine* 1999; **21**(40):439–46.

Department of Health. *Immunization against infectious disease – 'The Green Book'.* London: Department of Health, 2006. Access website for regular update: http://www.dh.gov.uk/.

Department of Health. *Health clearance for tuberculosis, hepatitis B, hepatitis C and HIV: New healthcare workers.* London: Department of Health, 2007.

Health Protection Agency. *Guidance on Viral Rash in Pregnancy. Investigation, Diagnosis and Management of Viral Rash Illness, or Exposure to Viral Rash Illness in Pregnancy.* London, Health Protection Agency, 2011.

Henderson DK, Dembry L, Fishman NO, *et al.* SHEA Guideline for management of healthcare workers who are infected with hepatitis B virus, hepatitis C virus, and/or human immunodeficiency virus. *Infection Control and Hospital Epidemiology* 2010; **31**(3):203–32.

Herwaldt LA, Pottinger JM, Carter CD, *et al.* Exposure workshops. *Infection Control and Hospital Epidemiology* 1997; **18**:850–71.

NICE Guidelines 33. *Tuberculosis: Clinical diagnosis and management of tuberculosis, and measures for its prevention and control* London: National Institute for Health and Clinical Excellence, 2011. Access website for regular update: http://www.nice.org.uk/.

PHLS Hepatitis Subcommittee. *Communicable Disease Review* 1992; **2**:R97–R101.

SHEA Guideline for management of healthcare workers who are infected with Hepatitis B virus, Hepatitis C virus, and/or Human immunodeficiency virus. *Infection Control and Hospital Epidemiology* 2010; **31**(3): 203–232.

Chapter 17

Primary and community health care facilities

I doubt if God has given us any refreshment which, taken in moderation, is unwholesome, except microbes.

Mark Twain

Primary and community health care facilities include GPs' surgeries, long-term facilities (e.g. nursing and residential homes), hospices, etc. The level of care provided to the clients/patients in these facilities varies greatly. For example, patients may visit their GP for a one-off consultation while the residents living in long-term facilities are elderly and may have chronic underlying conditions with multiple comorbidity. Some of these residents may have a mental illness and have a diminished immune response due to old age and malignant disease and are therefore more susceptible to infections. This chapter outlines the general principles of infection prevention and control in the community and the individuals' health care facilities should take relevant sections which are applicable to the level of care they provide.

Management responsibilities

The owners of the primary and community health care facilities are responsible for the health and safety of their clients/patients/residents, staff, and visitors. They should ensure that *all* staff and HCWs have a clear understanding of their responsibilities in relation to IPC. They should apply standard infection control precautions for the care of *all patients at all times*. It is important to emphasize that it is also the responsibility of each individual member of staff employed in these facilities to be familiar with, and adhere to IPC policies and procedures for their own safety and for the safety of their clients/patients and visitors.

Each community health care facility should have a designated person who should be responsible for overseeing that all IPC programmes are implemented, coordinated and monitored as per local guidelines. It is essential that they should undertake specific training in IPC so that this role can be performed efficiently, and effectively.

Policies and procedures

Appropriate IPC policies and procedures should be easily accessible (in hard copy and/or electronic format) and should be updated on an annual basis or earlier, if required.

They must be clearly labelled with issue and review dates. Adequate resources should be made available to staff to implement these policies and procedures effectively. The policies and procedures should address the following key areas:

- Hand hygiene.
- Use of Personnel Protective Equipment.
- Aseptic technique for clinical procedures.
- Decontamination of re-usable items and equipment.
- Environmental cleaning and management of spillage of blood/body fluids.
- Waste management.
- Safe handling and management of sharps injuries.
- Safe handling of linen.
- Wound management.
- Antimicrobial prescribing guidelines.

Communication

Health care facilities should ensure that the patients/clients and their carers/visitors should be given relevant information on IPC so that they can take appropriate precautions to reduce the risk of infection to themselves and to others. In addition, sharing of information between primary/community care and secondary care in patient transfers is an essential aspect in the prevention and control of HCAIs. HCWs have a responsibility to ensure that all relevant information is transferred with any patient moving within/between health care facilities and social services, this must include information on any HCAIs and this should be accompanied by the appropriate relevant documentation.

Training and education

All members of staff must be familiar with, and receive regular training on content of policies and procedures that are relevant and applicable to their area of work. It must be part of the induction programme for *all* new staff. IPC training should also be included in all *ongoing staff training programmes*. Records of all IPC training should be maintained, these should be stored and readily available for review and for inspection if required. Mandatory compliance with all best practice IPC policies and procedures should be included in job descriptions, personal development plans, and appraisal exercises for all staff.

Audits

The aim of infection control audit is to carry out systematic review of the local policies and procedures to ensure that what *should* be done is *being* done (see 'Audit in infection control', Chapter 1). Regular audits are essential as they will highlight gaps, issues, and level of compliance with the written policies and procedures on a day-to-day basis and help the health care facility manager to identify the areas of non-compliance.

General principles of infection control

Hand hygiene

Hand hygiene is the single most important procedure in prevention of cross-infection and must be implemented all the time (see Chapter 8 for details). Hand washing facilities must be provided and hand-wash basins should be accessible within the area of care. The hand-wash basin/sink should be designated for hand washing and should *not* be used for cleaning equipment, disposing of specimens, etc. In order to minimize hands contamination after hand washing, installation of either elbow operated or automated sensor-operated taps should be installed in the hand-wash basin. Supplies of liquid soap and good quality disposable paper towels in a dispenser should be available. Alcohol hand rub preparations are more effective than hand washing with soap and water and can be used on physically clean hands. However, non-medicated soap and water is recommended to decontaminate hands if the hands are visibly soiled with blood and/or body fluids, patient gasteroentritis, or suspected/confirmed case of *Clostridium difficile* infection.

Personal protective equipment

The selection of PPE should be based on the risk assessment (see Chapter 9 for details). Gloves should be worn during patient care activity which may involve exposure to blood and/or body fluids. They must be removed *immediately after use* and dispose of as clinical waste. *Hands must be washed after the removal of gloves.* Gloves must be changed both *between patient contacts* and *between separate procedures* on the same patient. Single-use disposable plastic aprons are recommended for general use and should be worn when there is a risk that clothing or uniforms may become exposed to blood and/or body fluids. Facemasks and eye protection must be worn where there is a risk of blood, body fluid, secretions, and excretions splashing into the face and eyes. Uniforms should *not* be worn outside of the workplace. A clean uniform should be available for each shift and changing facilities should be provided for all staff.

Aseptic technique for clinical procedures

The principles of asepsis using non-touch aseptic technique must be applied when undertaking any clinical and/or aseptic procedure. In addition, it is important that each facility should have a dedicated area for the storage of sterile goods. This area must be kept clean, dry, and free from clutter. Sterile packages must be protected from moisture, damage, and sources of heat (from either direct sunlight or radiators). Appropriate shelving should be fitted to facilitate off-the-floor storage and easy access to sterile goods (see Chapter 6, Box 6.1). A nominated person should have responsibility for setting and maintaining stock levels to avoid overstocking.

Urinary catheterization: UTIs are a major problem for elderly, debilitated residents who have long-term catheterization. Therefore, it is essential that insertion and maintenance of urinary catheters should follow the guidelines outlined in Chapter 13 to reduce the risk of infection and other related problems, including stricture formation and encrustation.

Intravenous catheter care: the principles of asepsis must be applied for the insertion and continuing care of IV catheters which are used for administration of fluids, medications, and/or total parenteral nutrition. Please refer to Chapter 12 for more details.

Enteral feeding: this is becoming a more common form of nutritional support for the elderly or those with swallowing difficulties. It is essential that all necessary steps are taken to reduce the risk of contamination of feeds and the administration equipment. Patients and carers should be educated and trained in the techniques of hand hygiene, enteral feeding, and the management of the administration system before the patient is discharged from hospital.

Decontamination of medical equipment and devices

The Medical Devices Regulations require the manufacturers of medical devices to supply information on decontamination so that items and equipment can be re-used. The *manufacturer's guidance should be used* to develop local written policies and procedures for the decontamination/sterilization of all types of medical equipment and devices. Every effort must be made to reprocess items that require sterilizing in a SSD. Please refer to Appendix 6.1 for guidance on disinfection procedures for individual items and equipment. Items which are marked single-use items should not be re-used.

Environmental cleaning and management of spillage

The environment must be visibly clean, free from dust and soilage. The cleaning schedule should include the cleaning of all equipment, fixtures, and fittings and be specific to the method and frequency of cleaning. Where a piece of equipment is used for more than one patient (commode, bath, hoist, etc) it must be suitably cleaned/disinfected following each use. Spillage of blood and body fluids must be cleaned up as soon as possible, as they are a potential source of infection. Refer to Chapter 6, Box 6.5 for methods on how to deal with spillage of blood and body fluids.

Waste management

All community health care facilities should have a written waste management policy that details the identification, segregation and safe handling and disposal of all waste arising from health care facilities. This policy should be in accordance with the local guidelines, and should include safe use, handling and disposal of sharps and risk assessment of waste. It is important that clinical waste bins and sharps boxes should be located wherever clinical waste is generated. For details please refer to the section 'Management of clinical waste', Chapter 18.

Safe handling and management of sharps injury

Employers must have a detailed local policy on the safe use, handling and disposal of sharps. Incidents causing exposure to blood and body fluids are associated with the risk of transmission of blood-borne viruses such as hepatitis B, hepatitis C or HIV. Every effort must be made to minimize the use of sharps whenever possible and every effort should be made to prevent such exposures. Best practice in the handling and disposal of sharps are outlined in 'Safe use, handling, and disposal of sharps', Chapter 18.

All sharps injuries must be managed correctly as per local policy and appropriate support must be made available to staff who may sustain a sharps injury.

Safe handling of linen

If linen is used in the health care facility, an appropriate commercial laundry contract should be arranged to collect and deliver linen. Clean linen *must* be stored within a suitable clean dedicated area.

Used linen must be handled with care at all times and must be laundered at 71°C for 3 min or 65°C for 10 min as a minimum. Thorough washing or rinsing is required at a lower temperature for heat-labile materials (see 'Laundry process', Chapter 18, for further details).

If the linen is infectious and/or contaminated, it is important that suitable PPE (e.g. gloves and plastic aprons) should be worn and linen must be handled gently to avoid contamination of the environment. They must be segregated into appropriate laundry bags as per local guidelines and hands must be thoroughly washed after removal of gloves. For details please refer to the section 'Linen and laundry services', Chapter 18.

Antimicrobial prescribing guidelines

In the UK, 80% of the antibiotic prescribing takes in primary care. Therefore medical practitioners managing the patients in the community play a key role in controlling the inappropriate use of antibiotics and should take responsibility for rational prescribing not only to prevent emergence of antibiotic resistant microorganisms (MRSA, ESBL,VRE, etc.) but also to prevent *C. difficile*-associated diarrhoea (see Chapter 11) . Therefore it is essential that local antibiotic prescribing guidelines should be developed in consultation with the local medical microbiologists and compliance with the guidelines should be monitored and audited on a regular basis.

Special problems
Clostridium difficile-associated diarrohea

C. difficile is a toxin-producing organism carried in the intestinal tract. Infection occurs most frequently in the elderly, especially after the use of broad-spectrum antibiotic therapy. Infected patients should be nursed in a single room with standard and contact infection control precautions. The spores survive in the environment and have been found on floors, bedpans, and the hands of staff. Therefore thorough cleaning of the environment with hot water and detergent followed by decontamination by hypochlorite (bleach) solution (1000 ppm) should be used to reduce spores in the environment. Hand washing by staff before and after handling patients and their environment is the most important control measure. Refer to Chapter 11 for details on the management of diarrhoea-associated with *C. difficili*.

Meticillin resistant *Staphylococcus aureus*

The basic principles of MRSA infection control in the community are the same as those for hospitals. The single most important factor is good hand hygiene. If standard and contact infection control precautions are followed, patients who are colonized with MRSA are not a risk to other residents, staff, visitors, or members of their family.

GPs who are seeing patients with known cases of MRSA, must make every effort to see the patients as soon as they arrive, rather than have them waiting in a reception room with other patients who may be susceptible to infection. In residential and nursing homes, these patients should be cared for using standard and contact infection control precautions which will prevent the transmission of MRSA. As long as these precautions are followed, residents who have MRSA are at minimal risk to other residents, staff, or visitors. Single-room isolation is not usually required although most residents are cared for in single rooms in the normal course of events. A patient with MRSA may share a room with other residents so long as they have intact skin (i.e. no open wounds) and do not have an invasive device such as PEG (percutaneous endoscopic gastrostomy) feeding tube or a urinary catheter *in situ*. There is no justification for discriminating against people who have MRSA by refusing them admission to a nursing or residential home or by treating them differently from other residents. Refer to Chapter 10 for details.

Outbreaks of infection

Outbreak of infection—especially gastrointestinal, respiratory, and scabies—are not uncommon in long-term health care facilities. It is essential that as soon as an outbreak of infection is suspected, the person in charge of the health care facility must inform the appropriate medical officer (e.g. GP and CCDC in the UK) by telephone. A record of all residents affected should be compiled to include the name, age, diagnosis, symptoms, and the date and time of the onset of symptoms. The medical officer and/or community infection control will advise of any immediate action necessary to control the outbreak.

Key references and further reading

APIC. *Infection Prevention Manual for long term Facilities*, 2nd edn. Washington, DC: Association for Professionals in Infection Control and Epidemiology, 2007.

CDC Guideline: *Guide to infection prevention in outpatient settings: Minimum Expectations for Safe Care*. Atlanta: Centre for Diseases Control and Prevention, 2011.

NICE guidelines. *Infection control. Prevention of healthcare-associated infection in primary and community care*. London: National Institute for Clinical Excellence, 2003. Available on: www.nice.org.uk

Scottish Executive. *Infection Control Standards in adult care home care: Final Standards*. Edinburgh: Scottish Executive, 2005.

Chapter 18

Support services

Some little bug is going
to find you some day,
some little bug will creep
behind you some day.

Roy Atwell, 1878

Management of clinical waste

The most practical approach to clinical waste management is to identify waste that represents a sufficient risk of causing infection during handling and after disposal and for which some precautions are necessary to prevent any significant potential risk of infection. It is essential that all health care facilities have clearly defined guidelines to ensure the safe identification, packaging, labelling, storage, transport, treatment, and disposal of waste, from the point of generation to the point of final disposal. Management of clinical and related waste must conform to the appropriate national guidelines. It is generally thought that clinical waste, unless in the form of a contaminated sharp, poses a substantially lower risk of infection than many other forms of contaminated waste and the legal approaches are commonly as much about a public and political perception of risk than actual risk of infection. For sharps waste, the disposal method *must* both render the sharps safe and also prevent their reuse in uncontrolled settings.

It is essential that all employees who are required to handle and move clinical waste should be adequately trained in safe procedures. If the waste is not contained, they must be provided with appropriate PPE, e.g. water-repellent clothing, heavy-duty gloves, and protective footwear, and be trained in how to use the PPE. Spillages and other incidents must be dealt with according to written protocols. All accidents and incidents involving clinical waste, particularly those resulting in injury to or contamination of handlers, must be dealt with according to local policy.

Definition and categorization of clinical waste

The definition and categorization of clinical or medical waste varies from country to country. Terms such as 'hospital waste', 'clinical waste', 'infectious waste', 'medical waste', 'biomedical waste', and 'biohazard waste', have been used synonymously and often inappropriately in many situations.

Infectious waste

In England and Wales infectious health care waste is defined as 'substances containing viable microorganisms or their toxins which are known or reliably believed to cause disease in man or other living organisms' and therefore subject to special requirements for handing, collection, and disposal to prevent infection.

Infectious waste is categorized in to **Category A waste** which is highly infectious waste and must be transported in a form that, when exposure to it occurs, is capable of causing permanent disability, life-threatening or fatal disease to humans or animals. Example of this type of waste includes patient-derived health care waste contaminated with haemorrhagic fever viruses, monkeypox or variola as well as laboratory cultures of hazard group 3 or 4 pathogens (HTM 07-01; Department of Health, 2011). **Category B** is any infectious substance that does not fall into category A, i.e. all other routine infectious waste should be included in this category.

Special waste

Special waste is defined as waste that is dangerous to life and difficult to dispose of by its nature, for example, cytotoxic and cytostatic, radioactive, and other pharmaceutical waste. Disposal of this type of waste is subject to strict regulations.

Offensive waste

This is health care waste that may cause offence (e.g. incontinence waste) but presents no hazard as listed in the categories above. It is handled and disposed of to minimize any offence but this can be done at a substantially lower cost than hazardous wastes.

Non-clinical

Non-clinical or household waste is defined as other waste not in the categories of either clinical, special, or offensive waste. It is non-toxic, non-infectious, or its basic nature is unlikely to prove a health hazard or give offence in its existing form. Disposal of this type of waste is suitable for landfill in a permitted or licensed site.

Safe handling of clinical waste

Clinical waste should be placed in a robust plastic bag marked according to locally agreed colour code (yellow, red, or orange are commonly used) (Table 18.1). The thickness should meet the appropriate local standard. It is recommended that the clinical waste bag should be a minimum gauge of 225 (55 µm thickness) if high density, or a minimum gauge of 100 (25 µm thickness) if low density. To avoid contamination, plastic bags should be secured in a foot-operated lidded bin or carrier frame. General principles for safe handling of clinical waste are:

- Clinical waste should be placed into the plastic waste bag at the point of generation.
- Bags should be replaced if they become offensive (e.g. smell) or when three-quarters full and should be securely closed by tying or sealed by plastic. Staples must *not* be used as they do not provide secure closure and may puncture the bag and may cause a sharps injury to the handler.
- Bags should be suitably identified with the name of the health care facility and the department that generated the waste, which clearly identifies their point of origin

Table 18.1 Colour coding of waste containers and sharp boxes and recommended methods of disposal

Colour coding	Methods of disposal
Yellow	Requires disposal by incineration
Orange	Requires disposal by incineration or may be treated by alternative treatment methods e.g. heating or microwave-based treatments. Alternative treatments methods are usually less expensive than incineration
Purple	For cytotoxic and cytostatic drugs. Requires disposal by incineration
Yellow and black stripes	Offensive waste require disposal by landfill in a permitted or licensed site
Black	Domestic waste is suitable for landfill in a permitted or licensed site
White	Waste requires recovery of ingredients e.g. metals from dental amalgam, photography and x-ray waste
Sharps boxes methods of disposal	
Yellow with a yellow lid	Partially discharged sharps including those contaminated with medicines other than those that are cytotoxic and cytostatic. Requires disposal by incineration
Yellow with a orange lid	Fully discharged sharps that are not contaminated with cytotoxic and cytostatic medicines. Requires disposal by incineration or alternative treatment
Yellow with a purple lid	Sharps including those contaminated with cytotoxic and cytostatic medicines. Requires disposal by incineration

Adapted from Department of Health. *Health Technical Memorandum 07-01: Safe management of healthcare waste.* London: Department of Health, 2011.

in case of improper disposal. Closing the bag with pre-printed coded clips should be considered as part of the traceability process.

◆ Bags should be handled by the neck only and kept upright. To avoid injuries by improperly disposed sharps, the hand should *not* be put underneath the waste bag while lifting.

◆ Waste should be stored within a designated collection area of each ward or department, which must be secured against unauthorized access and be removed from clinical areas daily or more frequently if necessary. The area should be cleaned when necessary and kept dry.

◆ When removed from this area to await collection for disposal, it should be stored in a cleanable area that keeps the waste safe from scavenging animals, people seeking to reuse items from the waste, or from playing children.

◆ Local laws or policy may require bagged waste to be put into robust rigid containers for bulk transport.

◆ Bulk waste transport vehicles are the responsibility of the transport manager. Loaded vehicles leaving the health care facility or hospital site must be properly secured. Spillage should be dealt with safely as per local protocol and vehicles should have a regular cleaning and disinfection schedule.

◆ All employees who are required to handle and move clinical waste should be adequately trained in safe procedures and in dealing with spillages or other incidents in their particular area of work (i.e. those who handle waste in bulk may be trained differently from those who place small amounts into plastic bags). A record of such training should be kept.

◆ Staff who regularly have to handle, transfer, transport, or incinerate clinical waste containers must be provided with appropriate PPE, i.e. heavy-duty gloves, appropriate footwear, an industrial apron or leg shields, waterproof clothing, face visors, or respiratory equipment as required.

◆ Spillages of waste should be treated according to the local policy.

◆ All accidents and incidents involving clinical waste, particularly those resulting in injury to or contamination of handlers, must be reported without delay to the line manager.

Safe use, handling, and disposal of sharps

Sharps are any medical items or devices which are contaminated with blood, tissue, and high-risk body fluids that can cause laceration or puncture wounds. Examples include discarded hypodermic needles and instruments used in invasive procedures (blood sampling, surgery and dentistry, acupuncture, ear-piercing, tattooing, etc.).

Contaminated sharps represent the major cause of accidents involving potential exposure to blood-borne diseases, and must be handled with care at all times. In clinical settings, sharps injuries are predominantly caused by needle devices and associated with venepuncture, administration of medication via intravascular lines, and recapping of needles. It is vital that the person who uses a sharp is responsible for putting it in a sharps bin and does not leave it around with the expectation that someone else will do this for them unless locally agreed (e.g. in an operating theatre). The vast majority of sharps injuries are from improperly disposed sharps.

The safe handling and disposal of needles and other sharp instruments form part of an overall strategy of clinical waste disposal to protect staff, patients, visitors, and people outside the hospital from exposure to blood-borne pathogens. The person in charge of the ward or department is responsible for ensuring sharps users within their own area dispose of the sharps correctly and the sharps bins are collected for proper disposal.

Health care facilities should provide documented operating procedures for safe handling of sharps, and ensure that health care workers are fully trained in the recommended handling techniques. General principles for handling and use of sharps are:

◆ Avoid sharps usage wherever possible and do not administer medication via sharps if there is no clinical need.

◆ Handling should be kept to a minimum. Needles should *not* be bent or broken by hand, removed from disposable syringes, or otherwise manipulated by hand. Sharps must not be passed directly from hand-to-hand. *Never* leave sharps lying around; dispose of them properly.

- Do not keep syringes, needles, or any other sharps object in your pockets. Since many needlestick injuries happen during re-sheathing, used needles must therefore *not* be re-sheathed unless there is a safe means available for doing so. Syringes/cartridges and needles should be disposed of intact. However, in certain situations, where re-sheathing of needles is necessary, it is essential that a safe method is used, i.e. one-handed scoop technique should be used. A mechanical device for holding or disposing of needles should be considered. Alternatively, the needle can be destroyed at the point of use using a mechanical device.
- *Do not use* needles or any sharps if there is any suspicion of a broken seal or other indication that it may have been used previously.

Guidance on proper use of sharps boxes

- All sharps boxes must be correctly assembled and used according to the manufacturer's instructions. They *must be puncture resistant* and should comply with appropriate standards (e.g. UN 3291, British Standard BS 3720).
- Sharps boxes *must not be used* for any other purpose, e.g. storage of ward items.
- They should be readily available wherever blood samples are taken and must be kept in a location that excludes injury to patients, visitors, and staff. To avoid damage by heat, sharps boxes should not be placed near radiators or in direct sunlight.
- Particular attention should be paid to the need for the provision of sufficient sharps boxes in a number of areas where use of sharps is high, e.g. operating theatres, A&E, and outpatient departments.
- Sharps containers must be *properly closed when three-quarters full* and stored at a designated secure point whilst awaiting collection. The sharps container must never be overfilled since used sharps protruding from overloaded containers constitute a very significant hazard to those who have to handle them.
- Used sharps boxes must be suitably marked for identification from wards or departments of the hospital or the health care facility. This enables the exact location and responsibility for any offending container to be determined.
- The staff responsible for the transport of the sharps boxes must take special care and should wear heavy-duty gloves when collecting sharps containers.

Guidance on proper disposal of sharps

- It is the *personal responsibility of the individual using a sharp* to dispose of it safely as soon as possible after use. Where the specific clinical procedure prevents the user from doing this, the user still retains overall responsibility for ensuring the safe disposal of used sharps.
- Used needles and syringes *must not* be disposed of in domestic waste. Health care staff who treat patients at home should place any sharps and syringes that they generate in appropriate containers for disposal through their employer's clinical waste disposal system or via collection as appropriate.
- Needles and syringes should be discarded as a single unit into a designated sharps box. Glass slides, glass drug ampoules, razors, disposable scissors, and IV cannulae must be discarded into a sharps box.

- When syringes containing arterial blood are to be sent to the laboratory, needles should be removed and the nozzles of the syringes sealed by means of a luer rubber cap or a blunt hub on the syringe nozzle.

- If a sharp has been accidentally dropped, it must be recovered and disposed of properly. If the search is unsuccessful, the individual should ensure that other people using the area are informed so that they can take care. It is particularly important to notify cleaning staff of the possible danger. The person in charge of the area should be notified and a record kept until the sharp has been found and disposed of properly.

- When an injury occurs with a contaminated sharp, bleeding should be encouraged and the site should be washed under running water. The injury must be reported to the line manager without delay and should be dealt with according to the written protocols (see Chapter 16, 'Management of Sharps injuries').

Management and disposal of clinical waste

Of all the categories comprising clinical medical waste, microbiological waste and sharps waste pose the greatest risk for infections. On-site incineration should be considered for microbiological, pathological, and anatomical waste (see below), provided the incinerator is engineered to completely burn these wastes and stay within local emissions standards. Improper incineration of waste with high moisture and low energy content (e.g. pathology waste), can lead to polluting emission problems. Contaminated sharps and related waste can be disposed of by incineration or by 'alternative technologies' to incineration—this can be less costly and less polluting (see below).

Some clinical waste may be considered for disinfection and subsequent transfer to landfill. Laboratory waste known or likely to contain Hazard Group 3 and 4 pathogens should be made safe either by autoclaving within the laboratory or in the case of an autoclave malfunction, should be packaged in accordance with the approved requirements for carriage, and transferred to an incinerator as soon as possible. Laboratory waste should not be allowed to accumulate for more than 24 hours.

The contents of disposable items such as bedpans and urinals may be discharged to the sewer via the sluice, WC, or purpose-built disposal unit. These items do not normally fall within the definition of infectious waste for transport purposes and therefore do not have to be packaged in UN type approved containers. Offensive waste should be transferred to landfill.

Household waste is disposed of by landfill or other locally acceptable means and may be compacted. Infectious or other hazardous health care waste must not be compacted prior to disposal. Anatomical waste (e.g. human tissue, limbs, and placentas) must be disposed of by incineration or according to the local legislative requirements.

Clinical waste is treated or decontaminated to reduce the microbial load and to render the by-products safe for further handling and disposal by landfill. Historically, treatment methods involved steam-sterilization (autoclaving), incineration, or interment (for anatomical waste). Alternative treatment methods developed in recent years include (but are not limited to) chemical disinfection, grinding/shredding/disinfection methods, energy-based technologies (e.g. microwave or radiowave treatments), and disinfection/encapsulation methods. Whatever method is used, it should render waste safe and render sharps un-reusable.

Kitchen and catering services

Food service establishments are frequently identified as places where mishandling of food has led to outbreaks of food poisoning. Hospitals and other health care facilities represent a special case of food service operation. The need for adequate food hygiene facilities is of paramount importance, since the consequences of an outbreak of food poisoning in a health care facility can be life threatening for susceptible patients. Therefore, particular care must be taken to minimize the risk of infection or intoxication through the food service system.

The catering manager has the responsibility for catering services. Conformance to safety systems (see 'Hazards analysis critical control point' below) is a constant requirement and aspects should be audited according to the schedule within the components of that system. Hospital administrators are responsible for food hygiene in hospitals and should ensure that a full independent audit is carried out at least twice yearly. Full reports of these inspections should be submitted to the health care facility administrator and the hospital infection control committee.

Preparation of food requires attention to raw materials, personal hygiene, kitchen hygiene, and especially time/temperature control of all food-handling operations including cooking, cooling, reheating, and distribution (see Box 18.1). Assuring safe food requires management and control of microbiological, chemical, and physical hazards.

Hazards analysis critical control point

It is recommended that food service departments in health care establishments take the hazards analysis critical control point (HACCP) approach to the food safety programme instead of the traditional approach based only on cooking procedures (recipe-based), as the latter may not address all the steps that a food product passes through, including receipt of goods, meal service, and distribution. The HACCP approach has been used widely in the food industry and this concept evolved at NASA (the US National Aeronautics and Space Agency) laboratories with the aim of guaranteeing that the food provided for astronauts was not contaminated microbiologically, chemically, or physically in a way that would lead to either a space mission failure or catastrophe. HACCP is a powerful process which focuses control at seven points in a process which are critical to the safety of the end product. The systematic approach of HACCP helps analyse potential hazards and identifies the points where hazards may occur. Once the changes are implemented, it must be *reviewed periodically*. An integral part of a properly constructed HACCP plan is the existence of good manufacturing practice throughout the food service chain. This includes factors that have become known as prerequisite or support programmes, including supplier control, cleaning and sanitation, personal hygiene, and staff training. All food must comply with relevant local food safety acts and the food hygiene regulations of the country involved.

Box 18.1 The commonest causes of food poisoning

- ◆ Preparing food too long in advance.
- ◆ Storing perishable food at ambient temperatures.
- ◆ Cooling food too slowly before placing in refrigerator.
- ◆ Not reheating food to temperatures at which food poisoning bacteria can be destroyed.
- ◆ Using contaminated food.
- ◆ Undercooking meat, meat products and poultry.
- ◆ Not thawing frozen poultry and meat for long enough.
- ◆ Cross-contamination between raw and cooked food.
- ◆ Keeping hot food below 63°C.
- ◆ Infected food handlers.

With permission from Barrie D. The provision of food and catering services in hospital. *Journal of Hospital Infection* 1996; **33**:13–33.

General measures

Hospital kitchen

The kitchen should have an agreed cleaning procedure and schedule for all items that may need cleaning. Methods, materials, and occurrence should be defined locally. Cleaning materials should be stored in a designated area. Good practice includes the use of separate bays for each task, colour-coded cloths, and satisfactory cleaning of colour-coded knives and chopping boards, and preparation surfaces. Food stores should be generally clean, uncluttered, and with good access to allow cleaning (no items stored on the ground and sufficient space under shelving to permit cleaning underneath). Shelving should be easy to clean. Any food capable of supporting microbial growth should be stored either *below* 8°C or *above* 63°C. Cook-chilled food should be stored *below* 3°C. Deep frozen food should be at −18°C or below; chilled food should be between 0°C and +3°C (see Box 18.2).

Food handlers

All food handlers should complete a pre-employment questionnaire, which should be reviewed by a person competent to assess the implications of any positive answers and decide if examination of faecal specimens is necessary. Pre-employment stool testing is not generally required in the absence of a history of enteric fever. All food handlers with infections (e.g. boils on the fingers) or suspected gastrointestinal infection *must stop working* and report to their manager *immediately*. Return to work depends on whether it is considered safe, usually by the occupational health department, but the opinion of the microbiologist and/or IPC doctor may also be sought.

Box 18.2 General rules of food hygiene

Delivery	◆ Accept frozen food below −18°C
	◆ Accept chilled food below +13°C
	◆ Check 'within date' code
	◆ Check state of packaging
Storage	◆ Practice stock rotation
	◆ Provide clean, dry, pest-free conditions
	◆ Keep at correct temperatures
	◆ Keep covered until required
	◆ Keep raw food separately from cooked items
	◆ Use separate utensils, surfaces
	◆ Wash hands between different food
Thawing	◆ Thaw below 15°C
	◆ Thaw completely
	◆ Cook within 24 h
Cooking	◆ Ensure centre of food reaches 70°C for 2 min
	◆ Cook on the day of consumption or chill rapidly and refrigerate within 1.5 h. Consume within 3 days
	◆ Hold below 10°C or above 63°C
Reheating	◆ Avoid, if possible
	◆ Reheat rapidly
	◆ Attain 70°C (use temperature probe)
Distribution	◆ Hot food above 63°C
	◆ Cold food below 10°C
	◆ Check with temperature probe
Waste	◆ Discard unwanted food after 1h
	◆ Always cover food waste
Cleaning maintenance	◆ Observe schedules for all items
	◆ Ensure good state of service and repair

With permission from Barrie D. The provision of food and catering services in hospital. *Journal of Hospital Infection* 1996; **33**:13–33.

Although catering staff are mainly responsible for providing food in hospitals, nursing and domestic staff are also involved in distributing or serving meals to patients. Everyone who handles, prepares, processes, and distributes food *must understand* the principles of basic food hygiene and *should be trained* in personal and catering hygiene methods.

Refrigerators

Under any circumstances, refrigerators used for storage of food items *must not* be used for storage of other items, e.g. contaminated material, including clinical specimens, or for storage of medical products such as drugs, vaccines, or blood and blood products. Medications and vaccines should be stored in accordance with manufacturers' instructions.

Vaccines (and other medications) requiring refrigeration should be stored in a refrigerator dedicated to vaccine storage. Blood and other clinical specimens requiring refrigeration should also have a dedicated refrigerator for storage.

Food trolleys

In hospitals and large health care establishments, mechanical transport can make it easier to distribute equipment and also reduce the movement of people, thus minimizing the spread of infection. Food trolleys should be of suitable height to allow good visibility during use, be appropriate for the type of transport, and should be enclosed or draped. They should be cleaned daily or more frequently if contamination occurs.

Ward kitchen

Ward kitchens or food-handling areas and the staff using them should observe the same levels of food and personal hygiene as other food handlers. There should be specific written cleaning and waste disposal policies. These should comply with written codes of practice for food handling in ward kitchens. Ward refrigerators, dishwashers, microwave ovens, and ice-making machines are used by nursing staff, domestic staff, and visitors, and are often used incorrectly. Ward kitchen refrigerators should be used solely for patients' food and never for medicines and other products. Ice-making machines should be purchased in consultation with the IPC team and a planned maintenance and cleaning protocol should be drawn up (see Box 18.3).

Texture-modified products

Texture-modified meals, which are provided to people with chewing and/or swallowing problems, also have a greater risk of bacterial contamination. This includes all food that has been pureed or minced *after* cooking. Where possible, food should be pureed *before* cooking. Where this is not possible, for example with pureed fruit, particular care must be taken to minimize cross-contamination. Strict time and temperature control must also be maintained.

Cook-chill food production systems

There has been an increasing trend in health care establishments to use 'cook-chill' food service systems to extend the life of prepared food products. The time and temperature control of product chilling and subsequent storage and handling is critical in cook-chill systems because bacteria can grow in the extended time between food production and consumption. The storage temperature for cook-chill systems should be 0°C, which is lower than that required for conventional cold storage. The storage time (shelf life) also needs to be closely monitored and may vary according to the production method used as well as the storage temperature (storage below 0°C controls the growth of most pathogenic bacteria).

Ice machines

Ice from contaminated ice machines has been associated with patient infection. Microorganisms may be present in ice, ice storage chests and ice-making machines.

The two main sources of microorganisms in ice are: 1) the potable water from which it is made, and 2) transfer of microorganisms from hands during dispensing of ice.

Currently, there are no microbiological standards for ice, ice-making machines, or ice storage equipment. However, it is important to clean ice storage chests at least monthly, with more frequent cleanings recommended for open chests. Portable ice chests and containers require cleaning and low-level disinfection before the addition of ice intended for consumption. Ice-making machines may also be contaminated via improper storage or handling of ice by patients and/or staff. Suggested steps to avoid this means of contamination include:

◆ Minimizing or avoiding direct hand contact with ice intended for consumption.

◆ Using a hard-surface scoop to dispense ice.

◆ Installing machines that dispense ice directly into portable containers at the touch of a control.

All ice machines must regularly be maintained and steps should be taken to clean and disinfect the ice machines and log book should be maintained for service and repair. General steps to maintain ice machines are summarized in Box 18.3.

Culturing of ice machines is not routinely recommended but may be useful as part of an epidemiological investigation. If the source water for ice in a health care facility is not faecally contaminated, then ice from clean ice machines and chests should pose

Box 18.3 General steps to maintain ice machines

◆ Disconnect the ice machine from the power supply.

◆ Remove and discard the ice.

◆ Disassemble the removable parts of the machine that make contact with water to make ice.

◆ Thoroughly clean the machine and all the parts.

◆ Check for any needed repair.

◆ Ensure the presence of an air space in the tubing that leads from the water inlet into the water distribution system of the machine.

◆ Inspect for rodent or insect infestations under the machine and treat if necessary.

◆ Check door gaskets (open compartment models) for evidence of leakage or dripping into the storage chest.

◆ Clean the ice-storage chest.

◆ Disinfect the machine by circulating with a diluted hypochlorite (50–100ppm av Cl_2) solution through the ice-making and storage systems (suggested contact time: 4 h for 50 ppm av Cl_2 solution, 2 h for 100 ppm av Cl_2 solution).

◆ Drain the chlorine solution, and flush with fresh tap water.

◆ Allow the ice-storage chest to dry, and return to service.

no special hazard for immunocompetent patients. Some waterborne bacteria found in ice could potentially be a risk to immunocompromised patients if they consume ice or drink beverages with ice.

Linen and laundry services

UK National Health Service guidelines (NHS Executive, 1995) recommend that linen (defined as all articles for laundering) should be divided into three categories:

- **Used linen** (which has been used) which can include fouled and blood stained linen from patients not considered to have infectious organisms or communicable diseases.

- **Infectious linen** is contaminated with microorganisms that represent an infection hazard to those workers who may come into contact with it. Within infectious linen, it is possible to identify a 'high-risk' group where the diseases involved are transmitted through a low infectious dose of organisms, e.g. *Escherichia coli* 0157, shigellosis, etc. Infested linen from patients infested with lice, fleas, etc. should be handled as infected linen. It is important that the laundry is notified to ensure special arrangements are instigated.

- **Heat-labile**. Linen which is made from fabrics likely to be damaged by the normal heat disinfection process, usually personal clothing

In addition, linen originating from patients with anthrax, viral haemorrhagic fevers and other category 4 pathogens should be bagged in yellow clinical waste bags and incinerated.

Although soiled linen may be contaminated with microorganisms, the risk of disease transmission is negligible if it is handled, transported, and laundered in a manner that avoids dispersal of microorganisms. Infection in laundry workers after handling soiled linen has only rarely been reported, and is usually ascribed to improper handling practices. However, it is essential that all personnel involved in the collection, transport, sorting, and washing of soiled linen should be *adequately trained and wear appropriate PPE*. All workers must cover all lesions on exposed skin with waterproof plasters and wear appropriate gloves. Gloves used for the task of sorting laundry should be of sufficient thickness to minimize sharps injuries. They *must* have access to hand washing facilities.

Inadvertent disposal of objects that may harm laundry workers or damage laundry items or machines (sharps and non-laundry items such as surgical instruments) in linen is a common problem. Therefore all staff are urged not to let these objects become mixed with laundry at the point of packaging and to search for and safely remove these items before processing.

If the health care facilities have decided to outsource provision of laundry services, then it is important that the IPC team should be involved in the contract-setting process for provision of such services.

General considerations

Laundry bags

Single bags of sufficient tensile strength are adequate for containing laundry; leak-proof containment is needed if the laundry is wet and can soak through a cloth bag. They must only be two-thirds filled to allow secure closure. Bags containing soiled laundry should be clearly identified with labels; colour-coding should meet the local policy so that HCWs may handle these items safely, regardless of whether the laundry is transported within the facility or destined for transport to an off-site laundry service. The recommended colour coding is white bags for used linen, red bags (or white bags with a red stripe for patients' clothing) for infected linen, and orange bags for heat-labile linen.

Infected linen should be placed in an impervious bag that can be emptied into a washing machine with no or minimal handling and the bag either decontaminated in the washing process or disposed of as infectious health care waste.

Segregation

Infectious linen should be *segregated at the point of generation* and care should be taken to ensure that only this type of linen is placed in the container. Bags containing infectious linen should be sealed, with a label indicating the point of origin attached.

Sorting

After removal, soiled and infected linen must be handled with care at all times. It should be placed into bags (or other appropriate containers) at the point of generation as soon as possible. Bags must be securely tied or otherwise closed to prevent leakage. Rinsing soiled laundry at the point of generation should not be done. Used linen can be sorted by staff using safe methods of work and appropriate PPE before washing. Infectious linen must not be sorted and loaded into a washing machine with no or only minimal handling. Both these categories of linen receive identical thermal disinfection; the designation of some linen as 'infectious' is only to minimize workers' contact with it.

Transport

Clean and used linen should *never* be transported or moved around a ward in the same bag or storage receptacle. There should be separate, designated bags and storage receptacles for clean and used linen.

Soiled linen in bags can be transported by cart or chute. Loose, soiled pieces of laundry should not be tossed into chutes. Clean laundry should be transported *such that it is not contaminated by used or infectious linen.* Clean linen must be wrapped or transported in a closed container specifically for clean linen prior to transport to prevent inadvertent contamination from dust and dirt during loading, delivery, and unloading, but the same vehicle can be used to both collect and deliver clean linen if suitable internal separation is used.

Storage

Clean linen should be stored in a clean area of the ward in closed cupboard. They *must* be stored separate from used/soiled linen and must not be stored within the sluice or bathroom.

Laundry process

Linen and clothing used in health care facilities are disinfected during laundering and generally rendered free of vegetative pathogens (hygienically clean), but they are not sterile. Washing machines in health care facilities can be either washer/extractor units or continuous batch machines. A typical washing cycle consists of three main phases, i.e. pre-wash, main wash, and rinse cycle.

The antimicrobial action of the laundering process results from a combination of cleaning (removal by dilution) and microbiocidal components. Dilution and agitation in water removes significant quantities of microorganisms. Soaps and detergents loosen soil allowing efficient dilution. Heat from the washing machine and from drying and ironing are effective in destroying microorganisms.

For used and infected linen, the washing process should have a disinfection cycle in which the temperature in the load is maintained at 65°C for not less than 10 min or, preferably, at 71°C for not less than 3 min. Additional time is recommended to allow mixing and heat penetration. Heat-labile linen is likely to be damaged by these temperatures and is processed in a cooler wash with the addition of certain chemicals, e.g. sodium hypochlorite.

In the absence of agreed standards, routine microbiological sampling of cleaned linen is not recommended. Sampling may be used as part of an outbreak investigation if epidemiological evidence suggests linen or clothing as a vehicle for disease transmission. Hygienically clean linen is suitable for neonatal intensive care units. The use of sterile linen in burns units remains unresolved.

Low-temperature wash

Although hot-water washing is an effective laundry disinfection method, the cost can be significantly high. Laundries are typically the largest users of hot water in hospitals, consuming between 50–75% of the total hot water. Several studies have shown that lower water temperatures can satisfactorily reduce microbial contamination when the cycling of the washer, the wash-detergent, and the amount of bleach are carefully monitored and controlled.

Low-temperature laundry cycles rely heavily on the presence of chlorine or oxygen-activated bleach to reduce the levels of microbial contamination. Regardless of whether hot or cold water is used for washing, the temperatures reached in drying and especially during ironing provide additional significant microbiocidal action.

Dry cleaning

The dry cleaning process involves organic solvents such as perchloroethylene for soil removal and is used for linen that might be damaged in conventional water and detergent washing. A number of studies have shown that dry cleaning alone is relatively ineffective in reducing the numbers of microorganisms on contaminated linen.

Although a number of microorganisms are significantly reduced when dry cleaned articles are heat pressed, dry cleaning should not be used routinely. It should be reserved only for fabrics which cannot be safely cleaned with water and detergent.

Home washing machine

The recommended standard for hospital laundering cannot be applied to domestic laundering as the majority of domestic washing machines operate at 40–60°C. However, it has been judged to be suitable for staff uniforms as these are only used to identify staff and are not personal protective equipment. If staff uniforms do become grossly contaminated, they should be washed with 'used' or 'infected' hospital linen as appropriate and not washed domestically.

Pest control

Every effort must be made to achieve a reasonable level of control of or the eradication of pests. Hospital management is responsible for ensuring that the premises are free from pests. Each health care facility should have a pest control programme. This may be contracted to an *approved* pest control contractor.

Cockroaches, flies, maggots, ants, mosquitoes, spiders, mites, midges, and mice are among the typical arthropod and vertebrate pest populations found in health care facilities. Insects can serve as agents for the mechanical transmission of microorganisms, or as active participants in the disease transmission process by serving as vectors. Arthropods recovered from health care facilities have been shown to carry a wide variety of pathogenic microorganisms.

Apart from the possibility of disease transmission, food may be tainted and spoiled, fabric and building structure damaged. Pharaoh's ants have been responsible for the penetration of sterile packs and the invasion of patients' dressings, including those in use on a wound. Cockroaches can carry a wide variety of pathogens including food poisoning bacteria. Cockroaches, in particular, have been known to feed on fixed sputum smears in laboratories. Insects need to be kept out of all areas of the health care facility, but this is especially important for the operating rooms and any area where immunosuppressed patients are located.

Hospital kitchens, boiler rooms, ducts, and drains provide warmth, water, food, and shelter for cockroaches, pharaoh's ants and other pests. In addition, insects also feed on food scraps from kitchens/cafeterias, foods in vending machines, discharges on dressings either in use or discarded, medical waste, human waste, and routine solid waste. Both cockroaches and ants are frequently found in the laundry, central sterile supply department, or anywhere in the facility where water or moisture is present (e.g. sink traps, drains, cleaning staff closets).

From a public health and hygiene perspective, it is reasonable to control and eradicate arthropod and vertebrate pests from all indoor environments, including health care facilities.

Modern approaches to institutional pest management usually focus on:

◆ Eliminating food sources, indoor habitats, and other conditions that attract pests.

◆ Excluding pests from the indoor environments.

- Monitoring for the presence of pests.
- Applying pesticides as needed.

Sealing windows in modern health care facilities helps to minimize insect intrusion. It is essential that older buildings should be of sound structure and well maintained. Cracks in plaster and woodwork, unsealed areas around pipe work, damaged tiles, badly fitted equipment and kitchen units are all likely to provide excellent points of entry or refuge for pests. The drains should be covered, and any leaking pipe work repaired.

Close-fitted windows and doors, fly screens, and bird netting will help to exclude pests from hospitals and other health care facilities. When windows need to be opened for ventilation, ensuring that screens are in good repair and closing doors to the outside can help with pest control. Pests require food, warmth, moisture, refuge, and a means of entry; hospital staff should be encouraged to keep food covered, to remove spillage and waste, and to avoid accumulations of static water.

Prevention of infection after death

The overall principle of after-death procedures is to present the body in an aesthetically acceptable state for the bereaved to pay their last respects and to proceed with their after-death procedures or ceremonies. As a general rule, standard infection control precautions should be continued after death. If the person has died of a communicable disease, the risk of transmitting infection is less from droplet and/or airborne transmission as the deceased person is no longer breathing, sneezing, or coughing. The risk of transmission occurs mainly from contact with the infected body or when procedures such as postmortem or embalming are carried out, therefore these procedures should be avoided if possible (see Table 18.2).

If a person is known or suspected to have died of a communicable disease, it is the duty of those with knowledge of the case to ensure that those who need to handle the body, including mortuary staff, postmortem room, and funeral personnel are aware that there is a potential risk for transmission of infection. There should be an effective mechanism to ensure that this *confidential information* is communicated *only* to appropriate staff who are at risk.

Last offices should be performed according to the local hospital guidance and the following infection control guidance should be incorporated to prevent transmission of infections:

- Standard infection control precautions must be observed by clinical staff in the performance of last offices.
- Where there is a danger of infection, a notification as to any additional infection control precautions should be attached to the body in a way which is clearly visible and also to the outside of the body bag and with the identification forms.
- **Body bags:** body bags should *not* be used routinely for the transport of bodies as the bodies cool more slowly inside a body bag, which increase the rate of decomposition and making hygienic preparation more difficult and render a body unpleasant to view. However, their use should be considered to contain leakage of blood and body fluids in transit which cannot be contained by any other method.

Table 18.2 Guidelines for handling cadavers with infections

Degree of risk of Infection	Infectious diseases	Bagging	Viewing	Embalming	Hygiene preparation
Low	Acute encephalitis	No	Yes	Yes	Yes
	Chickenpox/shingles	No	Yes	Yes	Yes
	Cryptosporidiosis	No	Yes	Yes	Yes
	Dermatophytosis	No	Yes	Yes	Yes
	Legionellosis	No	Yes	Yes	Yes
	Lyme disease	No	Yes	Yes	Yes
	Measles	No	Yes	Yes	Yes
	Meningitis (except meningococcal)	No	Yes	Yes	Yes
	Mumps	No	Yes	Yes	Yes
	Meticillin-resistant *Staphylococcus aureus* (MRSA)	No	Yes	Yes	Yes
	Ophthalmia neonatorum	No	Yes	Yes	Yes
	Orf	No	Yes	Yes	Yes
	Psittacosis	No	Yes	Yes	Yes
	Rubella	No	Yes	Yes	Yes
	Tetanus	No	Yes	Yes	Yes
	Whooping cough	No	Yes	Yes	Yes
Medium	Acute poliomyelitis	No	Yes	Yes*	Yes
	Cholera	No	Yes	Yes*	Yes
	Diphtheria	Adv	Yes	Yes*	Yes
	Dysentery	Adv	Yes	Yes	Yes
	Food poisoning	No	Yes	Yes	Yes
	Hepatitis A	No	Yes	Yes	Yes
	HIV/AIDS	Yes only if bleeding	Yes	No	Yes
	Leptospirosis (Weil's disease)	No	Yes	Yes	Yes
	Malaria	No	Yes	Yes	Yes
	Paratyphoid fever	Adv	Yes	Yes	Yes
	Q fever	No	Yes	Yes	Yes

(continued)

Table 18.2 (*continued*)

Degree of risk of Infection	Infectious diseases	Bagging	Viewing	Embalming	Hygiene preparation
	Relapsing fever	Adv	Yes	Yes	Yes
	Meningococcal septicaemia	Adv	Yes	Yes*	Yes
	Scarlet fever	Adv	Yes	Yes*	Yes
	Tuberculosis	Adv	Yes	Yes*	Yes
	Typhoid fever	Adv	Yes	Yes	Yes
	Typhus	Adv	No	No	No
High	Anthrax	Adv	No	No	No
	CJD and TSE	Yes	Yes	No	Yes
	Group A streptococcal infection (invasive)	No	Yes	Yes*	Yes
	Hepatitis B and C	Yes	Yes	No	Yes
	Plague	Yes	No	No	No
	Rabies	Yes	No	No	No
	Smallpox	Yes	No	No	No
	Viral haemorrhagic fever	Yes	No	No	No
	Yellow fever	Yes	No	No	No

Adapted with permission from Healing TD, Hoffman PN and Young SE. The infection hazards of human. Cadavers. *Communicable Diseases Reviews* 1995; **5**(5):R61–68. With corrections published in *CDR Review* **5**(6):R92.

*Requires particular care during embalming

Adv: advisable and may be required by local health regulations

Bagging: placing the body in a plastic body bag

Viewing: allowing the bereaved to see, touch and spend time with the body before disposal;

Embalming: injecting chemical preservatives into the body to slow the process of decay. Cosmetic work may be included

Hygienic preparation: cleaning and tidying the body so it presents a suitable appearance for viewing (an alternative to embalming)

♦ For aesthetic it is necessary that the body must be kept in cold conditions. This can be achieved by keeping the body in refrigeration and it is essential to minimize the number of times the remains are removed from cold storage. This can be done by minimizing and controlling the viewing times. If refrigeration is not available, the body can be kept cool using a cold table and instilling air chillers. Storage of bodies at 6°C is recommended provided that the bodies are to be held for less than 48 hours; for longer-term storage, the bodies should be kept at 5°C or lower.

♦ In certain circumstances, infectious diseases (e.g. cases of anthrax and smallpox) which may survive for significant periods of time in the deceased and burial site may act as a source of infection and records of such bodies should be kept in the parish.

◆ **Postmortem examination:** the principles of safe practice for the mortuary must be adhered to irrespective of the infective state of the body. A full postmortem should not be done merely to confirm the cause of death. When a postmortem is carried out on such patients, all those concerned must be suitably informed and trained in safe procedures. They must follow local written protocol. Strict banning of eating, smoking or drinking *must be enforced* within work areas.

◆ **Funeral parlours:** the workrooms of funeral parlours must be of a standard acceptable as per local regulations. Strict banning of eating, smoking, or drinking must be enforced within work areas. Staff with broken skin/lesions (e.g. abrasions, cuts, severe eczema, or other skin conditions) should report to their supervisor and use impermeable waterproof dressings to cover the lesions. Staff with uncovered skin lesions or cuts should not work on bodies where infection is likely. Any action that will bring a staff member's hands in contact with their face whilst undertaking an embalming procedure should be avoided.

◆ **Routine hygienic preparation** of the body after death includes washing the face and hands, closing the eyes and mouth, tidying the hair, and sometime shaving the face. It also includes plugging orifices to prevent discharges, or covering any wounds. In some cultures, relatives expect to carry out the ritual preparation before burial and this can be permitted under supervison and use of appropriate precautions should be agreed with religious authorities.

◆ **Visitors** should be subject to the same rules of hygiene and must be supervised if in the workroom. Viewing and touching the face may also be permitted except where there is a risk of infection and appropriate advice should be given.

◆ **Embalming** is done for preservation of the body from decay by injecting solutions containing formaldehyde. This is an invasive procedure as it involves replacing blood with a preservative (embalming) solution. Since this procedure involves extensive contact with blood and body fluids and use of sharps instruments, it therefore carries a risk of infection and should be avoided in patients with infectious diseases (See Table 18.2 for guidance).

Environmental procedures and issues

◆ Body fluids and other contaminated liquids may be discharged into the drainage system, but as far as practical, this should be disinfected before discharge. However, it is important to note that due to very high organic load of these liquids, any disinfection process will be of poor quality.

◆ All non-liquid waste should be put into hazardous infectious waste (yellow) bags, transported, and disposed of by incineration or an acceptable licensed company.

◆ All instruments should be cleaned in warm (not hot) water and detergent. Running water should *not* be used as it facilitates splashing. Instruments should then be cleaned and disinfected according to local policy.

◆ All *spills of blood or other body fluids* should be cleaned up promptly and steps must be taken to minimize the risk of splashes and droplets and appropriate PPE e.g. face shield, gloves, and plastic apron should be used. Blood spills should be soaked up by using hypochlorite granules and the spillage mopped up promptly with disposable paper towels (see Chapter 6, Box 6.5). The granules or towels should be scraped/soaked up and placed in a yellow clinical (infectious) waste bag. The area should then be cleaned with general purpose detergent and hot water. For general cleaning of the environment, a general purpose detergent and hot water is preferred.

◆ Hypochlorite (bleach) is corrosive to metals and should *not be used* in the presence of formaldehyde as there is evidence that hypochlorites can react with formaldehyde to produce bis-chloromethyl ether which is a carcinogen. In addition, chlorine-releasing granules must not be used as when they come into contact with urine, chlorine fumes may be released which may lead to respiratory problems. In this situation, an absorbent substance *without hypochlorite* should be used.

◆ Appropriate national regulations (e.g. Control of Substances Hazardous to Health [COSHH] in the UK) must be followed at all times both by those who handle and prepare the body for burial or cremation and by those who have contact with or view the body.

Key references and further reading

Management of clinical waste

CDC/HICPAC. Guidelines for environmental infection control in health-care facilities: recommendations of CDC and the Healthcare Infection Control Practices Advisory Committee. *Morbidity and Mortality Weekly Report* 2003; **52**(RR-10):1–48.

Department of Health. *Health Technical Memorandum 07-01*: *Safe management of healthcare waste*. London: Department of Health, 2011.

Hoffman P. Laundry, kitchens and healthcare waste. In: Fraise AP, Bradley C (eds). *Ayliffe's Control of Healthcare-associated Infection*, 3rd edn, pp.150–68. London: Hodder Arnold, 2009.

Kitchen and catering services

Barrie D. The provision of food and catering services in hospital. *Journal of Hospital Infection* 1996; **33**:13–33.

CDC/HICPAC. Guidelines for environmental infection control in healthcare facilities: recommendations of CDC and the Healthcare Infection Control Practices Advisory Committee. *Morbidity and Mortality Weekly Report* 2003; **52**(RR-10):1–48.

Department of Health. *Chilled and Frozen. Guidelines on Cook-Chill and Cook-Freeze Catering systems*. London: HMSO, 1989.

Department of Health. *Food handlers: Fitness to work*. London: Department of Health, 1995.

Hoffman P. Laundry, kitchens and healthcare waste. In: Fraise AP, Bradley C (eds). *Ayliffe's Control of Healthcare-associated Infection*, 3rd edn, pp.150–68. London: Hodder Arnold, 2009.

Hoffman P. Disinfection and cleaning. In: McLauchlin J, Little C (eds). *Hobbs' Food Poisoning and Food Hygiene*. 7th edn, pp.233–44. London: Hodder Arnold, 2007.

McLauchlin J, Little C (eds). *Hobbs' Food Poisoning and Food Hygiene*, 7th edn. London: Edward Arnold, 2007.

WHO. *Hazard Analysis Critical Control Point Evaluation. A guide to identifying hazards and assessing risks associated with food preparation and storage*. Geneva: World Health Organization, 1992.

Linen and laundry services

Barrie D. How hospital linen and laundry services are provided. *Journal of Hospital Infection* 1994; **27**:219–39.

British Standards Institution. *EN 14065:2002. Textiles – laundry processed textiles- biocontamination control system.* Milton Keynes: British Standards Institution, 2002.

Department of Health. *Uniforms and workwear. Guidance on uniform and workwear policies for NHS employers.* London: Department of Health, 2010.

NHS Executive. *HSG (95)18. Hospital laundry arrangements for used and infected linen.* London: NHSE, 1995.

Patel SN, Murray-Leonard J, Wilson AP. Laundering of hospital staff uniforms at home. *Journal of Hospital Infection* 2006; **62**:89–93.

Wilson JA, Loveday HP, Hoffman PN, *et al.* Uniform: an evidence review of the microbiological significance of uniforms and uniform policy in the prevention and control of healthcare-associated infections. Report to the Dept. of Health. *Journal of Hospital Infection* 2007; **66**:301–7.

Prevention of infection after death

Healing TD, Hoffman PN, Young SE. The infection hazards of human cadavers. *Communicable Diseases Reviews* 1995; **5**(5):R61–68. With corrections published in *CDR Review* 5(6):R92.

Health & Safety Executive. *Safe working and the prevention of infection in the mortuary and post-mortem room,* 2nd edn. Norwich: HSE, 2003.

Health & Safety Executive. *Controlling the risks of infection at work from human remains. A guide for those involved in funeral services (including embalmers) and those involved in exhumation.* Norwich: HSE, 2005.

Hoffman PN, Healing TJ, Young SEJ. The infection hazards of human cadavers. In: Wenzel R, Brewer T and Butzler J-P (eds) *A Guide to Infection Control in the Hospital.* 3rd edn. Boston, MA: International Society for Infectious Diseases, 2008.

Chapter 19

Health estates

A hospital can be a very dangerous place to be sick.

Curtis Donskey

The provision of a safe environment within health care premises is a statutory obligation and must be part of the risk management strategy of the hospital. The environment in which patients are nursed must be designed to reduce the risk of transmission of infection to a minimum.

Advances in medical treatment have changed the types of patients being admitted to hospital. Currently patients with impaired host defences represent an increasing proportion of admissions to hospital and to reflect that, the design of health care facilities has undergone substantial changes. From an infection control perspective, the primary objective of hospital design should be to ensure that patients are at no greater risk of infection within the hospital than outside. Microbial flora within a health care facility can be influenced by its design and the IPC team plays a major role in this.

It is essential that along with the physicians and nurses from the units, and the designated members of the projects teams, the IPC team must also be involved in the design, construction, and commissioning of any new or upgraded building or health care facility at an *early stage*. Equally important is the engagement of the IPC team when major renovation or demolition work is being planned as such situations can represent a risk to patient safety through the heavy release of fungi into the air. Therefore input from the IPC team at the planning stage and through the entire life of the project is essential to ensure that the new health care premises meet with infection control requirements. Early involvement of the IPC team in the process is essential to identify potential infection control issues early and provides an opportunity to design solutions prospectively. The IPC team also plays an important role in educating architects, engineers, and construction workers about potential infection control risks and appropriate methods for reducing them. It is also important that the IPC team should visit the construction site on a regular basis to ensure that agreed plans are being adequately implemented. It is the responsibility of the project team to ensure that the policies and procedures set forth by the IPC team are incorporated into the contract.

The general hospital environment

Functional design of health care facilities should allow routine cleaning to be carried out efficiently. Surfaces, including walls, must be smooth, easy to clean, and protected from damage. Unnecessary horizontal, textured, and moisture-retaining surfaces, or inaccessible areas where moisture or soil will accumulate, *should be avoided*. Where possible, all surfaces should be smooth and impervious.

To prevent dust accumulation, *cupboards* rather than open shelves are recommended and cupboard doors should be easily washable. Consideration must be given to the design of radiators and other fixed or relatively immovable items, e.g. computer stations and their wiring, to ensure that all surfaces are accessible for cleaning. When furnishings and fittings are being selected, it is essential that they *must be durable enough* to withstand cleaning and disinfectant use in the health care facilities. Items intended for domestic use are frequently inappropriate for the hospital setting. In equipment-processing areas, work surfaces should be non-porous, smooth, and easily cleaned.

Walls and ceilings

Ideally, walls and ceilings should have a smooth, impervious surface that is easy to clean with minimal likelihood of dust accumulation. In general, pathogenic microorganisms do not readily adhere to walls or ceilings unless the surface becomes moist, sticky, or damaged. Little evidence exists that walls and ceilings are a significant source of HCAIs. Wall coverings should be fluid resistant and easily cleaned, especially in areas where contact with blood or body fluids may occur, i.e. delivery suite, operating rooms, laboratories, etc. Finishing around plumbing fixtures should be smooth and water resistant. In addition, pipe penetrations and joints should be tightly sealed. If the tiles are used then they should not get wet as wet tiles support microbial growth and therefore they must be replaced as soon as possible. False ceilings may harbour dust and pests that may contaminate the environment if disturbed and should be avoided in high-risk areas unless adequately sealed.

Floor

Bacteria on hospital floors predominantly consist of skin microorganisms, e.g. coagulase-negative staphylococci, *Bacillus* spp., and diphtheroids; however, *Staphylococcus aureus* and *Clostridium* spp. can also be cultured. It is important to note that the infection risk from contaminated floors is small. Gram-negative bacteria are rarely found on dry floors, but may be present after cleaning or a spill when the floor is wet. All floors should have non-slip finishes. In clinical areas, floors should be made of smooth, impermeable, seamless materials, such as welded vinyl. Flooring should be able to be easily cleaned, in good repair, and water resistant.

Carpet

Carpet harbours large numbers of microorganisms, e.g. coagulase-negative staphylococci, *Bacillus* spp., fungi, vancomycin-resistant enterococci (VRE), and MRSA. Therefore, their use in clinical areas should be avoided. In addition, carpets are expensive to clean and maintain, difficult to disinfect, and become smelly with time.

If carpets are used in the health care facility, then they must be fitted with a moisture impermeable barrier. They should be well maintained to ensure that they are vacuumed daily and periodically steam cleaned. An appropriate choice of vacuum cleaner is important to minimize airborne dispersal of microorganisms (see 'Vacuum cleaner', Chapter 6).

Fixtures and fittings

All fixtures and fittings should be designed to allow easy cleaning and to discourage the accumulation of dust. When choosing material it is important to *avoid* porous or textured material. It must be *durable, easy to clean, washable* and able to withstand cleaning and disinfectant products used in the health care facilities.

Furniture

Various microorganisms have been recovered from furniture. Therefore, it is important that the furniture used by patients (beds, mattresses, chairs, tables, etc.) *must be durable enough* to withstand cleaning and disinfectant use in health care facilities. Fabrics should be avoided, especially if soiling with blood and body fluids is possible. Upholstery and protective covers must be in good repair at all times and breaches in the material must be repaired or replaced immediately.

Room curtains and blinds

Curtains must be easily washable and of a design that does not attract accumulated dust. Sufficient curtains must be purchased to enable single curtains to be replaced when soiled. There must also be a laundering programme in place, and the laundering process must not compromise the fire retardant finish. There is no evidence to show that frequent changing produces any benefit, therefore curtains need not be changed after discharge of every patient. All blinds (especially horizontal blinds) should be avoided as they have a large surface area with the potential for dust accumulation and are very difficult to clean.

Patient accommodation

Outpatient accommodation

Patient waiting areas should have provision for separating patients who may be highly infectious. A triage system should be in place to identify such patient especially in A&E departments and all suspected/confirmed infectious cases must be isolated in the A&E in a single room with an en suite toilet facility until they are transfered to other wards or department. Outpatients should have a separate room for patients with known or suspected infection. Every effort should be made to see these patients as quickly as possible to minimize contact with other patients in the waiting area.

Inpatient accommodation

To minimize the risk of cross-infection, wherever possible, restrict the number of beds per room/bay to a minimum number possible as this will greatly assist in the prevention of cross-infection. Ideally there should be only four beds per room/bay and they should act as a 'separate unit' with doors so that they can be used to cohort patients in cases of an outbreak. There should be sufficient space such that a HCW caring for one patient can do so without encroaching into another patient's bed space and allow room for hoists and other patients care items and equipment. UK NHS Estates recommend 3.6 metres between the centres of adjacent beds (NHS Estates, 2002).

Design, accessibility, and space in patient areas all contribute to ease of cleaning and maintenance and the spacing must take account of access to equipment around the bed and access for staff to hand wash facilities. Consideration can be given to permanent screens between bed spaces as an aid to prevent frequent traffic and thus avoid the potential for microorganism transfer. Shared patient accommodation should include facilities such as toilets, baths, and showers that are easy to clean and conveniently located to minimize unnecessary patient movement. Staff hand-wash basins should always be readily accessible in patient areas. Depending on the type of hospital, there should be sufficient single rooms with en suite toilet facilities, as single rooms without en suite toilet facilities are *not* ideal for isolation of infected patients.

Hand washing facilities

Hand washing is the single most important method of prevention of cross-infection in hospital. Health care facilities should have an adequate number of hand-wash basins. Each patient room, examination room, and procedure room needs at least one sink. There must be a minimum of one sink per single room and one sink per 4–6 bedded cubicles. They should be located conveniently (i.e. preferably near the entrance) for easy access by the HCW.

The hand-wash basin should be large enough to prevent splashing and splash backs should be included to prevent wall damage. They should be sealed to the wall or placed sufficiently far away from the wall to allow effective cleaning of all surfaces. The surrounding area should be made of non-porous material to resist fungal growth. The tap outflow should not point directly into the sink outlet as Gram-negative bacteria colonize 'U bends' and can be dispersed by splashing if disturbed by a stream of water. Contaminated tap water in health care facilities can be a source of cross-infection. Location of hand-wash basins in clinical areas is important to ensure that they are *not very close to the patients* to prevent contamination with microorganisms with splashes which are generated when the tap is open.

Hand-wash basins should be fitted with soap dispensers. They should be supplied with both hot and cold water (preferably with a mixer tap) to achieve the correct temperature. The tap should be fitted with a hands-off control (e.g. elbow operated or automated sensor-operated taps) to avoid contamination. If a hand-wash basin is used, then the water should be turned off using a paper towel rather than bare fingers or hands to avoid recontamination of hands. Electronically operated systems may be an acceptable option in specialized areas such as theatres. Plugs are *not* necessary, since hands should be washed only under running water.

Isolation rooms

In an acute hospital, it is essential that adequate numbers of single rooms are available for the isolation of patients with suspected/confirmed infection. It is recommended that there is at least one single room for every 4–6 beds. However, some new-build hospitals are aiming for greater than 50% single rooms, all with hand-wash basins and an en suite toilet and bathroom/shower facilities. Isolation rooms should have an anteroom which should be a minimum of 7 m². The purpose of the anteroom provides a controlled environment for donning/removal of PPE and to provide hand washing facilities.

Currently the option of having switchable ventilation from source (negative pressure) to protective (positive pressure) is *not* recommended because of the inherent difficulty of providing failsafe mechanisms and the risk of user error. Patients requiring source (negative pressure) isolation have been mistakenly placed in a protective (positive pressure) room with a subsequent spread of infection. These dual action rooms have been implicated in outbreaks when the incorrect air pressure was selected for a specific infection or patient. This design should *not* be used in new builds or refurbishments.

Source isolation room

The aim of source isolation is to prevent exogenous infections, i.e. the transfer of microorganisms from an infected/colonized patient to other staff, patients and visitors (see 'Chain of infection', Chapter 1). Most infected patients can be nursed in single rooms with en suite toilet facilities but some patients with infectious diseases which are spread by an airborne route, e.g. patients with open tuberculosis (esp. M/XDR-TB) measles and chickenpox require negative pressure ventilation. It is recommended that a *minimum* of six air changes per hour (ACH) is required for the protection of staff and visitors. However, in new buildings 12 ACHs are advised. In addition there should be adequate temperature and humidity regulation, so that windows cannot be opened and doors can be kept closed when the room is in use. The ventilation system should be designed to maintain a 15 pascal (Pa) pressure differential between rooms. The supply air system should provide 100% fresh air and *no recirculation* should be permitted. The exhaust air from isolation rooms should be vented to the exterior and extracted air should terminate in a safe location *away* from the fresh air supply inlet and ideally 1.2 metres above the highest part of the building. Where this is not possible or there are other buildings in close proximity, pre- and HEPA (high efficiency particulate air) filters should be used.

Regular maintenance and monitoring programmes must be established for ventilated rooms to ensure that the design criteria are met. Pressure and airflow must be monitored and filters must be replaced on a periodic planned basis according to written protocols. These rooms should be self-closing and the walls, windows, ceiling, floor, and penetrations are well sealed.

Patient nurse-call systems should have the capacity for direct speech between the nurse and patient. Hand-wash basins should be fitted in the anteroom and bedroom. The door of the anteroom and bedroom should be fitted with a type window to allow for visual observation of the patient. The bedroom windows should be of a double skinned, non-openable type with an electrically or manually operated blind sandwiched between the inner and outer panes of glass. The inner window panel should be lockable. The ceiling should be of a solid, non-porous type construction with no service inspection hatches. Floor finishes should be easily cleaned with a continuous coved skirting and welded joints. The surfaces should be smooth, easy to clean, and durable to appropriate hospital cleaning protocols and resistant to damage due to use of disinfectants.

Protective isolation room

The aim of *protective isolation* is the reverse of source isolation—to prevent ingress of fungal spores in the air supply system and to ensure that the only air available to breathe has been supplied via the mechanical supply system with its HEPA filter to immunosuppressed patients and therefore these rooms require positive pressure ventilation. Most immunocompromised patients can be nursed in single rooms with en suite toilet facilities; only severely immunocompromised patients, e.g. solid organ and bone marrow transplant patients, require isolation in positive pressure ventilation rooms to prevent infection especially from *Aspergillus* spp. These rooms should have a HEPA filter with the air pressure in the room positive in relation to the corridor. In addition, rooms should be tightly sealed, especially around windows. The door of the anteroom and bedroom should be fitted with a glass window to allow for visual inspection of the patient. The ceiling should be of a solid, non-porous type construction with no service inspection hatches. Floor finishes should be easily cleaned with a continuous coved skirting and welded joints. All doors should be self-closing.

Ventilation and air-conditioning

A clear distinction must be made between ventilation provided as part of environmental patient comfort and that as part of the control of infection. Air-conditioning or ventilation systems in critical areas such as operating theatres, respiratory isolation rooms, bone marrow transplant units, as well as in special treatment or procedural areas should maintain the inflow of fresh air and allow the temperature, humidity, and purity (from dust, infectious agents, and gases) of the air to be maintained within prescribed limits. Hospital air-conditioning systems must be monitored regularly and serviced by the hospital estates department and/or other accredited service technicians. Maintenance schedules must be documented and carried out according to manufacturers' recommendations.

Construction, renovation, and demolition

The association between construction and the development of aspergillosis in immunocompromised patients and the association between hospitalization and legionellosis have been known for decades. Therefore it is essential that as part of the planning process for renovation and constructing of a health care facility, an infection control risk assessment should be conducted to determine the potential risk of transmission of microorganisms within the hospital. In general, the risks can be categorized as infections transmitted by air, water, or the environment.

Environmental disturbances caused by construction, renovation, and demolition activities in and around hospitals markedly increase the airborne *Aspergillus* spp. spore counts in the indoor air, thereby increasing the risk of acquiring aspergillosis among immunocompromised patients. *Aspergillus* spp. is are ubiquitous environmental fungi and disease follows exposure to airborne fungal spores. Environmental spore counts are seasonal and large fluctuations may be observed in the outside air. Although one case of health care-associated aspergillosis is often difficult to link to a specific environmental exposure, the occurrence of temporarily clustered cases increase the likelihood that an environmental source within the facility may be identified and corrected. Therefore it is essential that all the activities related to construction, renovation, and demolition should be planned and coordinated by a multidisciplinary team to minimize the risk of airborne infection both during projects and after their completion. The IPC team should carry out a risk assessment before initiating the project to identify potential exposure of susceptible patients to dust and moisture and determine the need for dust and moisture containment measures. Microbiological sampling of air in health care facilities remains a controversial issue because of currently unresolved technical limitations and the need for substantial laboratory support. For details please consult the APIC *Toolkit: Construction and Renovation* (APIC, 2007).

Operating theatres

The purpose of mechanical ventilation in operating theatres (OTs) is to meet the following requirements:

1. **Supply of clean air:** this is achieved by supplying large amounts of clean air at positive pressure to prevent entry of contaminated air from surrounding clinical areas around the theatre. The suggested outlined of the design of operating suite areas in the descending order of cleanliness is illustrated in Figure 19.1.

2. **Dilution and removal of microorganisms:** individuals continuously shed skin scales (squamous epithelial cells) and they contain colonies of microorganisms. The main source of airborne contamination in the OT is skin scales which are constantly dispersed from the theatre personnel and these microcolonies can either settle in and around the surgical wound or on exposed sterile instruments. Wound exposure to microorganisms by contaminated instruments by airborne bacteria is the major source of surgical site infection, thus preparation rooms used

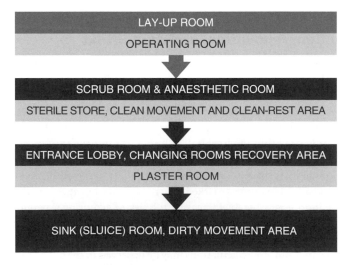

Fig. 19.1 Operating suite areas in the descending order of cleanliness.

for laying-up instruments is very important to prevent contamination of sterile instruments. Since the dispersal of microorganisms will increase with the number of people present in the OT, it is therefore essential that the number of theatre personnel *must be kept to an absolute minimum* and theatre discipline must be imposed. Due to immobility, the dispersal of microorganisms from the patient is very minimal. Mechanical ventilation in the OT helps dilute and remove microorganisms shed by the personnel present in the theatre. Similarly, the area of the operating suite may itself generate airborne contamination which mainly originates from the dirty utility/sluice area. Therefore it is essential that air *must be* mechanically extracted from this area and this is achieved by putting the sluice room under negative pressure so the air from this area should flow inward from the surrounding clean areas of the theatre suite.

3. **Provide a comfortable climate:** provision of a comfortable climate for the operating team is essential. Therefore the temperature of the OT should be maintained at 18–25°C and the humidity should be maintained between 40–60% both for comfort of staff and to inhibit microbial growth. Additional ventilation units to create comfortable environment, such as mobile air cooling devices or fan, *must not* be introduced into the OT without consultation with the IPC team.

4. **Removal of anaesthetics and other gases:** removal of anaesthetic gases is important for the safety of HCWs who are working in the OT. In addition, ventilation helps remove smells generated mainly during gastrointestinal surgery.

The pressure between rooms can be measured in pascals, but robust flow in the desired direction is more important than its precise value (Taylor et al., 2009). Theatre ventilation must be checked regularly and maintained by an appropriate engineer. The works and maintenance department must keep written records of all work on the ventilation system. Coarse and fine air filters must be replaced regularly according to the manufacturers' instructions or when the pressure differential across the filter indicates that a change is required. Remember that the preparation room (where the sterile instruments are prepared) and the main operating room where the surgery is performed are the most important areas to prevent surgical site infections.

For economic reasons, operating suites can be ventilated at a reduced rate ('setback'), or the ventilation turned off, when not in use. If this happens, the ventilation status should be clearly indicated and if the ventilation was turned completely off, one hour of full ventilation before use has been recommended and this time provides a good safety margin (Clarke et al., 1985).

Types of operating theatres

Conventionally ventilated theatre

The recommend air supplied to a new OT and refurbished old OT should have 25 air changes per hour (i.e. air equivalent to 25 times the volume of the theatre should be supplied every hour; Department of Health, 2007). This is a new recommendation and in most of the old theatres the requirement was 20 air changes per hour, therefore in older or pre-existing theatres 20 air changes per hour is acceptable. However it is essential that the air supplied to preparation rooms used for lay-up of surgical instruments should have *at least 25 air changes per hour* and preferably higher. Figure 19.2 outlines the layout of the conventional theatre suite ventilation with supply and extract of air, and recommended pressure differential in the OT.

Ultraclean ventilated theatres

In ultraclean ventilated (UCV) theatres, sometimes referred to as 'laminar flow' theatres, highly filtered air descends in an organized flow from a canopy in the theatre ceiling over the centre of the theatre. This unidirectional downward flow rapidly removes contamination generated by the surgical team working within this area and resists ingress of contamination from outside, resulting in very low bacterial counts in this area. UVC theatres are commonly used for orthopaedic prosthetic surgery where the consequences of wound infection are substantial and can be catastrophic for patients. It is accepted that ultraclean air (<10 cfu/m^3) reduces the risk of infection in implant surgery.

For UCV theatres, the commissioning engineers should supply data showing ventilation status (full or setback) is functioning adequately. The data includes downward air-velocity measurements at multiple points under the UCV canopy, particle

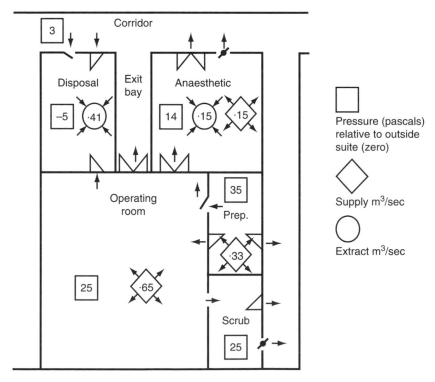

Fig. 19.2 The layout of the conventional operating theatre suite ventilation with supply and extract of air, and recommended pressure differential in various rooms to achieve positive pressure and air flow from clean to dirty area. Direction of air flow can be confirmed by a microbiologist using the smoke test.

challenging of the filters in the canopy to show they prevent passage of all particles, and showing absence of ingress into the area under the canopy from the theatre periphery. Air movement between rooms in a UCV suite is unimportant but, if air flows from the preparation room into the theatre, it should not interfere with the UCV flow. The routine monitoring or verification of operating theatre ventilation is a matter of periodic engineering assessments: inspection every 3 months and verification annually and there is no requirement for microbiological sampling of the air entering an ultraclean theatre (Department of Health, 2007).

Commissioning and microbiological monitoring

Guidance on sampling methods and infection control aspects of commissioning of both conventionally ventilated and UC OT are outside of the scope of this book and they have been described fully elsewhere (Holton and Ridgway, 1993; Hoffman et al., 2002; Department of Health, 2007).

The IPC team should be part of the design and the commissioning process. The commissioning or 'validation' is a process that assesses a facility has been supplied and functions to the required standard. The monitoring or 'verification' is the ongoing assessment that an OT continues to function within acceptable limits. A conventionally ventilated theatre requires microbiological checks at commissioning, immediately after commissioning, and at any major refurbishment. This is done by the microbiologist or a member of the IPC team. Routine bacteriological testing of operating room air is not necessary but may be useful if there is an outbreak of surgical site infections. Microbiological sampling of air supplied to the theatre, usually established by sampling the air using an air sampler in a clean, unoccupied theatre, should show 10 cfu/m^3 or less (Department of Health, 2007). Settle plates used to evaluate air-borne contaminants are *not* useful.

Key references and further reading

American Institute of Architects. *Guidelines for Design and Construction of Hospital and Health Care Facilities*. Washington, DC: The American Institute of Architects and the Facilities Guidelines Institute, 2010.

APIC. *Toolkit: Construction and Renovation* 3rd edn. Washington, DC: Association for Professionals in Infection Control and Epidemiology, 2007.

Clarke RP, Reed PJ, Seal DV, *et al*. Ventilation conditions and air-borne bacteria and particles in the operating theatres: proposed safe economies. *Journal of Hygiene* 1985; **95**:325–35.

Department of Health. *Health Technical Memorandum 03-01. Heating and ventilation systems: Specialised ventilation for healthcare premises. Part A: Design and validation. Part B: Operational management and performance verification*. London: The Stationery Office, 2007.

Hoffman P, Williams J, Stacey A, *et al*. Hospital Infection Society Working Party Report: Microbiological commissioning and monitoring of operating theatre suites. *Journal of Hospital Infection* 2002; **52**:1–28.

Holton J, Ridgway GL. Commissioning operating theatres. *Journal of Hospital Infection* 1993; **23**:153–60.

NHS Estates. *Infection Control in the Build Environment (HFN 30)*. London: The Stationery Office, 2002.

NHS Estates. *HFN 30. Infection Control in the Build Environment. Isolation facilities in acute setting (Supplement 1).* London: The Stationery Office, 2005.

Stockley JM, Constantine CE. Association of Medical Microbiologists' New Hospital Development Project Group. Building New Hospitals: a UK perspective. *Journal of Hospital Infection* 2006; **62**:285–99.

Taylor EW, Hoffman P. Operating Theatre. In: Fraise AP, Bradley C (eds). *Ayliffe's Control of Healthcare-Associated Infection – A practical handbook,* pp.375–94, 5th edn. London: Edward Arnold, 2009.

Woodhead K, Taylor EW, Bannister G, *et al.* Hospital Infection Society Working Party Report: Behaviors and rituals in the operating theatre. *Journal of Hospital Infection* 2002; **51**:241–55.

Chapter 20

Internet information resources

Knowledge is of two kinds. We know a subject ourselves,
or we know where we can find information on it.

Samuel Johnson

Evidence-based practice

Cochrane Collaboration	http://www.cochrane.org/
Joanna Briggs Institute	http://www.joannabriggs.edu.au/
National Guideline Clearing House	http://www.ngc.gov
National Institute for Clinical Evidence (NICE)	http://www.nice.org.uk
National Resource for Infection Control (NIRC)	http://www.nric.org.uk/
Scottish Intercollegiate Guidelines Network (SIGN)	http://www.sign.ac.uk/

Journals and newsletters

American Journal of Infection Control	http://www.ajicjournal.org/
Antimicrobial Resistance and Infection Control	http://www.aricjournal.com/
Australian Journal of Infection Control	http://www.aica.org.au/
Canadian Journal of Infection Control	http://www.chica.org/inside_cjic_journal.html
Communicable Disease Newsletter (WHO)	http://www.searo.who.int/
Communicable Diseases and Public Health	http://www.hpa.org.uk/cdph/
Communicable Disease Report Weekly	http://www.hpa.org.uk/cdr/
Emerging Infectious Diseases	http://www.cdc.gov/ncidod/EID/
Eurosurveillance	http://www.eurosurveillance.org/
Infection Control and Hospital Epidemiology	http://www.journals.uchicago.edu/ICHE/home.html
Infection Control Resource	http://www.infectioncontrolresource.org/
International Journal of Infection Control	http://www.ijic.info/
Journal of Hospital Infection	http://www.journalofhospitalinfection.com/

Journal of Infection Prevention	http://bji.sagepub.com/
Morbidity & Mortality Weekly Report (MMWR)	http://www.cdc.gov/mmwr/
WHO weekly Epidemiology Record	http://www.who.int/wer/

Organizations and regulatory bodies

Advisory Committee on Dangerous Pathogens	http://www.hse.gov.uk
American College of Occupational and Environmental Medicine	http://www.acoem.org/
American Society for Microbiology	http://www.asm.org/
Association of Peri-Operative Registered Nurses (AORN), USA	http://www.aorn.org
Association for Professionals in Infection Control and Epidemiology (APIC), USA	http://www.apic.org
Australian Infection Control Association	http://www.aica.org.au/
Baltic Network Infection Control	http://www.balticcare.org/Links.htm
British Travel Health Association	http://www.btha.org
Centre for Disease Control & Prevention (CDC) USA	http://www.cdc.gov
Communicable Disease Surveillance & Response (WHO)	http://www.who.int/csr/en/
Community and Hospital Infection Control Association (CHICA), Canada	http://www.chica.org
UK Department of Health (reducing HCAI)	http://hcai.dh.gov.uk/
European Centre for Disease Prevention and Control (ECDC)	http://www.ecdc.europa.eu/
European Operating Room Nurses Association (EORNA)	http://www.eorna.org
European Society of Clinical Microbiology and Infectious Diseases (ESCMID)	http://www.escmid.org
Global Infectious Diseases and Epidemiology	http://www.gideononline.com/
Health Canada Disease Prevention and Control Guidelines	http://www.hc-sc.gc.ca/
Health Protection Agency (HPA), UK	http://www.hpa.org.uk/
Health Protection Agency, Scotland	http://www.hps.scot.nhs.uk/scieh.asp
Healthcare infection Society, UK	http://www.his.org.uk
Hospital in Europe Link for Infection Control through Surveillance (HELICS)	http://helics.univ-lyon1.fr/helicshome.htm
Infection Prevention Society (IPS)	http://www.ips.uk.net
International Nosocomial Infection Control Consortium (INICC)	http://www.inicc.org/

Infectious Diseases Research Network (IDRN)	http://www.idrn.org/
Infectious Diseases Society of America	http://www.idsociety.org/
Infectious Diseases Societies Worldwide	http://www.idlinks.com/
Institute of Health Improvement, USA	http://www.ihi.org/
International Federation of Infection Control (IFIC)	http://www.theific.org
International Scientific Forum for Home Hygiene (IFH)	http://www.ifh-homehygiene.org/
International Sharps Injury Prevention Society	http://www.isips.org/
International Society for Infectious Diseases	http://www.isid.org
International Society of Travel Medicine	http://www.istm.org
Medicine and Healthcare products Regulatory Agency (MHRA)	http://www.mhra.gov.uk
National Disease Surveillance Centre, Republic of Ireland	http://www.hpsc.ie/hpsc/
National electronic Library of Infection (NELI)	http://www.neli.org.uk/
National Foundation for Infectious Diseases, (USA)	http://www.nfid.org/
National Prion Clinic	http://www.nationalprionclinic.org
Occupational Safety & Health Administration (OSHA), USA	http://www.osha.gov
Pan American Health Organization	http://www.paho.org
Public Health Agency of Canada	http://www.phac-aspc.gc.ca/
Public Health Agency, N. Ireland	http://www.publichealth.hscni.net/
Society for Healthcare Epidemiology of America (SHEA), USA	http://www.shea-online.org
Webber Training	http://webbertraining.com
World Forum for Hospital Sterile Supply	http://www.wfhss.com
World Health Organization (WHO)	http://www.who.int/

Index